THE Breast Cancer Prevention PROGRAM

Macmillan Publishing books may be purchased for business or sales promotional use. For information please write: Special Markets Department, Macmillan Publishing USA, 1633 Broadway, New York, NY 10019

THE Breast Cancer Prevention PROGRAM

Samuel S. Epstein, M.D., and David Steinman
with Suzanne LeVert

Macmillan • USA

For my mother and grandmother, both breast cancer survivors

Samuel S. Epstein, M.D.

For my wife, Teri, my mother and my sisters

David Steinman

Macmillan
A Simon & Schuster Macmillan Company
1633 Broadway
New York, NY 10019-6785

Book Design: Scott Meola

Library of Congress Cataloging-in-Publication Data
Epstein, Samuel S.
   The breast cancer prevention program / Samuel S. Epstein and
David Steinman ; with Suzanne LeVert.
      p.   cm.
   Includes bibliographical references and index.
   ISBN: 0-02-536192-9
   1. Breast—Cancer—Prevention. 2. Breast—Cancer—Risk factors.
3. Breast—Cancer—Popular works.   I. Steinman, David.   II. LeVert,
Suzanne.   III. Title.
   [DNLM: 1. Breast Neoplasms—prevention and control—popular works.
2. Breast Neoplasms—etiology—popular works. 3. Risk Factors—\
popular works.   Not Acquired]
RC280.B8E66   .   1997
616.99'449052—dc21
DNLM/DLC
for Library of Congress   97-22253
                                                              CIP

10 9 8 7 6 5 4 3 2 1
Printed in the United States of America

ACKNOWLEDGMENTS

We thank the following for reviewing portions of this book: John Bailar, University of Chicago Health Sciences Center; H. Leon Bradlow, Strang Cornell Cancer Center, New York; John Burlington, Food and Drug Administration; Kenneth Cantor, Robert Hoover and Sheilah Hoar Zahm, Environmental Epidemiology Branch, National Cancer Institute; Graham Colditz and Rose E. Frisch, Harvard School of Public Health; Walter Willett, Harvard School of Nutrition; Aaron Folsom, University of Minnesota Medical School; John Gofman, University California, Berkeley; Hershel Jick, Boston University Medical Center; Matthew Longnecker, University of California, Los Angeles; Ernest Sternglass, University of Pittsburgh; Michael Wisner and Mary S. Wolff, Mount Sinai Medical Center, New York, and Barbara Seaman.

We thank Drs. John Gofman, Devra Davis, World Resources Institute, Leon Bradlow, Strang Cornell Cancer Center, New York, and John Spratt, University of Louisville Health Sciences Center, for publications on the causes of breast cancer.

We thank Mark M. Methner, National Institute for Occupational Safety and Health, for important information on workplace exposures, Nancy Evans, Breast Cancer Action, San Francisco, for helpful comments; and Sandra Steingraber and Kathryn Patton for fresh perspectives. We thank Terry Zeyen and Robert Basile for their research assistance, and the University of Illinois School of Public Health, Chicago, for research support.

Finally, we thank Emily Epstein for her insightful review; Corinne Brophy for stylistic advice; our agent Madeleine Morel, 2-M Communications, for invaluable assistance in seeing this project through; and Natalie Chapman, Macmillan, for her patience, editing, and unflagging faith in our objectives.

Contents

INTRODUCTION

The Politics of Risk

What you don't know CAN hurt you.

Breast cancer rates continue to climb, with this disease striking more women every year, and yet information about known risks and prevention strategies is not reaching you. The cancer establishment has a vested interest in keeping you focused on early detection, treatment, and basic genetic research rather than on reducing the risks for developing the disease in the first place.

For the first time, this book provides all the medically sound and scientifically documented information currently available about known risk factors for this devastating disease and offers equally sound advice about how to avoid these risks in your own life.

Breast cancer: Few words in the medical lexicon arouse as much fear in the average woman as do these two. Potentially fatal, often disfiguring, breast cancer strikes at the heart of a woman's sexuality and vitality as no other disease does. Yet this book is not just for women, but for their partners, parents, children, and siblings as well, for breast cancer affects every aspect of a woman's life, including her relationships, in the most intimate ways.

Breast cancer is frightening, too, because it appears to be so random and unavoidable, a disease that is claiming more victims every day. At the same time that we hear how many more women are being diagnosed with breast cancer every year—now more than 186,000—news reports and magazine articles are telling us how little science knows about what causes cancer and how to prevent it, implying that our only hope is to find better ways to diagnose and treat the disease. Not a day goes by, it seems, without an announcement of a new avenue of genetic research or developments in diagnostic or treatment strategies.

The most important story—the story that could truly save lives—is not being told, at least not by the mainstream press. What's missing is the almost universally ignored information that currently exists about *prevention*, that is, information about the risks women can and should avoid in their everyday lives to protect themselves against cancer. By prevention we mean reduction in avoidable risks, most but not all of which are already known. Ironically, much of the blame for the lack of attention to prevention must be laid directly at the feet of the medical "experts" most women count on to provide them with accurate information about cancer: the American Cancer Society (ACS), the National Cancer Institute (NCI), and the twenty or so comprehensive cancer centers funded by the ACS and NCI that together make up the powerful lobby known as the *cancer establishment.*

During the past two decades alone, the cancer establisment has spent more than $20 billion trying to win the "War on Cancer" that it nevertheless continues to lose. As cancer rates climb ever upward, the ACS and NCI remain focused on basic molecular research, screening techniques, diagnostic tests, and treatment strategies— avenues of research that have yet to stem the rising tide of cancer incidence or make more than a slight dent in mortality rates—while relegating prevention to an afterthought at best.

Expressing the view held by many of his colleagues in the establishment, cancer expert Walter Willet, M.D., wrote in a 1996 *Nutrition* newsletter: "Breast cancer is definitely a tough problem to crack. We've done a lot of research, but most of what we've learned doesn't translate into public health advice for women."

We do not agree, and we have written this book to give you

information that the cancer establishment has failed to publicize. There is a host of known and well-documented prevention strategies that women can use to protect themselves from breast cancer, strategies that the cancer establishment continues to ignore despite repeated urging by concerned scientists throughout the United States and around the world. We will cite study after study implicating medical and environmental factors in the development of breast cancer and explain why organizations such as the ACS and NCI ignore or downplay these very same studies. We will also provide you with practical tips on avoiding these risks and, by doing so, significantly reducing your chances for developing this devastating disease.

First, however, you must get past the rhetoric you have heard so often in the media: Contrary to popular belief, you do have significant control over your risks of breast and other types of cancers, and there are steps you can take to protect yourself and your family from cancer. There is also a great deal of information out there—on your bookstore shelf as well as in the medical journals we cite throughout this book—that supports what you will read. Indeed, excellent books that focus somewhat narrowly on certain aspects of breast cancer prevention—for instance, diet, estrogen replacement therapy, or radiation—are now available to supplement what we offer you here. In this book, you will receive a thorough overview of *all* known and suspected causes of breast cancer and the most effective techniques available to avoid or counter those causes.

The information you will receive in this book is based on a critical review of more than 2,500 publications and documents, largely from well-known and respected medical journals. In many cases, however, misleading interpretations of these studies by the cancer establishment and the media have prevented you from receiving the information you need to protect yourself against known medical, environmental, and life-style risk factors for breast cancer.

Interpreting Study Results

As you will see throughout this text, media stories about study results published in medical and scientific journals are not always accurate or comprehensive. That's why it is vital you follow these tips whenever you read or hear new information on breast cancer and other health issues:

1. Consider the source with skepticism. It is important to look at both who conducted the study or analysis and who is interpreting and publishing the results. Studies conducted or funded by the cancer establishment tend to trivialize or dismiss many risk factors because of its mind-set against preventive strategies or its financial ties to industries that benefit from breast cancer, including the cancer drug and mammography (radiology) industries. If an industry with financial ties to the subject under investigation conducts or sponsors the study, you should treat its results with skepticism as well. For instance, if a major manufacturer of breast implants funds a study that finds no risk associated with implants, it is appropriate to question the basis, methods, and alleged results of that study (chapter 6).

2. Keep in mind that major news sources tend to follow the lead of the cancer establishment and downplay evidence for risk. This bias in reporting reflects the media's reliance on the cancer establishment for information. This practice is particularly undermining when the media release results of unpublished studies funded by a particular industry or studies published in nonpeer-reviewed journals (and thus not evaluated for their scientific integrity and accuracy). In addition, some reporters may be biased because they themselves have indirect financial or personal links to the cancer establishment or simply because they are innately conservative.

3. Learn to read between the lines—and that means reading the original study whenever possible. Whenever you read only media summaries or general conclusions of studies, you may miss important facts that could apply to your own risks. Whenever you read a study, look for answers to these questions:

    a. How many individuals participated in the study? In general, the more healthy persons (controls) and persons with disease (cases) who took part in the study, the more accurate the results are likely to be.

b. How long did the study last, and how long was the follow-up period? Breast cancer tends to develop very slowly, over many years and even decades. To be accurate and conclusive, studies about risks should take place over an extended period of time, and then follow-up should occur many years later.

c. Did the study look at overall populations only, while ignoring high-risk subgroups? A common but misleading method of intepreting studies is to apply the results to the "average" woman while ignoring higher risks to certain subgroups of women, such as smokers or those who did not exercise on a regular basis. Such epidemiological studies (studies of how cancer affects certain populations) are crucial to understanding the risks of breast cancer.

d. Do other studies confirm the results? Be wary of drawing conclusions from a single study, even a large and well-controlled one, that totally breaks away from earlier studies showing different results on the same issue. Furthermore, the weight of the evidence of human (epidemiological) studies is still further strengthened by experimental animal studies on carcinogenicity.

e. Do studies on animals support results of the study? Decades of research point to the strong likelihood that chemicals that cause cancer in well-designed animal studies will also cause cancer in humans. All twenty-five chemicals now known to cause cancer in humans have also been shown to do the same in animals—and generally involving the same organs. In fact, about half of these carcinogens were first identified in animal studies, and were only confirmed as human carcinogens decades later. Federal regulatory agencies consider the predictive value of animal tests to human cancer firmly established enough to base their regulations on them, and the International Agency for Research on Cancer of the World Health Organization uses animal studies as the basis for evaluating cancer risks to humans.

In addition, and most importantly, we offer sensible and practical strategies every woman can implement to reduce her risk for developing this disease. Here are just a few of the questions about breast cancer we answer in the chapters that follow:

- How important is a family history of breast cancer to my own risk?

- Why does having children—or not having children—affect my risk?

- Should I breast-feed my child and for how long?

- Will taking the birth control pill increase or decrease my risk of breast cancer?

- Will taking estrogen replacement therapy increase or decrease my risk?

- Should I get a mammogram? If so, when should I begin, and how often should I get one?

- Are there other medical procedures I should avoid? Are there ones I should pursue?

- How does what I eat and drink affect my risk?

- How does smoking cigarettes affect my risk?

- Will regular exercise help me decrease my risk?

- Does mental depression or excess stress affect my risk?

- Are food contaminants dangerous? If so, what are they and how can I avoid them?

- Will having breast implants increase my risk?

- Will coloring my hair increase my risk?

- What is the relationship between where I live and work and my risk for developing breast cancer?

- What are electromagnetic fields, or EMFs, and should I avoid them?

- What can I do to raise the flag for breast cancer prevention in my community?

Each chapter opens with a brief overview of its main theme followed by a thorough description of all known or suspected risks. We also outline in the Personal Protection sections the practical steps you can take to reduce your risks.

In addition to offering you a holistic plan for healthful living and a comprehensive strategy to reduce your risks for developing breast cancer, *The Breast Cancer Prevention Program* provides new and provocative information. Did you know that:

- Routine mammography of premenopausal women increases breast cancer risk?

- Some nonhormone-related prescription drugs may pose largely unpublicized risks to women?

- Confidential government and industry files reveal that there are high levels of estrogen and other hormones in beef, while ignoring the lifelong breast cancer risks that they pose?

- Milk products from cows injected with genetically engineered growth hormone contain high levels of another hormone that may put infants and young children at higher risk for developing breast and other cancers later in life?

- Synthetic industrial chemicals expose more than one million women in the workplace to a higher risk of breast cancer?

- Cancer-causing chemicals carried home on the clothes of men working in certain industries pose significant risk to their mothers and sisters, and wives and daughters?

We know that this book may make you angry when you realize how many lives might have been saved had a greater effort been made to make this information public before now. However, we also hope reading this book makes you feel stronger, more capable, and more empowered to take action to protect your own health.

PART I

Understanding Breast Cancer Risks

1

Determining Your Risk

More is known about the causes and prevention of breast cancer than you may realize. Knowing the Twelve Common but Unpublicized Risks for Breast Cancer, or the "Dirty Dozen," on page 9 is your first step toward preventing breast cancer from developing in the future.

The current statistics about breast cancer are shocking:

- Breast cancer is the leading cause of death in women between the ages of 35 and 54.

- Breast cancer is the second largest cause of cancer deaths (after lung cancer) among women of all ages.

- In 1971, when President Richard Nixon declared the "War on Cancer," a woman's lifetime risk for contracting breast cancer was one in fourteen. Today it is one in eight.

- American women are now twice as likely to develop breast cancer than they were a century ago, and most of this increase in incidence has occurred over the past thirty years.

- From 1950 to 1992 the incidence of breast cancer rates among white women (data from black women were not compiled until the 1970s) increased by 55 percent.

- From 1973 to 1992 the incidence of breast cancer among white women increased by 34 percent, and among black women by 47 percent.

- In 1996 alone, 186,000 women learned they had breast cancer and about 46,000 died from it.

- Since 1960, more than 960,000 American women—double the number of Americans (male and female) who died in World Wars I and II and in the Korean, Vietnam, and Persian Gulf wars combined—have died from breast cancer.

It would be comforting if a statistical anomaly or glitch could explain away such frightening figures. Unfortunately, these numbers reflect a stark truth: Today, more people are at risk for developing cancer—and more women are at higher risk for developing breast cancer—than ever before in history. Indeed, the general cancer statistics are at least as alarming as are those of breast cancer: One or another type of cancer now strikes more than one in three Americans, and kills more than one in four. Without question, cancer represents the greatest and most urgent medical challenge of the late twentieth century.

Yet many Americans—even well-meaning physicians—mistakenly believe that we are winning the war on cancer, that we have gotten a handle on increasing rates, and that mortality rates are actually decreasing rapidly because of improved diagnostic and treatment methods. Nothing could be further from the truth. Although there is some good news on the mortality front (from 1990 to 1995 the mortality rates for breast cancer decreased by 6.6 percent in white women and 1.6 percent in black women), most of the improvement is due to better health care access and earlier diagnosis rather than to any success in preventing the disease. In fact, the incidence rates—the numbers of older women being diagnosed with breast cancer—increased steadily during this same period. The truth is that until prevention becomes the top priority, breast cancer will continue to damage the lives of increasing numbers of women.

Before we delve further into the very real risks you may face, there are several other myths worth exploding about our perception of breast cancer.

MYTH #1: Breast cancer rates are increasing only because women are living longer.

You may have heard that the increase in breast cancer rates merely reflects an increase in life expectancy. Because most women who develop breast cancer do so after menopause, it is possible that a longer life span might explain today's marked increases in breast cancer rates. It is true that women now live approximately thirty-five years longer than they did at the beginning of this century. In fact, up until about 1920, most women died before or shortly after reaching menopause.

Unfortunately, increased longevity is not the explanation. We know this because while life expectancy rates have remained relatively stable since 1950, the incidence of breast cancer has increased by about 55 percent. Furthermore, rates of cancer and other diseases are *age-adjusted*, meaning that epidemiologists—scientists who study diseases, their causes, and their trends over time—reconcile changes in rates to reflect and exclude longevity factors.

MYTH #2: Breast cancer rates are increasing only because the disease can be detected sooner and better than ever before.

Although it is impossible to completely discount the contribution improved screening methods have made to the increase in breast cancer rates, this claim, too, fails to hold up under scrutiny. Much of the increase in breast cancer rates preceded 1980, before large-scale mammography screening began in the United States. In addition, similar increases in breast cancer rates exist in countries that still do not conduct large-scale screening programs, such as Great Britain and France.

MYTH #3: Breast cancer rates are leveling off.

The opposite is true: Today, one in eight women in the United States will develop breast cancer in her lifetime—a risk that was one in twenty in 1960. Next year, about 1 percent more women will develop breast cancer than did this year, and unless we find ways to prevent breast cancer the rates will continue to increase.

MYTH #4: Breast cancer cannot be prevented.

It is time to dispel conclusively this dangerous yet deeply entrenched myth. To do so means refuting the position taken by the cancer establishment represented by the American Cancer Society (ACS) and the National Cancer Institute (NCI). In their 1997 publication, *Cancer Facts and Figures*, for instance, the American Cancer Society wrote:

> *To date, knowledge about risk factors has not trans-*
> *lated into practical ways to prevent breast cancer. Since*
> *women may not be able to alter their personal risk fac-*
> *tors, the best opportunity for reducing mortality is*
> *through early detection.*

The cancer establishment has long insisted that the only risk factors known to cause breast cancer are hereditary (genetic) and biological (early menses and late menopause), both discussed in chapter 2, as well as dietary (a high-fat diet, discussed in chapter 9). We now know, however, that these so-called traditional risk factors account for less than 30 percent of breast cancer cases. With pervasive ties to the pharmaceutical and radiological industries, however, the ACS has a financial incentive to continue this policy of ignoring preventive strategies, and both the ACS and the NCI have an ingrained conservative mind-set against exploring environmental and dietary contaminants as causes of cancer—a mind-set reflected in their publications that blanket waiting rooms in hospitals, clinics, and doctors' offices across the country.

This leaves the average woman with the mistaken impression that scientists know nothing about the causes of breast cancer or how to prevent it (which, as you will see throughout this book, is untrue), and that the only subjects worth studying are those perceived to be ones with more attainable goals: better detection, early treatment, and genetic screening methods. Unfortunately, this attitude sets a vicious cycle in motion: Urged by the establishment's rhetoric, the public continues to fund research into genetic causes, chemoprevention (the use of drugs to prevent breast cancer), and diagnostic and treatment methods. The media then faithfully report the results of this research, which only encourages more funding for similar studies. Meanwhile, investigation into the more avoidable causes of breast cancer fails to receive proper funding or attention, and the rates of breast cancer continue to increase year after year.

In chapter 13, "The Politics of Breast Cancer," you will learn more about why this bias in research and reporting exists, how it leads to countless human tragedies every year, and what you can do to make other women and men aware of the truth. For now, you can start to reverse the cycle by gaining an understanding of your own risks and how to reduce them.

BREAST CANCER RISK FACTORS: THE WHOLE STORY

Thanks to advances in the biological sciences, we now have an increasingly clearer picture of our most dreaded and pervasive enemy: the cancer cell. In the wide range of diseases called cancer, a cell—the smallest unit of living matter in the body—becomes deranged and begins to grow abnormally. This corruption can occur spontaneously through some internal malfunction of the cell itself, or it can occur when the cell comes into contact with a carcinogen that triggers a disruption of the cell's normal activity. (The tar in cigarettes contains one such group of carcinogens; ultraviolet rays from the sun are carcinogenic as well.) By definition, a cancer is a group of malignant cells that multiply uncontrollably, invade local tissues, and sometimes spread (or metastasize) to other sites in the body.

What happens to a cell when something triggers it to grow uncontrollably? Normally, every cell in the body "knows" how often and under which circumstances it is to reproduce and the rate at which it will be destroyed or lost in the body. Most cells have a finite life span that is part of their genetic code. When a carcinogen or internal malfunction alters this genetic code, the cells lose their innate control over growth processes and divide without internal restraint. These cells also fail to die at a normal time, but instead continue to live and divide until a cancer forms.

Breast cancer is a malignant tumor that arises in the breast. It may also invade nearby tissues (such as the lymph glands) and then metastasize through the bloodstream, most often to the lungs, bone, liver, and brain. Scientists continue to search for the identity of the cancer-causing *triggers* (carcinogens), the substances or conditions under which a breast cell becomes deranged and starts to reproduce without control.

Without question, the story that receives the most press when it comes to breast cancer is the search for a genetic cause of the disease. During the 1980s, advances in molecular biology techniques triggered an explosion in genetic research, leading to several breakthroughs in the 1990s. One reason public funds are used to continue such research is the hope that when genetic therapy techniques become more sophisticated, doctors may be able to dismantle breast cancer genes and thus prevent women born with them from developing the disease.

As vital and exciting as this research is, it represents just a small part of the breast cancer picture. Indeed, as we will explain further, *only a very small percentage of all breast cancer cases have a direct genetic cause.* Genetic factors obviously cannot account for the startling increases in breast cancer incidence over the past few decades. By concentrating on genetic research, then, the cancer establishment takes the hope of prevention out of the hands of most women. By far the vast majority of breast cancer cases are linked to one or more environmental, medical, or personal risk factors over which you have far more control than you might think (the Dirty Dozen).

The Dirty Dozen:
Twelve Common but Unpublicized Risks for Breast Cancer

MODERN MEDICAL RISKS

- Oral contraceptives, with early and prolonged use

- Estrogen replacement therapy, with high doses and prolonged use

- Premenopausal mammography, with early and repeated exposure

- Nonhormonal prescription drugs such as some anti-hypertensives

- Silicone gel breast implants, especially those wrapped in polyurethane foam

DIETARY AND ENVIRONMENTAL RISKS

- Diet high in animal fat contaminated with undisclosed carcinogens and estrogenic chemicals

- Exposure in the home to household chemicals or pollution from neighboring chemical plants and hazardous waste sites

- Workplace exposure to a wide range of carcinogens

LIFESTYLE RISKS

- Alcohol, with early or excessive use

- Tobacco, with early or excessive use

- Inactivity and sedentary life-style

- Dark hair dyes, with early or prolonged use

Are you surprised at the risk factors on this list? Did you believe that the birth control pill and estrogen replacement therapy (ERT) were perfectly safe and always beneficial? Were you under the impression that scientists have never been able to identify chemical contaminants in the air, water, and workplace that can cause breast cancer? Or that the food you eat is safe for you and your children?

If so, no doubt you would be surprised to learn that these substances and conditions are the leading causes of breast cancer among women today. We also hope you will be heartened by the knowledge that you have the power to avoid these substances and conditions— called risk factors—and thus significantly reduce your chances of developing breast cancer.

Although scientists still cannot pinpoint the exact cause of breast cancer in any specific individual who develops the disease, they have identified a number of risk factors related to the cause of breast cancer. Risk factors are those conditions, substances, or habits associated with the development of a disease. No doubt you are aware, for instance, that smoking cigarettes is a major risk factor for lung cancer. Not everyone who smokes develops lung cancer, nor does everyone with lung cancer have a history of smoking; however, an individual's risk for developing lung cancer skyrockets if he or she inhales the cancer-causing substances in cigarette smoke.

As you can see from the Dirty Dozen list of risks, many of the risk factors identified for breast cancer—and for most other types of cancer as well—involve modern chemical technology and its by-products. Indeed, for the past fifty years or so, science and industry have moved forward with incredible speed, introducing one new product, substance, drug, or treatment after another, hailing each one as a terrific advancement. Although these technological advances have made twentieth century life possible, their reckless use—without regard to any adverse consequences to humans or the environment—has led to serious health problems. Every day, new drugs and procedures emerge out of our medical research facilities, often providing relief for one illness, only to trigger the development of another. Science even labels a natural event such as menopause a disease and then encourages women to take medication to treat it. Birth control pills and breast implants are two other modern so-called conveniences that may only be putting more women at higher risk for developing breast cancer.

In an effort to produce more and cheaper food, the agrichemical industry has developed toxic pesticides to protect crops and sex growth hormones to fatten cattle for slaughter, without taking into account their long-term effects on humans. Daily life becomes ever faster, more efficient, and comfortable, with electricity surging into every household, providing power for microwave ovens, hair dryers, and electric blankets. Millions of men and women find employment in the factories and laboratories that manufacture synthetic or other carcinogenic chemicals and radioactive products, or in the industries that use them.

At the same time, these runaway technologies and the industries responsible have encouraged us to develop some unhealthy habits. Fat- and chemical-laden convenience foods line our grocery store shelves, adding pounds to our frames and toxic contaminants to our bodies. The automobile, television set, and personal computer form a deadly triumvirate of human energy- and time-savers, keeping more and more of us from getting the exercise we need to stay healthy.

The truth is, we now understand that cancer has at least one thing in common with other deadly diseases such as heart disease and stroke: It usually does not strike at random but instead requires certain conditions, exposure to toxic substances, or both, to occur. In the same way that most cases of heart disease, for instance, are triggered by a combination of intake of high-fat foods and lack of physical activity, most cases of breast cancer can be traced to one or (more often) a combination of the Dirty Dozen risks. Just as improving diet and exercise habits reduces our risks of heart disease, avoiding exposure to damaging X rays, carcinogenic medications, and food contaminants lowers the risks for breast cancer.

EXAMINING THE RISKS

Most forms of cancer, including breast cancer, are what epidemiologists call *multifactorial diseases*, diseases having many different risk factors or potential causes that may interact with one another in ways that are still not completely understood. In most cases, genetic, familial, environmental, and life-style factors all work together to create the conditions necessary for cancer to develop. A woman born with a familial predisposition for breast cancer, for instance, may not develop the disease unless she encounters other risk factors. And the reverse is equally true: Someone without any genetic history of breast cancer can be "hit" by so many environmental carcinogens that her cells develop the genetic mutation that causes breast cancer.

In this book, we concentrate on those risk factors that are—or should be—avoidable, specifically the Dirty Dozen risks. We explain in careful detail the risks and benefits involved with each potential trigger for breast cancer, so that you can make rational, well-informed decisions about those over which you have personal control. We expose the larger, less controllable risks, including the carcinogenic contaminants present in your foods (without your knowledge or permission) and the toxins in the air you breathe and the water you drink discharged by industries who answer to no one but underfunded and undermotivated (and sometimes even complicit) government regulatory agencies.

Apart from the Dirty Dozen risks, other risk factors include your family history, age, and reproductive history. These are risk factors over which, at least at this point in your life, you may have less control. Let us examine these other risk factors first.

FAMILY HISTORY

In recent years, reports of familial and genetic links to breast cancer have made the front pages of newspapers around the world. To date, scientists have identified at least three genes with mutations related to the development of breast cancer. Two genes, called BRCA1 (which was first identified among Jews of Eastern or

Central European decent) and BRCA2, are tumor suppressers. When working properly, they keep cells from dividing abnormally. Women who have abnormalities in these genes, however, run a very high risk of developing breast cancer. A National Institutes of Health study, the largest study to date on cancer susceptibility genes in the general population, showed that, on average, a woman carrying one of three alterations in BRCA1 and BRCA2 genes has about a fourfold increased risk for developing breast cancer. Scientists now estimate that these genetic mutations cause about 4 percent of breast cancer cases increasing a woman's risk by about 56 percent by the age of 70.

Another gene affects breast cancer through its influence on estrogen production. In 1997, researchers linked increased breast cancer risk to a very common variation of this gene, called CYP1. Carried by about 40 percent of women, the CYP1 gene may be involved in some way in 30 percent of all cases of the disease. The variation causes women to enter puberty and start producing estrogen approximately five months earlier than do women without the variation. As we will see further in chapter 2, increased exposure to estrogen raises the risk of breast cancer at all ages. Furthermore, researchers found that among women with breast cancer, those with the genetic variation CYP1 were two and one-half times more likely to have disease that had spread than were women without this variation. Yet another way genes might affect breast cancer involves breast density and size. The cancer risk for women with the densest breast tissue is significantly higher than the risk for women with less dense breasts. Scientists have not yet identified the genes responsible for controlling density.

Apart from these recently discovered genes, about 1 to 2 percent of American women carry a rare gene, ataxia-telongiectasia (A-T), which markedly increases their sensitivity to X rays, including mammography, and thus their risk for breast cancer.

Despite these compelling findings, at this point, genetic research does not offer women much practical help when it comes to protecting themselves against the disease, nor is it relevant to the striking increase in breast cancer incidence in recent decades.

The National Breast Center of Australia published a concise overview of genetic risks in the Spring 1995 issue of *BreastNEWS*, dividing these risks into three general categories:

1. **At or slightly above average risk:** Women who have (a) no family history, or (b) a first- or second-degree relative diagnosed with breast cancer after the age of 50. Most women (95 percent) fall into this category. Their lifetime risk is between 1 in 13 and 1 in 8.

2. **Moderately increased risk:** Women who have (a) one or more first- or second-degree relatives diagnosed with breast cancer before the age of 50; or (b) two first- or second-degree relatives on the same side of the family with breast cancer, especially those diagnosed before the age of 50. Less than 4 percent of women fall into this group. Their lifetime risk is between 1 in 8 and 1 in 4.

3. **Potentially high risk:** Women who have three or more first- or second-degree relatives on the same side of the family diagnosed with breast or ovarian cancer. Less than 1 percent of women fit in this category. Their lifetime risk is between 1 in 4 and 1 in 2.

As you can see, the vast majority of breast cancer cases are not genetically linked. However, you should understand that if you have a strong family history of breast cancer, you may have a risk about three times greater than a woman without this history.

At the same time, even the 4 percent of women who do inherit a predisposition are not necessarily fated to develop breast cancer. Geneticists have long known that environmental influences have an impact on genes. Using techniques to examine the structure of the genes in fine detail, researchers now know that DNA is hardly stable but instead exquisitely sensitive to environmental influences. One researcher notes:

What we're seeing is a molecule in a dynamic state of damage and repair, undergoing constant change. Rather than thinking of DNA as a rigid structure, like the Eiffel Tower, that barely bends in the wind, DNA is more like a chemical chameleon, constantly altering its fine structure in response to changes in the cellular environment. It's a whole new way to look at DNA.

Another recent study in the *Journal of the National Cancer Institute* confirms that it is not who you were you born to, but where you live that matters most. For instance, immigrant women who arrive in the United States (or in other countries with high breast cancer rates), from countries with much lower rates of breast cancer rather quickly develop higher and higher risks until they match the rate of those of American women—no matter what their genetic history.

AGE

Your risk for developing breast cancer changes dramatically with age: The older you are, the higher your risk. More than 80 percent of breast cancer occurs in women over 50 years of age. To date, the median age for breast cancer diagnosis is about 64 years, which means that half of women who will get breast cancer will get it before the age of 64 and half will get it after that age. To understand your risk at your current age, look at Table 1.1 on page 16.

A given percentage increase creates very different risks at any particular age. For instance, a 100 percent increase at the age of 35 increases risks from 1 in 622 to 1 in 311. However, a 100 percent increase at the age of 80 increases risks from 1 in 10 to 1 in 5. Whenever you read about the way certain factors increase the risk for developing breast cancer, you can refer back to Table 1.1 to calculate your own risk at your current age, and thus what any percentage increase then means to you.

TABLE 1.1: AVERAGE RISK FOR DEVELOPING BREAST CANCER BY AGE		
Age	Risk per Year	Risk Resulting from 100% Increase
25	1 in 19,608	
30	1 in 2,525	
35	1 in 622	1 in 311
40	1 in 217	
45	1 in 93	
50	1 in 50	1 in 25
55	1 in 33	
60	1 in 24	
65	1 in 17	
70	1 in 14	
75	1 in 11	
80	1 in 10	1 in 5
85	1 in 9	
Over 85	1 in 8	

Data from the National Cancer Institute reported in Science, *1992. 259:618.*

REPRODUCTIVE HISTORY

In chapter 2, "Estrogen: The Common Link," you will see that the main culprit usually involved directly or indirectly in breast cancer is estrogen, the primary female sex hormone. In general, the longer you are exposed to estrogen, and the greater the amount of estrogen that flows through your bloodstream, the greater is your risk for developing breast cancer. If you menstruate for more than forty years, for instance, your risk is much higher than is that of someone who menstruates for thirty years or less. Because pregnancy influences the amount of estrogen your body produces, it also has an impact on breast cancer risk. Women who never become pregnant, for example, have a higher risk than do those who have a child before the age of thirty, whereas women who get pregnant for the first time after the age of thirty have a greater risk than do those who never get pregnant.

At first glance, you may think that the amount of estrogen to which your body is exposed and the way it affects breast tissue are matters over which you have little control. In fact, one of the reasons that breast cancer rates are rising may be the amount of "reproductive engineering" and extra exposure to estrogen that now occurs, thanks to the widespread use of the birth control pill and estrogen replacement therapy after menopause.

And that brings us to the focus of this book, specifically the medical, dietary, and environmental risk factors that promote breast cancer largely by influencing either the amount of estrogen to which women are exposed or the way estrogen behaves in their bodies.

MODERN MEDICINE AND RISK

In Part II of this book, you will read about the ways that some advances in medical technology have increased risks of breast cancer. Chapter 3, "The Pill: Assessing Your Risks," and chapter 4, "Estrogen Replacement Therapy: Pros and Cons," discuss how the direct manipulation of the amount and duration of estrogen exposure experienced by women has increased breast cancer rates to skyrocket over the past forty years.

Three other medical advances also pose serious risks of breast cancer. Hailed by the cancer establishment as the most promising avenue of breast cancer "prevention," the radiographic technique of mammography may, in fact, offer far more risks than benefits to premenopausal women. In addition, receiving radiation for diagnosis or treatment of other diseases is likely to increase your risk, especially if these exposures occurred during childhood, as we discuss in chapter 5, "The Case Against Mammography." Breast implants, explored in chapter 6, may also significantly increase a woman's risk of breast cancer under certain circumstances. Although the drug tamoxifen may help treat breast cancer in some women, it poses critical risks (though not for breast cancer) when used in attempts to prevent breast cancer in healthy women, as we explore in chapter 7, "The Case Against Chemoprevention."

In addition, your risks do not end with drugs and procedures directly linked to the breast. Did you know that certain non-hormone-related prescription drugs, including some high blood pressure medications and tranquilizers, may put you at increased risk for developing breast cancer? We explain these risks in chapter 8, "Common Medications and Your Risks.

We must stress that in citing these examples of medical risks we do not intend to make a sweeping condemnation of modern professional medicine, as some proponents of alternative and natural medicine have done. Some alternative medicine advocates virtually dismiss the many triumphs and life-saving miracles of modern medicine and medical biotechnology, including coronary bypass surgery, blood-cholesterol-lowering drugs, blood-clot-dissolving drugs, and combination therapy with protease inhibitors for AIDS patients, to name just a few.

DIETARY AND ENVIRONMENTAL RISKS

Part III of this book focuses on several other the Dirty Dozen risks, namely, the damage industrial technology and modern lifestyles may inflict on the human body and, specifically, on estrogen production and breast cells. Today, most supermarkets are laden with meats tainted with carcinogenic and estrogenic chemicals and vegetables and fruits sprayed with toxic pesticides. Even the water from your kitchen faucet may contain carcinogenic substances.

In addition, most Americans now come into daily contact with everything from microwave ovens to fax machines, dry cleaning chemicals to computer modems, electric toothbrushes to super-strength household cleaners. As we marvel at the convenience and efficiency of these modern wonders, we must also realize that the pace at which this technology has developed has far surpassed our ability to control it and has led to myriad health problems, including increased cancer rates. We must increase our awareness of the hazards to our health that are found in our homes, neighborhoods, and workplaces.

In chapter 9, "Eating for Health and Longevity," we outline the facts about the dangers that the toxic, carcinogenic, and estrogenic contaminants in our foods pose to all women. First, we explain how your own daily diet—the amount of fat, fiber, and other nutrients you consume—affects your risk for developing breast cancer, and then we give you tips on how to improve your diet to reduce those risks. Second, we explain the important roles that pesticides, other industrial chemicals, and sex hormones contaminating meat, dairy, and other foods play in breast cancer risk. We show you how to avoid these chemicals as much as possible.

Tobacco is the most dangerous and commonly used legal drug in the world, and its consumption has been linked to breast cancer. The use of alcohol, especially in women undergoing hormone replacement therapy, has also been implicated in breast cancer risk. Inactivity (which often leads to obesity) is yet another factor in breast cancer development, as may be the way you cope with stress in your life. In chapter 10, "Lifestyle Risk Factors and Coping Strategies," we will give you tips on how to assess and reduce your own risks in your day-to-day life.

Studies show that there are links between risks of breast cancer and living near chemical plants, hazardous waste sites, and—possibly—nuclear facilities. We also know that simply living in the United States puts you at higher risk than does living almost anywhere else in the world, and that in the United States, the farther northeast you live, the greater are your chances of developing breast cancer. The factors involved in these geographical distinctions are complex, with industrial, ethnic, socioeconomic, and cultural components.

In chapter 11, "Where You Live," we analyze current research and provide practical suggestions about choosing a safe place to live and making your home as safe as possible. Scientists have identified four different classes of indoor pollutants as potential causes of breast cancer: household cleaning products, home lawn and garden pesticides, fumes from cooking and heating appliances, and contaminated work clothes. In addition, electromagnetic field (EMF) radiation from hair dryers, electric blankets, and televisions may also have an impact on your risk of breast cancer. Even the amount of nighttime electric light to which you are exposed may be a factor in your risk profile.

Your workplace, too, may harbor potential hazards. The manufacturing and chemical industries, which have attracted women in great numbers since World War II, expose more than four million women to chemicals well recognized as causes of occupational cancer in men, some of which also may cause breast cancer. Are you one of them? In chapter 12, "Hazards in the Workplace," we outline the risks associated with the petrochemical, cosmetology, and pharmaceutical industries, as well as the risks metals, asbestos, art supplies, and radiation pose to the women who work with them.

As discussed in the introduction, by the time you finish this book you may wonder why warnings about everyday and easily controllable hazards have not been plastered across the front pages of every newspaper in the country and why the cancer establishment has failed to publicize this information. For these reasons we have included chapter 13, "The Politics of Breast Cancer: Setting a New Agenda," along with information on how you can get involved.

No one is helpless against the medical, environmental, and lifestyle risks of breast cancer. Once you have identified the specific risks you face, you then have the power to eliminate or at least radically reduce them. Chapter 2 lays the groundwork for understanding your risks by explaining the connection between breast cancer and estrogen.

2

Estrogen: The Common Link

Understanding the effects of hormones on the health of your breasts is crucial to assessing and reducing your risk of breast cancer. You can control many of the factors that influence your exposure to estrogen throughout your life cycles by making informed decisions about childbearing, breast-feeding, and other reproductive issues.

Almost all of your body's functions—from sleep to appetite to sexual desire to heart rate—depend on the actions of a group of body chemicals called hormones. Glands and organs that together make up the endocrine system secrete these chemical messengers, which deliver instructions to other organs and tissues through the bloodstream. Among the hormones directly affecting your breasts are the female sex hormones, estrogen and progesterone. The ovaries, two glands located in the lower abdomen, act as the primary secretors of female hormones. Other body tissues also produce some estrogen, including the adrenal glands and abdominal fat, but in much smaller quantities.

The evidence is overwhelming that estrogen is intimately connected to the development of most breast cancer. Estrogen encourages breast cells to divide more often and more rapidly. Thus if a mutation (inherited or triggered by a carcinogen) lies embedded in the DNA, cancer cells are more likely to proliferate when high estrogen levels are present. (The main reason men—who also have breasts and breast tissue—rarely develop breast cancer is that their exposure to estrogen is minimal.) This also may help to explain why breast cancer rates have increased in tandem with the widespread use of birth control pills and estrogen replacement therapy, both of which increase the amount of estrogen circulating in a woman's body over her lifetime.

Indeed, we now know that two distinct types of breast cancer exist: the far more common estrogen-dependent breast cancer influenced primarily by estrogen, and the less common nonestrogen-dependent breast cancer. More than two-thirds of women with breast cancer have estrogen-dependent cancers, and that number is increasing at a particularly alarming rate: According to a study published in 1990 by the *Journal of the National Cancer Institute*, the incidence of estrogen-dependent breast cancers, particularly among postmenopausal women, increased by 130 percent from the mid-1970s to the mid-1980s, in contrast to only a 27 percent increase in nonestrogen-dependent cancers. A 1997 study in the same journal confirmed these findings.

UNDERSTANDING ESTROGEN

From birth to adolescence, ovarian activity is fairly dormant. Although a little girl grows and changes in many other ways, the first signs of physical sexual development usually do not appear until she reaches the average age of 10. At that time, an internal alarm clock in the brain—a regulating area at the base of the brain called the hypothalamus—signals the start of puberty by stimulating the ovaries to produce the sex hormones. A young girl's activity, weight, and percentage of body fat appear to be what triggers the hypothalamus to stimulate ovarian activity. The younger the girl is when she reaches a certain weight, the sooner puberty begins.

Estrogen and progesterone are powerful hormones that prompt several physical changes to take place. Known as secondary sex characteristics, these developments include the budding of the breasts, the growth of pubic and underarm hair, increasing height and weight, and skin changes. Recent research indicates that another hormone, called dihydroepiandrosterone (DHEA), is also involved in the onset of puberty. A weak precursor of the male hormone testosterone and secreted by the adrenal glands, DHEA levels sharply

The Estrogen Connection

Why is estrogen-dependent breast cancer so much more common today than it was just a few decades ago? Plainly speaking, the average woman is exposed to more estrogen over a longer period of time than ever before and at the same time, she is exposed to the more carcinogenic or "bad" type of estrogen than women were in the past. This overexposure to estrogen is occurring for a variety of reasons:

- The widespread use of oral contraceptives and estrogen replacement therapy not only lengthens the amount of time women are exposed to additional estrogen, but also increases the total amount of estrogen that circulates in the bloodstream over a woman's lifetime (chapters 3 and 4).

- Contamination of the food we eat by estrogens and estrogen-mimicking industrial chemicals (pseudoestrogens) increases the levels of estrogen in the body and exposes the body to the bad carcinogenic forms of the hormone (chapter 9).

- Poor eating habits, lack of exercise, and other detrimental lifestyle habits, such as the consumption of large amounts of alcohol, also increase the amount of estrogen circulating in the body (chapter 9).

- Certain reproductive choices more commonly made today, such as deciding not to have any children, bearing a first child late in life, and choosing not to breast-feed, also affect estrogen levels.

increase after the age of 6, a time referred to as the adrenarche, and reach adult levels around age 18. About two years after the very first changes begin to occur, a young girl reaches menarche and menstruates for the first time, usually at about the age of 12. From that time onward, in an average healthy woman, varying amounts of estrogen flow through the bloodstream on a cyclical basis until menopause. At menopause a natural reversal of the changes that occurred at puberty begins, and the ovaries and other tissues produce estrogen in much lesser quantities.

All humans are born with breast tissue that is highly sensitive to hormones. In fact, in many infants, both male and female, a little liquid is discharged from the breasts (commonly known as *witches' milk*) on the second or third day after birth owing to stimulation by their mother's hormones.

Female breast tissue and male breast tissue, however, then develop in significantly different ways. Containing from fifteen to twenty lobules, or sections, the female breast has milk-producing glands and a network of ducts to collect milk from the glands and deliver it to the nipple. Fibrous connective tissue and fat support the glands, ducts, and lobules, giving the breast its size and shape. Chest muscles also support the breasts, which are nourished by a rich supply of blood and lymphatic vessels.

Once a woman begins to menstruate, estrogen affects breast tissue in very specific ways. During the first half of the menstrual cycle, the ovaries secrete estrogen, which causes new cells to grow in glands, ducts, and other breast tissue. Estrogen is, in essence, the "build-up" hormone. Under its influence, cells multiply and swell in preparation for possible milk production. The ducts, in particular, lengthen and enlarge. During the second half of the cycle, glands in the breasts become flooded with progesterone (the other female hormone). Progesterone plays an equally important role in the female cycle, acting to oppose the actions of estrogen. Whereas estrogen causes breast (and other estrogen-sensitive) tissue to proliferate, progesterone limits cell division and thus protects against estrogen-dependent cancers. If pregnancy does not occur, the levels of both hormones decrease, the body absorbs the new cells, the blood supply to the breasts diminishes, and the cycle begins again.

If pregnancy occurs, the breasts enlarge considerably. The duct system, stimulated by an estrogen surge produced by the placenta and the pituitary gland, grows and branches. By the end of the pregnancy, under the influence of estrogen, progesterone, and other hormones, the breasts become milk-producing organs. In fact, almost all the tissue is now glandular. Once childbirth occurs, other hormones stimulate milk production.

In the context of breast cancer risk, it is important to note that only when a woman goes through a full-term pregnancy do her breasts reach full development. Until then, the immature breast cells are more susceptible to abnormal changes stimulated by estrogen, as well as by a wide range of cancer-causing pollutants. Studies show that breast tissue is especially sensitive to exposures to environmental carcinogens that occur between a woman's first period and her first pregnancy. If that pregnancy occurs before the age of 30 or so, the hormones of pregnancy mature the breast tissue. These same hormones after the age of 30 could stimulate breast cells that have already been mutated by earlier carcinogenic exposure.

Before we move on to a discussion of the types of estrogens, it is important to mention that the "other" female hormone, progesterone, also comes in different forms. Natural progesterone, produced by the ovaries and adrenal glands, works as a counterbalance to oppose the action of estrogen on breast tissue and throughout the body. Additionally, synthetic progesterone (called progestins) are used for oral contraceptives and hormone replacement therapy.

TYPES OF ESTROGEN

Although we use the word estrogen in the singular, several types of the hormone exist. Some are produced by the body, others are found as food contaminants, and others are prescribed as medications. Still others are found naturally in plants. Each type of estrogen acts to varying degrees on breast tissue and thus influences the risk of breast cancer.

Natural Estrogen

The ovaries, adrenal glands, and fatty tissues produce three types of estrogen: estrone, estriol, and estradiol. All three have feminizing effects, which means they play a role in maintaining fertility and influencing female characteristics. Estradiol is the most potent and plentiful form of estrogen; estrone and estriol are relatively weak and are produced in much smaller quantities.

In addition to the three main types, scientists have discovered that the body produces two different chemical types of estradiol: 2-hydroxyestrone, a "good estrogen" that reduces the risk of breast cancer, and 16-alpha-hydroxyestrone, a "bad estrogen" that can trigger or stimulate the development of cancer. The same factors that influence the total amount of estrogen in the body—diet, medication, reproductive patterns, and life-style—also influence the balance between good and bad estrogens in the bloodstream.

Synthetic Estrogen

The pharmaceutical industry has developed a wide variety of synthetic estrogens, and many are more powerful, more active when taken by mouth, more potentially carcinogenic, and longer-lasting in the body than are the natural estrogens. Ethinyl estradiol is used in oral contraceptives and is one example of a synthetic estrogen. Prolonged exposure to synthetic estrogens significantly increases the risk for developing breast cancer.

Estrogen Drugs Increase the Risk of Breast Cancer

Despite recent news reports to the contrary, taking the birth control pill or estrogen replacement therapy increases your risk of breast cancer. Many studies have confirmed that fact, as Carol Ann Rinzler points out in her excellent book, *Estrogen and Breast Cancer: A Warning to Women*. Here is just a sampling (we discuss others in chapters 3 and 4):

- In 1991, pooled results from sixteen previous studies found that users of the estrogen replacement therapy for fifteen years increased their risk of breast cancer by 30 percent.

- In 1995, a National Cancer Institute study found that a few months' use of oral contraceptives could increase the risk of breast cancer by 30 percent; ten years' use doubled the risk to 100 percent.

Pseudoestrogen

Several dietary contaminants, including some industrial chemical and pesticides, act like estrogen in the body but are much less potent. Although chemically quite different from estrogen, they affect menstrual and reproductive cycles as well as trigger both normal and abnormal cell divisions in the breast, as estrogen does. In addition, pseudoestrogens, or xenoestrogens, as these chemicals are known, can intensify the effects of natural estrogen, mainly by stimulating the production of "bad estrogen" and lengthening the duration of exposure to estrogen.

Phytoestrogen

Certain plants also contain different chemicals that act like estrogen in the body, and some are chemically related to natural human estrogen. Some phytoestrogens can reduce overall estrogen levels while stimulating production of "good estrogen." In fact, some researchers on the cutting edge now believe that phytoestrogens (which are found in some common foods such as soy beans) may be a safe alternative to estrogen replacement therapy. However, other phytoestrogens (such as zeranol, which is found in some fungi and used to fatten cattle before slaughter) increase production of "bad estrogen." In chapter 9, you will learn more about both types of phytoestrogen and their effect on breast cancer risk.

ESTROGEN AND YOUR BREASTS

As your body produces estrogen and you constantly ingest natural, synthetic, pseudo-, or phytoestrogens, these hormones travel through your body in the bloodstream. Up to about 97 percent of estrogen ends up being scavenged by proteins, called estrogen-binding proteins, that carry estrogen to the liver, where it can be metabolized and excreted via the gall bladder to the gut, and thus divert it away from sensitive breast cells. How much of this protein there is in the blood and how effective it is in binding to estrogen depend to a large degree on the same factors that influence other aspects of breast cancer risk: diet, medications, exercise habits, reproductive choices, and environmental contaminants. By controlling these factors as much as possible, you can boost your body's ability to metabolize estrogen and thus decrease the hormone's potentially harmful effects on breast tissue.

The estrogen that reaches the liver stimulates the release of other proteins and substances the liver produces. Some of these substances benefit the body, such as high-density lipoproteins, or HDLs (the "good" cholesterol), which help lower the risk of cardiovascular disease. Other substances produced by the liver after estrogen stimulation produce negative effects. One such substance is angiotensinogen, which elevates blood pressure in some women. In addition, estrogen stimulation of the liver may exacerbate liver disease, gall bladder disease, and certain blood clotting disorders. These effects, both negative and positive, only intensify when more potent synthetic forms of estrogen are ingested.

The estrogen that continues to circulate in the bloodstream, particularly estradiol, binds itself tightly to breast and other cells by way of estrogen receptors on the outer membranes of the cells. Once estrogen (or estrogen-like substances such as pseudo- and phyto-estrogen) attaches to the receptor cell, it triggers a change in the genetic makeup of the cell—or DNA—altering the way the cell behaves. In most cases, the change is a positive one: Estrogen stimulates the wall of the uterus to prepare for the implantation of an egg, for instance. Estrogen also helps keep a woman's skin supple, bones strong, and cardiovascular system less susceptible to disease.

The cells of the breast contain many estrogen receptors and are highly sensitive to the effects of this hormone. The presence of estrogen promotes the growth of glands, ducts, and other breast tissue. However, if some breast are abnormal, either because of an inherited malformation or because carcinogens have triggered a mutation, the presence of estrogen—particularly the "bad" type—may promote the growth of cancer by causing these abnormal cells to divide more quickly and more often.

As previously noted, the increasing incidence of breast cancer in recent decades has been seen mainly among postmenopausal women with estrogen-dependent tumors. In addition to this increase, there has been a steady increase in the levels of estrogen receptors in breast tumors. Exposure to estrogenic pollutants appears to be implicated in both of these increases.

THE "NATURAL ESTROGEN WINDOW" AND YOUR RISK

Although scientists are still uncertain as to exactly what causes the original mutation to occur, the influence of estrogen on the process of cancer development is clear. Two types of estrogen receptor proteins exist: the well-known alpha type found in the breast, uterus, and, to a lesser extent, other organs; and a more recent discovery, the beta type, found in the ovaries, bladder, and blood vessels. The beta type is probably involved in some of the protective effects of estrogen, including those on the heart and bone (chapter 7). It is now clear that estrogen receptors have profound influences on a wide range of metabolic effects in a wide range of organs in addition to the breast.

High levels of estrogen flow through your body from the time of your first period until you pass through menopause, for an average of about forty years. This time period is what we call your "natural estrogen window": The window opens wide when your ovaries first begin to produce estrogen at menarche and closes when your ovaries significantly reduce their production of estrogen at menopause (if you do not choose to take estrogen replacement therapy). In between, your estrogen window temporarily closes if you breast-feed, because the ovaries produce little or no estrogen during this period. (Other factors, including diet, exercise habits, environmental influences, and medications, also may open or close this window, as we will see in chapters 8 through 12.)

Three estrogen-related factors contribute to your risk for developing breast cancer:

- **Overall estrogen level**: The total amount of estrogen to which you are exposed over the course of your life, including natural, synthetic, pseudo-, and phytoestrogens.

- **Duration of exposure:** The length of time you are exposed to estrogen, which depends on how many children you bear, whether you breast-feed, and other reproductive factors.

- **Balance between the "good" and "bad" estrogens:** How much estrogen metabolizes into the more cancer-stimulating type of estrogen compared with the amount that metabolizes into a type that offers some protection against breast cancer development.

Table 2.1 on page 31 outlines the various dietary, medical, reproductive, and lifestyle factors that influence breast cancer risk by either promoting or inhibiting the presence, type, and activity of estrogen in your body.

REPRODUCTIVE PATTERNS AND YOUR RISK

A woman's fertile life, between menarche and menopause, is the period of her highest estrogen production. In this chapter on estrogen, we focus primarily on the way your reproductive history affects your estrogen window by increasing or reducing your risks of breast cancer. However, the causes of most cases of breast cancer are unrelated to natural reproductive issues, which, along with genetic vulnerability and a high-fat diet, were once thought to be the traditional risk factors of prime importance to the development of the disease. According to a November 1995 article in the *Journal of the National Cancer Institute*, epidemiologists can relate fewer than 30 percent of breast cancer cases to genetic or natural reproductive risk factors. Most women who have breast cancer, then, have few or none of the traditional risk factors.

Nevertheless, it is important to understand how your reproductive history may affect your risk. Among the factors you should understand are:

- When you enter puberty and menopause
- If you bear a child and at what age

TABLE 2.1: ESTROGEN AND BREAST CANCER: THE RISKS

Increased Risk	Decreased Risk
Hormonal Drugs	
Long-term oral contraceptive use	No oral contraceptive use
Long-term estrogen replacement therapy use	No estrogen replacement therapy use
Diet	
Industrial contaminants	Dietary protectants
High animal fat, high calorie	Low animal fat, low calorie
Lifestyle Factors	
Alcohol	Minimal or no use
Tobacco	Minimal or no use
Obesity	Normal weight range or leanness
Inactivity	Regular, vigorous exercise
Reproductive History	
Early menarche	Late menarche
Late menopause	Early menopause
No or late childbearing	Early childbearing
No breast-feeding	Breast-feeding

- If you decide to have one or more abortions and when
- If you decide to breast-feed

AGE AT MENARCHE AND MENOPAUSE

Estrogen levels are at their highest and most stimulating during the years your ovaries produce estrogen—the forty years or so between menarche and menopause. The longer you are fertile, the higher are your risks for breast cancer. At first glance, it might appear that the one risk factor for breast cancer you cannot control is your age at the onset of puberty and menopause. Most of us have been told (or have assumed) that such biological events are preprogrammed for us at birth or occur at "nature's will." However, we now know that two highly controllable lifestyle factors significantly affect the ages at which fertility begins and ends: the type and amount of food a woman eats (which directly affect her weight), and the amount of exercise she gets.

Puberty begins when the hypothalamus (a regulating area in the brain) signals the ovaries to begin estrogen production. Scientists believe that it is a young girl's body weight, percentage of body fat, level of physical activity, or a combination of these things that tells the hypothalamus to send out its signal. During the past two centuries, as the American diet has become more fat- and calorie-laden year by year, young girls have reached their "triggering weight" earlier and earlier. In fact, the average age of menarche has declined from about the age of 17 in the eighteenth century to about 12 years of age today.

Standard pediatric textbooks and earlier United States studies agree that, on average, Caucasian girls begin puberty by the age of 10 years and African-Americans between the ages of 8 and 9 years. However, a recent large-scale national survey of approximately 17,000 girls by 2,009 pediatricians, published in the April 4, 1997 issue of *Pediatrics*, reveals alarming evidence of precocious puberty. At the age of 3, 3 percent of African-American girls and 1 percent of Caucasian girls showed breast and/or pubic hair development, with proportions increasing to 27.2 percent and 6.7 percent, respectively, at 7 years of age. At the age of 8, 48.3 percent of African-American girls and 14.7 percent of Caucasian girls had begun puberty. The authors concluded that exposure to unidentified environmental estrogens may be responsible for the premature onset of puberty.

Many studies have confirmed the fact that the younger a woman is when she begins menstruating, the higher is her risk for developing both pre- and postmenopausal breast cancer. According to a study performed by cancer epidemiologist Walter Willet, the results of which were published in a 1989 article in *Nature* magazine, the risk associated with having an early menarche—for instance, one that takes place at the age of 10—is approximately twice that associated with a menarche that occurs much later, say at the age of 16 or so. Scientists estimate that for each additional year of menstruation—that is, for each year earlier that menarche begins—a woman's risk increases from 4 to 12 percent.

The same kind of risk profile exists at the other end of the fertility cycle: The younger a woman is at menopause, the lower her risk of breast cancer. For instance, a woman who stops menstruating at the age of 42 has half the risk for developing breast cancer as does a woman who stops at the age of 52.

The good news is that you do have some control over the length of time your body naturally produces estrogen: A recent study of some two hundred women between the ages of 17 and 22 years found that those whose diets were high in fiber and low in animal fat had a later menarche and subsequently fewer ovulatory and menstrual cycles than did those whose diet included more high-fat, low-fiber foods.

Vigorous exercise on a regular basis also works to delay the onset of menarche. Interestingly enough, a low-fat, high-fiber diet and regular exercise are the very same factors that influence the onset of an early menopause and thus reduce the risk of breast cancer by closing the estrogen window sooner than may have otherwise occurred.

PREGNANCY, CHILDBIRTH, AND YOUR RISK

To have a child, or more than one child, is an intensely personal decision that most women make without considering the impact childbirth may have on their risk for developing breast cancer. The truth, however, is that whether and when you decide to have a child influence the amount of estrogen in your bloodstream and thus the health of your breasts. In 1733, the famous Italian physician Bernardo Ramazzini related childbearing and breast cancer when he noted that nuns developed breast cancer far more frequently than did married women. More recent studies confirm these old findings: Breast cancer mortality is lowest in those United States counties with the highest birth rates.

Three major aspects that influence risk are deciding to have a child, the age at which you have your first child, and the number of children you have.

Deciding to Have a Child

Immature breast tissue is more vulnerable to estrogen stimulation than is breast tissue that has reached full maturity after a full-term pregnancy. That is one reason why bearing a child helps reduce the risk of breast cancer—particularly premenopausal cancer—for most women. In fact, childless women over the age of 45 run a risk from 20 to 70 percent higher than that of women who have given birth. A childless woman aged 45, for instance, increases her risks for developing breast cancer from 1 in 93 to as high as 1 in 37. In addition, experimental studies on rats show that mature breast cells are 50 percent less susceptible to the risk of breast cancer induced by a chemical carcinogen than are immature cells exposed to the same carcinogen.

Another reason pregnancy reduces the risk of breast cancer is that the period during and after gestation effectively closes the estrogen window. Although there is an initial estrogen surge at the very beginning of pregnancy (one that actually promotes the rapid growth and proliferation of breast tissue and cells and leaves breast cells more vulnerable to carcinogenic influences), estrogen levels decrease quickly and then progesterone levels soar. The presence of high levels of progesterone helps to mature the breast cells and bring them to a more stable and quiescent state as they prepare for milk production. These mature cells reproduce more slowly and thus are more resistant to carcinogenic influences. Another benefit of pregnancy regarding breast cancer is that during pregnancy and for several months after a full-term birth breast fluid contains much lower amounts of estrogen than are usually present. Finally, in childless women whose ovulatory cycle continues without interruption, the breasts go through many more cycles of estrogen stimulation. This prolonged level of exposure and estrogen-stimulated cell division increases the susceptibility of breast cells to carcinogenic influences.

Your Age at First Birth

During the past six decades, the incidence of breast cancer has increased at the same time that a rather striking sociological change in childbearing patterns has occurred: About 70 percent of women born in the 1930s bore their first child by the time they reached the age of 25, whereas only 50 percent of women born in the 1950s and 1960s had their first child by that age. More recent statistics, although not yet compiled, are certain to show that women are having their first child at later and later ages, especially professional women. Scientists believe that a strong connection exists between the later ages of childbearing and the increases in breast cancer rates.

Because breast cells do not mature until after a full-term pregnancy, woman are particularly vulnerable to breast cancer during the period between menarche and the birth of her first child. Therefore, the younger you are when you have your first child, the lower your risk of breast cancer, particularly if you have your baby before the age of 24. Conversely, having a first baby later in life may actually increase your risk: Women who have their first child after the age of 35, for instance, run a 30 percent higher risk for developing premenopausal breast cancer (a risk that may be reduced if they decide to breast-feed).

The reason for the increase in risk is that the immature breast cells of a woman with a late pregnancy are exposed to carcinogenic influences for many years longer—perhaps ten to fifteen years, or more—than are those of a woman who gives birth in her early twenties. Coupled with the surge of estrogen that comes with pregnancy, this longer exposure creates a climate for breast cancer development. Fortunately, the increased risk for women who choose to have a late first pregnancy is short-lived. Once she reaches the age of about 45, her risk decreases, especially during her postmenopausal years.

How Many Children You Have

Because each pregnancy you carry to term further matures your breast tissue, the more children you have the lower your risk of breast cancer. In fact, women who have at least five full-term pregnancies have half the risk of those who never bear children. An important exception to this protective effect is again for those women with a family history of breast cancer. Early repeated pregnancies seem to increase the risk in these women, and they remain at greater risk for much of their lives. In an important 1996 study published in the *Journal of the National Cancer Institute*, Dr. Graham Colditz of Harvard University and other co-investigators wisely counseled that "Women with a positive family history of breast cancer should not be counseled to have early and repeated pregnancies as a means of reducing their personal risk of breast cancer."

ABORTION AND BREAST CANCER RISK

As early as 1981, a study published in the *British Journal of Cancer* showed that women under the age of 33 who had never had a full-term pregnancy more than doubled their risk of breast cancer by having a first-trimester abortion. Then, in October, 1996, an analysis of twenty-three studies of abortion and breast cancer risk suggested that induced abortion can increase a woman's later risk for developing breast cancer more than about 30 percent. For example, if you were to have an abortion at the age of 25, your risk for developing breast cancer at the age of 60 would increase from 1 in 24 to about 1 in 18, especially if you have more than one abortion before your first full-term pregnancy.

The reason for this increase in risk is that a pregnancy terminated by a surgical abortion or miscarriage does not offer the same protection against breast cancer as does a full-term pregnancy. Again, estrogen levels lie at the heart of the issue. If a surge of progesterone fails to follow the initial increase in estrogen levels that occurs at the beginning of pregnancy, breast tissue both fails to fully mature (which leaves it more vulnerable) and receives additional estrogen stimulation.

However, it is important to note that a significant difference in risk exists between abortions performed early in the first trimester and those performed late in the pregnancy—and that difference is crucial. If an abortion is performed before estrogen surges, no increase in risk occurs. To test this hypothesis, scientists conducted a study on rats and published their findings in a 1980 issue of the *American Journal of Pathology*. The investigators injected the same known breast carcinogen into one group of rats that had had a single pregnancy and another into rats that had had an interrupted pregnancy. Those rats who had interrupted pregnancies suffered an accelerated breast cancer development compared with those who carried their young to term. However, if termination occurred before the progesterone surge, no increase in risk resulted.

In no way do we offer this information to alarm you unnecessarily or to make any political statement for or against abortion. Unfortunately, several so-called pro-life activist groups have tried to use the moderate breast cancer–abortion connection to frighten women into deciding against having the procedure, even though other influences, such as poor diet and exercise habits, appear to be more important risks of breast cancer than does abortion. In Japan, for instance, abortion is a common method of birth control, yet breast cancer incidence there is low. The decision to terminate a pregnancy is just as personal and intimate as is the decision to carry a baby to term. Without question, the emotional, financial, and medical risks connected with an unwanted pregnancy far outweigh the small to moderate increase in risk of breast cancer that surgical abortion appears to engender.

BREAST-FEEDING

In 1995, the latest in a long litany of studies (see page 39), this one published in an issue of *Cancer Causes and Control*, showed that women who breast-fed for seventeen months or longer had a reduction in risk of about 30 percent. Even those who breast-fed for only two weeks reduced their risk by about 13 percent. Clearly, a healthful way to reduce your chance of developing breast cancer is to breast-feed your baby. In addition to providing your baby with important nutrients, breast-feeding offers you some protection against breast cancer. It does so for two reasons: breast-feeding temporarily closes the estrogen window, and it reduces the levels of carcinogens in the breast.

When your baby suckles at your breast, that action sends a signal to the hypothalamus that helps control the release of hormones. The hypothalamus then inhibits the release of estrogen, progesterone, and other hormones, thus effectively stopping your menstrual cycle while you breast-feed and for a number of months afterward. How long your estrogen window remains closed after you stop lactating depends on how long you breast-feed, your weight, and other factors. The period usually lasts about a year or longer. Conversely, nonlactating women begin ovulating soon after childbirth. Nevertheless, women who breast-feed still can get pregnant, even if their estrogen levels remain lower than women who do not breast-feed.

In addition, studies show that breast-feeding reduces the levels of carcinogens that concentrate in the breast and other body fat, thus reducing the risk these carcinogens pose. In 1994, the *Journal of the National Cancer Institute* published a study of more than 500 Canadian women who breast-fed their babies, revealing something remarkable: The longer they had done so, the lower the levels of DDE (dichlorodiphenyldichloroethylene) in their breast milk. DDE is a by-product of the pesticide DDT (dichlorodiphenyltrichloroethane). Dichlorodiphenyldrichloroethylene concentrations

The Protection of Breast-feeding

Many studies have shown that breast-feeding will not only provide your baby with essential nutrients but also offer you protection against breast cancer. The following represents the most conclusive studies about this aspect of breast cancer prevention:

- In 1977, a study of women living in house boats in Aberdeen, Hong Kong—where traditionally infants nursed only from the right breast—reported the striking finding that risk of developing cancer was three times higher in the left breast, where milk would stagnate, than in the right breast.

- In 1986, a study in the *Journal of the American Medical Association* concluded that premenopausal women who had breast-fed had half the risk of breast cancer of those who had never breast-fed. This protective effect was enjoyed regardless of the woman's age, the number of children she had, or her age at first full-term pregnancy.

- In 1988, a Chinese study published in *Cancer* demonstrated a "clear beneficial effect on breast cancer risk of lactation in a population characterized by a long cumulative duration of nursing in the majority of women."

- In a 1989 issue of the *American Journal of Epidemiology*, scientists reported that they found a "modest" reduction among both pre- and postmenopausal Australian women who had breast-fed.

- In 1992, the *American Journal of Epidemiology* reported that Japanese women who breast-fed reduced their risk by about 40 percent. The longer they breast-fed, the lower their risk.

- In 1993, a United Kingdom study in the *British Medical Journal* found that the "risk of breast cancer fell with increasing duration of breast-feeding . . . and with the number of babies breast-fed."

- In 1994, the *New England Journal of Medicine* reported that women under the age of 20 who breast-fed for six months or longer had a 50 percent lower risk of premenopausal breast cancer than women who did not breast-feed.

in women who had never breast-fed were about twice those of women who had breast-fed for twelve months or longer. Other studies show that this reduction becomes more pronounced the more children a woman bears and breast-feeds.

Unfortunately, the protection a woman obtains from breast-feeding may come at the expense of exposing her baby to the carcinogens in her breast milk. This further stresses the need for women to choose diets low in carcinogen-contaminated meat and high-fat dairy products (chapter 9).

PERSONAL PROTECTION

Now that you have read about how your natural cycles of estrogen production affect your risk of breast cancer, you can make more informed choices in your reproductive life.

WHAT YOU CAN DO

- Avoid early menarche (or help your daughters to do so) and late menopause by exercising regularly and eating a high-fiber, low animal protein diet.

- Choose if, when, and how many children to have with care.

- Weigh the risks and benefits of abortion with care. If you choose to have an abortion, undergo the procedure as early as possible.

- Learn as much as possible about breast-feeding before you have your baby, and breast-feed your baby for as long as possible. Although even just a few months of breast-feeding offers protection, the longer you breast-feed, the more you lower your risk.

Avoid Early Menarche and Late Menopause

Although presumably you have reached puberty and thus cannot modify your own associated risks, you do have the power to help your younger sisters, daughters, and nieces postpone the onset of their menses by encouraging them to eat a low animal fat, high-fiber, low animal protein diet and exercise regularly (chapters 9 and 10).

If you have not yet reached menopause, you should consider following the same advice for two reasons. First, by making healthful eating and regular exercise a part of your life, you will help protect yourself against many diseases, including heart disease, diabetes, and arthritis. Second, if you maintain a normal weight and exercise regularly, chances are you will stop menstruating a year or two sooner than you might have if you had gained weight and had led a sedentary lifestyle.

Carefully Choose If, When, and How Many Children to Have

The younger you are when you have your first child and the more children you have, the lower your risk of breast cancer. Of course, deciding when and if to have a child is a uniquely personal issue.

For women with a family history of breast cancer, having children at an early age increases premenopausal and postmenopausal risks.

Carefully Weigh the Risks and Benefits of Abortion

Should you decide to have an abortion, the best way to avoid adding to your breast cancer risk is to terminate the pregnancy as early as possible. By doing so you will avoid flooding your breast tissue with the surge of estrogen that occurs by the beginning of the second month of pregnancy. Drug-induced abortions (as opposed to surgical abortions) in the form of RU-486 and other drugs should make early abortions easier to obtain and endure.

REDUCE YOUR RISKS BY BREAST-FEEDING

Most doctors now recommend breast-feeding for any number of reasons, including the fact that it offers some protection against breast cancer. Nevertheless, only 50 percent of American women breast-fed their babies in 1994 and only 30 percent were still nursing at six months. We believe that hospitals and insurance companies bear a great deal of responsibility for this turn of events because, until quite recently, they offered only minimal support to new mothers who wanted to breast-feed, often covering only a hospital stay of less than twenty-four hours. Unfortunately, such a short stay does not allow a woman and her baby to receive the necessary support and training they may need to become accustomed to breast-feeding during the first few days after childbirth. This is especially true for very young, low-income, less well-educated women, who also tend to receive even less encouragement, training, and support for breast-feeding than do their more economically advantaged sisters.

Doctors and nurses have long warned that this insurance industry policy is a major disincentive to breast-feeding. In response to such concerns, Maryland, New Jersey, and New York passed laws in the mid-1990s insisting that the health care insurers that operate in these states allow mothers and their newborns to remain in the hospital for more than twenty-four hours. Recent federal legislation, championed by President Bill Clinton, now requires all health care insurers, such as Blue Cross and Blue Shield, to cover at least a forty-eight-hour hospital stay for both mothers and infants. The next hurdle is to encourage employers to allow mothers who are breast-feeding some flexibility with their schedules until their babies are weaned. We discuss that issue at greater length in chapter 13. Meanwhile, in chapter 3 we outline one of the most important and avoidable risk factors related to estrogen: oral contraceptives.

PART II

Modern Medicine and Breast Cancer Risks

3

The Pill: Assessing Your Risks

> Oral contraceptives represent an avoidable cause of breast cancer. Oral contraceptives are unsafe, especially for women with benign breast disease, with a family history of breast cancer, or who began taking oral contraceptives in their teen years for prolonged periods. Safe and effective nonhormone contraceptives are available as alternatives to the birth control pill.

"No Link Is Found Between Pill and Breast Cancer" read a headline in *The New York Times* on September 25, 1996. This article, and many others like it in newspapers and popular magazines throughout the country, announced a new study published by the British medical journal *The Lancet*. Based on a collaborative reanalysis (known as a *meta-analysis*) of some fifty-four epidemiological studies involving a total of 150,000 women, the article claimed that a relationship between "breast cancer risk and hormone exposure is unusual" and that women who use or have used oral contraceptives are at only a "slightly" increased risk for developing breast cancer.

Unfortunately, this report and its media interpretations misled women about the very real risks associated with taking the Pill. In fact, there is no evidence that the Pill is safe to take, especially not for prolonged periods or starting in one's teenage years. Later in this chapter, we will outline in more depth the serious flaws in the interpretation of *The Lancet* study. In the meantime, it is important to understand how oral contraceptives work and how they may increase the risk of breast cancer.

UNDERSTANDING ORAL CONTRACEPTION

Since its introduction in the 1960s, the birth control pill, or oral contraceptive, has become one of the most popular and widely prescribed drugs in the United States and around the world. It is convenient, affordable, and up to 99 percent effective in preventing pregnancy. Unfortunately, by taking the Pill, you expose breast tissue to higher amounts of estrogen than your body would normally produce. The Pill works by maintaining high levels of estrogen in the body in order to prevent the ovaries from releasing eggs.

TYPES OF ORAL CONTRACEPTIVES

Believe it or not, the origin of the modern oral contraceptive is the Mexican wild yam (a plant unrelated to the yams we eat at Thanksgiving). During the 1930s, scientist Russell Marker discovered that the Mexican yam contains a chemical called diosgenin, from which he could synthesize estrogen, progesterone, and other hormones.

Ever since, industry scientists have been working to refine the makeup of oral contraceptives. The first oral contraceptives contained high doses of mestranol (ethinylestradiol methyl ether), a relatively weak synthetic estrogen (up to 0.15 milligrams or 150 micrograms), and synthetic progesterone or progestin (up to 10 milligrams). In the late 1970s, scientists developed a "second-generation" Pill, one that delivered lower doses of ethinyl estradiol, a highly potent synthetic estrogen (20 to 35 micrograms or less) and progestin (under one milligram). It should be noted that ethinyl estradiol is about forty times more potent than the most active natural estrogen, estradiol.

Because the doses of estrogen and progestin are lower in the second-generation Pill than in the first, the pharmaceutical industry hails them as being "safer." However, several factors indicate just the opposite—that the second-generation Pill actually poses higher risks for developing breast cancer:

- The type of estrogen (mestranol) used in the first-genera-tion Pill is half as potent as the type used in the second-gen-eration Pill (ethinyl estradiol). Also, unlike ethinyl estradiol, mestranol does not bind to estrogen receptors in the breast.

- Most women who used the first-generation Pill did so for a relatively short time and usually starting in their twenties, whereas women using the second-generation Pill tend to do so for much longer, sometimes starting in their teens and continuing to menopause, thus putting breast tissue under constant hormone stimulation.

Women used the so-called first-generation Pill from the early 1960s through the 1970s—and most of the studies that have been performed on the Pill were based on the first-generation form. Most women in the 1980s and today use the second-generation Pill. More recently, a third-generation Pill that uses progestin only has become popular in Europe and is slowly becoming accepted in North America. Other forms of hormonal contraceptives (such as the implant Norplant, or levonorgestrel, manufactured by Wyeth-Ayerst Laboratories; the injectable Depo-Provera, or medroxyprogesterone, manufactured by Upjohn; and "Morning-After Pills," which are taken orally shortly after unprotected sex) are also used in the United States and around the world. Each contains different amounts of estrogens, progestins, or both, having different poten-cies, and each has its own set of side effects, levels of breast cancer risk, and marketing history.

MARKETING OF THE PILL

In the late 1950s, a California-based company called Syntex began to manufacture hormonal drugs for birth control. Other companies such as Searle and Parke-Davis soon joined Syntex in a race to market the first generation of oral contraceptives based on a combination of estrogen and progesterone. By 1960, the Food and Drug Administration (FDA) approved the first oral contraceptive (called Enovid-10, which contained 10 milligrams of the progestin called norethynodrel along with mestranol), despite receiving reports of serious side effects and in the absence of any large-scale studies. Searle marketed Enovid-10, and within a few years the Food and Drug Administration (FDA) approved other oral contraceptives. Ortho Pharmaceutical, Upjohn, Mead Johnson, and Eli Lilly soon got into the game with Syntex, Searle, and Parke-Davis.

Both the medical establishment and the press enthusiastically and uncritically endorsed the FDA's approval of these new drugs, while the lines between professional medical groups and the pharmaceutical industry—supposedly regulated by the government—disappeared altogether. Magazine articles officially authorized by the FDA offered glowing accolades for the Pill, including one in the July 3, 1964, issue of *Life* magazine authored by the agency's top physician, Joseph F. Sadusk. (Sadusk later became a vice-president of Parke-Davis.) Nine days later, the American Medical Association placed their official stamp of approval on another enthusiastic article about birth control, this one published in the magazine *This Week*.

The Pill marked the beginning of the world's largest mass human experiment in commercial drugs. In 1960 alone, 800,000 American women used oral contraceptives. By 1965, one in four married women were or had been using the Pill, and by 1969, federal family-planning programs had become major distributors. By 1970, eight United States pharmaceutical companies were selling some thirty-six oral contraceptives under twelve brand names.

The Pill, however, had a few early vocal critics. In 1969, Barbara Seaman, who later founded the National Women's Health Network, investigated the industry and published her findings in the trail-blazing book *The Doctors' Case Against the Pill*. After revealing that

Searle had suppressed numerous reports of the Pill's serious side effects, including blood clots, Seaman warned that the pharmaceutical industry, government, and doctors routinely dismissed or trivialized evidence of the risks. By doing so, doctors violated the fundamental principles of informed consent.

Seaman's aggressive reporting triggered federal investigations. Senator Gaylord Nelson of Wisconsin chaired Senate hearings that received widespread and dramatic press coverage. A headline in the *New York Post* read "Senate Panel Told the Pill Can Kill," while one in the *San Francisco Chronicle* announced "Pill and Cancer—What Medicine Says." This article quoted Dr. Hugh Davis of Johns Hopkins University, in Baltimore, Maryland, who told the panel his disturbing opinion on the Pill:

> *Never in history have so many individuals taken such potent drugs with so little information available as to the actual and potential hazards. The synthetic chemicals in the Pill are quite unnatural with respect to their manufacture and with respect to their behavior once they are introduced into the human body. In using these agents, we are in fact embarked on a massive endocrinologic experiment with millions of healthy women.*

Despite these concerns, the popularity of oral contraceptives continued to surge. By 1986, more than 50 percent of British women aged 20 to 24 were taking the Pill. Today, 75 percent of United States women have used oral contraceptives at some time in their lives and more than eleven million are currently using the Pill. Of this eleven million, 33 percent are over the age of 30 and about 10 percent are over 40. In many cases, women begin taking the Pill in their teens and continue to take it, without stopping, into their fifties—despite the clear risks associated with its use over long periods of time. Moreover, women often go directly from taking the Pill to taking estrogen replacement therapy, further increasing their estrogen exposure and probably their lifetime cancer risk.

THE PILL AND BREAST CANCER RISK

To date, scientists have performed their most extensive and comprehensive tests on the first-generation Pill, mainly because it has been around for almost two decades longer than have its second- and third-generation counterparts (see the studies on pages 51–53). Although the results of studies performed on the first-generation Pill may not apply to later forms, it seems clear that some of the same risks and side effects remain. In fact, the risks are probably much greater with second-generation oral contraceptives because of their higher potency. The few studies that have been performed on the second- and third-generation Pills indicate an increase in breast cancer risk.

As early as the 1930s, experimental studies showed that estrogen induces breast and other cancers in a wide variety of rodent species. By the late 1960s, researchers overseeing studies at the National Institutes of Health in Washington, D.C., reported to the FDA that they had found precancerous changes in the breasts of monkeys given doses of oral contraceptives. As described in a 1969 article in the journal *Cancer*, six rhesus monkeys given standard doses of an oral contraceptive manufactured by Searle developed breast cancer after only eighteen months. The researchers concluded that the use of oral contraceptives had adverse effects: "Since tumors in general and carcinomas of the breast specifically seem very rare in monkeys, it appears possible that the lesion was causally related to the drug." Nevertheless, both the FDA and Searle claimed that the finding was random and inconclusive.

At the First National Conference on Breast Cancer in 1969, the chief of endocrine cancer at the National Cancer Institute, Roy Hertz, warned about the potential danger of birth control pills:

> *Our inadequate knowledge concerning the relationship of estrogen to cancer in women is comparable to what was known about the association between lung cancer and cigarette smoking before extensive epidemiological studies delineated this overwhelmingly demonstrated significant statistical relationship.*

Another set of animal studies conducted in the 1970s led to an article in the May 21, 1976, issue of the *Medical Letter*. The article emphasized that estrogen causes cancer of the breast, endometrium, cervix, pituitary gland, ovaries, testes, kidney, and bone in mice, rats, hamsters, squirrel-monkeys, and dogs. The *Letter* warned: "No other drug effect so readily reproducible in such a wide variety of test animals has been generally regarded as not potentially applicable to man."

Since that time, more than twenty well-controlled studies have demonstrated the clear risk of premenopausal breast cancer with the use of oral contraceptives. These estimates indicate that a young woman who uses oral contraceptives has up to ten times the risk for developing breast cancer as does a nonuser, particularly:

- If she uses the Pill during her teens or early twenties
- If she uses the Pill for two years or more
- If she uses the Pill before her first full-term pregnancy
- If she has a family history of breast cancer

Furthermore, several studies (cited in various sources such as a 1988 article in the *British Journal of Cancer*, a May 1989 article cited in the *New York Times*, and a 1990 article in *Cancer*) warned that the risk of breast cancer is long-lasting. This means that postmenopausal women are also at increased risk for developing breast cancer many years after first using oral contraceptives.

Hormonal Contraceptives and Breast Cancer: The Studies

- In 1977, a study published in *Cancer* found that the risk of breast cancer increased after two to four years of oral contraceptive use, and further increased in women with a history of benign breast disease and in women who had not yet had a full-term pregnancy.

- A 1981 study published in the *British Journal of Cancer* reported a nearly fourfold increased risk in women under the age of 33 who had used oral contraceptives for eight years before their first pregnancy.

(continued)

- In 1982, the *American Journal of Epidemiology* announced that women aged 35 to 54 who at any time used oral contraceptives before their first childbirth tripled their risk of breast cancer. The longer they had used oral contraceptives, the more their risk increased.

- In 1986, a joint study from Sweden and Norway published in *The Lancet* revealed that women under the age of 45 doubled their risk if they used the Pill for more than eight years before having their first child.

- A 1987 study published in the *British Journal of Cancer* reported that women under the age of 45 who had used the Pill for over four years before their first full-term pregnancy more than doubled their risk.

- A 1988 study from Slovenia published in *Neoplasia* reported that the overall risk of breast cancer increased significantly with duration of use, particularly for seven or more years. This risk increased to more than sevenfold in women with a family history.

- In 1988, the Cancer and Steroid Hormone Study published in the journal *Contraception* revealed that women who had used oral contraceptives for eight years or more, who had never given birth, and who had begun menstruating before the age of 13 were at increased risk for developing breast cancer before the age of 45. The risk was nearly threefold for eight to eleven years of use, and twelvefold for twelve or more years of use.

- In 1989, Swedish investigators reported to the *Journal of the National Cancer Institute* that using the Pill at a young age "significantly increases the risk of breast cancer. . . ." "Starting age and duration of OC use before the first full-term pregnancy as well as before age 25 were . . .associated with significant increases in breast cancer risk."

- In 1990, an analysis of some thirty-two studies published in the journal *Cancer* revealed a "statistically positive trend in the risk of premenopausal breast cancer for women exposed to OCs for longer duration." This risk was predominant among women who used oral contraceptives for at least four years before their first full-term pregnancy.

- In 1991, an eleven-nation study published in *Contraception* demonstrated a "small increase" in the risk of breast cancer in recent and current users. This risk increased with duration of use.

- In 1994, a large, well-controlled study published in the *Journal of the National Cancer Institute* reported a "small increased risk of breast cancer associated with long duration of oral contraceptive use." The increase in risk was about 30 percent but increased to 70 percent "particularly among women aged 35 years or younger." A 30-old-woman, then, increases her risk from 1 in 2,525 to 1 in 764.

- In 1995, a National Cancer Institute study found a definite link between the length of time oral contraceptives are used and breast cancer risk. A few months of use could increase a woman's risk by 30 percent. A more than twofold risk was found with ten years of use or longer. The same study showed that oral contraceptive use was associated with cancer in its most advanced stages at diagnosis in women under the age of 35.

In addition to stimulating breast tissue, the high levels of hormones found in the first-generation Pill caused a host of other side effects, some quite serious. According to many studies performed around the world and published in the 1970s in well-established medical journals such as *The Lancet, Annals of Internal Medicine,* and *Journal of the American Medical Association,* women who used the first-generation Pill risked the following:

- Stroke and blot clots, especially if the women also smoked or had concurrent high blood pressure

- Heart attack, particularly in women over the age of 35 who smoked

- Diabetic-type changes (some 5 percent of women on the Pill developed diabetes)

- Gallbladder disease

- Liver cancer

- Depression

- Increased susceptibility to venereal disease

- Possibly passing along an increased risk of breast cancer to their infant daughters through breast-feeding (because residues of oral contraceptive hormones are found to contaminate breast milk)

As more of the medical community finally became aware of these side effects and as these complaints began to influence the sales of oral contraceptives, industry scientists set about devising a Pill containing lower amounts of hormones. Their research led to the so-called second-generation Pill. Unfortunately, the efforts to diminish serious side effects, including increased risk of breast cancer, have not been successful. It is likely that we have jumped from the frying pan into the fire.

Risks of The Second-Generation Pill

Today, both the pharmaceutical industry and the medical establishment refute studies that link breast cancer and the Pill, claiming that the much lower doses of estrogen and progestin used in the second-generation Pill are safer. As discussed, however, several factors undermine this claim. In the 1995 revised edition of her landmark book *The Doctors' Case Against the Pill*, Barbara Seaman warned that "Women should be aware that the lower hormone doses have not solved all the problems surrounding the Pill." Others, such as the Public Citizen Health Research Group, expressed even stronger concerns in a 1991 report in *Women's Health Alert*:

> *If low doses allow women to use the Pill for a longer period of time, perhaps the accumulated effect by age 60 is worse. Without data, no one can be sure whether low doses are safer or not. For epidemiological evidence on the association between low dose Pills and breast cancer, we will have to wait quite a while, maybe 20 years, until the young women now taking lower doses of the Pill reach the age at which they may or may not develop breast cancer.*

The new Pill simply has not been around long enough for scientists to adequately assess its long-term safety. Moreover, the formula for the new Pill demands the use of progestin and the synthetic ethinyl estradiol, which is forty times more potent than natural estradiol; this means that although the amount is lower, the stimulatory effect is very much higher. Finally, women now tend to start using the Pill much earlier, and they use it for much longer—even until menopause—than women have in the past, partly because women become sexually active much younger and partly because doctors prescribe the Pill so readily.

Even the FDA has joined in with its own set of concerns. The author of the 1995 book *The Pill: A Biography of the Drug that Changed the World*, B. Asbell, quoted FDA officials as admitting the following:

> *Questions about the Pill's association with cancer, however, remain. Some widely reported recent studies support the hypothesis that in certain groups of women the risk of breast cancer increases with oral contraceptive use. . . . One of the major problems . . . is that all the data reflect the effects of the higher-dose Pills. . . . No studies have been done on the recent low-dose Pills, and none are under way. The cancer-Pill issue is very complicated and therefore difficult to study, and the research is expensive. . . .*

If information about the second-generation Pill seems scanty, the problems and dangers seem only to be compounded in the third generation of oral contraceptives.

RISKS OF THE THIRD-GENERATION PILL AND OTHER HORMONAL CONTRACEPTIVES

Evidence is growing that the third-generation Pill, which contains only synthetic progestin, may be just as dangerous, or even more so, than its predecessors. In 1986, a study in the *New England Journal of Medicine* reported that women taking progestin-only contraceptives run a 30 percent increased risk of breast cancer, a result confirmed by animal studies. In 1989 two researchers, J. Weisz and P.D. Stolley, wrote the following in a letter to the Commissioner of the FDA:

> *The incidence of breast cancer has long been known to be markedly increased in dogs exposed chronically to the action of diverse progestogens (synthetic version of progesterone). . . . Other studies find that progestins injected into rodents increase the effects of other chemical carcinogens.*

Despite these alarming findings, the pharmaceutical industry went on to develop alternatives to the traditional combination oral contraceptives that contain powerful progestins alone. One such alternative is Norplant (levonorgestrel), made with a progestin that the World Health Organization's International Agency for Research on Cancer warned is "one of the most potent progestational compounds." Consisting of small capsules filled with progestin that are implanted under the skin by a physician, Norplant is relatively inexpensive and easy to administer, and it prevents pregnancy for up to five years. At this time, most women who choose Norplant are low-income, African-American women who lack access to the kind of medical support and education other forms of birth control require.

Although its risks for breast cancer have not yet been studied specifically, mainly because it has been used for a relatively short time, Norplant has recently come under serious scrutiny by the FDA for other reasons. According to an anonymous source quoted in a 1995 issue of the newsletter *Breast Implants,* the FDA has received more than 6,000 complaints of adverse reactions to Norplant. Patients have complained of blistering and scarring at the implantation site, double vision, vomiting, severe migraine headaches, blood clots, heart attacks, respiratory failure, and stroke. By 1995, more than 180 lawsuits, including forty-six class action suits, had been filed against the maker of Norplant, Wyeth-Ayerst Laboratories.

Today, the manufacturer mandates that users of Norplant sign a "patient acknowledgment form," indicating that they received warnings from their doctors about these serious risks.

Another contraceptive option is Depo-Provera, an injectable form of progestin that protects against pregnancy for three months. Another birth control method used largely by low-income women in the United States and in less developed countries, Depo-Provera also increases the risk of breast cancer within a relatively short time after its use, as evidenced by studies in the *Journal of the National Cancer Institute*, the *British Medical Journal*, and *Lancet*, among others. In an article in a 1995 issue of *Journal of the American Medical Association*, researchers stated, "We found that women who started using [Depo-Provera] appeared to have an increased risk of breast cancer within 5 years. . . ."

Studies on animals also indicate an increased breast cancer risk. As early as 1973, studies showed that Depo-Provera induced breast cancer in beagle dogs when given in doses equivalent to those used for contraception. In 1989, the FDA acknowledged the breast cancer risk of Depo-Provera:

> *All oral contraceptives containing progesterone-derived progestogens, such as medroxyprogesterone acetate [Depo-Provera] and megestrol acetate, were taken off the market in the 1960s because all were found to induce tumors in beagle dogs.*

Despite these and other warnings, the FDA still allows doctors to prescribe and administer Depo-Provera.

A third major type of hormonal contraceptives in use today is Morning-After Pills used by women who have unprotected sex and do not wish to become pregnant. Morning-After Pills consist of very high doses of synthetic estrogens, progestins, or combinations that must be started within three days of unprotected intercourse. The most common brand of Morning-After Pill is Desogen, a combination of desogestrel and ethinyl estradiol, manufactured by Organon; however, no studies have investigated the risks of their short-term and infrequent use. Because these drugs subject the body to just one large "hit" of hormones instead of hormones on a daily basis, the risks they pose for breast cancer are possibly minimal.

ORAL CONTRACEPTIVES: THE WHOLE STORY

Without question, hormonal contraceptives are highly effective methods of birth control. They also offer other benefits, such as protecting against uterine and ovarian cancers, and lowering the risks of tubal pregnancies and childbirth-related mortality. Nevertheless, oral contraceptives pose serious risks including those of breast cancer, stroke, and blood clots. Another serious drawback to the Pill is its failure to protect against syphilis, gonorrhea, acquired immune deficiency syndrome (AIDS), and other sexually transmitted diseases, the incidences of which continue to increase, especially among teenagers and young adults.

The cancer establishment continues to dismiss the risks, despite clear evidence to the contrary that is well recognized by informed and independent experts. As early as January 7, 1989, a *New York Times* report emphasized the conclusion of leading experts that data linking oral contraceptives to breast cancer were so troubling that some women should be discouraged from taking oral contraceptives. The article quotes Marc Lippman, M.D., a prominent breast cancer specialist and director of the Vincent Lombardi Cancer Center of Georgetown University Medical School in Washington, D.C.:

> *I don't want to be inflammatory, but breast cancer is a disease for which 20 years or 30 years may be the time required to see the impact of long-term use. . . . Unfortunately, that's the time we're getting into now. It's worrisome. I would do what I could to encourage women to consider other forms of contraception.*

Craig Henderson, M.D., of the Dana Farber Cancer Center in Boston, Massachusetts, voiced similar misgivings. He, too, said that he would "discourage" young women from taking the Pill for longer than two years. He also criticized the medical establishment and family planning clinics for taking the risks of using the Pill so lightly. "Because we have perceived the Pill as being completely without danger, in our more sexually permissive society we have moved to saying a young girl can take birth control pills almost as soon as she reaches menarche."

There are many other ways in which the pharmaceutical industry and cancer establishment trivialize risks. The FDA, for instance, has taken little action to ensure that drug packaging inserts provide clear warnings. For instance, the package insert for the popular contraceptive Ortho-Novum (norethindrone, plus ethinyl estradiol or mestranol), manufactured by Ortho Pharmaceutical, reassures doctors and prospective users about the minimal increase in breast cancer risk:

> *Numerous epidemiological studies have been performed on the incidence of breast . . . cancer in women using oral contraceptives. While there are conflicting reports, most studies suggest that use of oral contraceptives is not associated with an overall increase in the risk of developing breast cancer.*

A Norplant brochure, frequently distributed by gynecologists, never even mentioned breast cancer. Instead, it simply suggested that women with a history of nodules, fibrocystic disease, an abnormal breast X-ray film or mammogram "may need to be checked more often by their health care provider." The 1997 *Physicians Desk Reference* is only slightly less dismissive of breast cancer risks in advising "no consistent pattern of findings has been identified." In none of their widely distributed literature does the American Cancer Society even discuss oral contraceptive risk factors for breast cancer—or any cancer, for that matter. The only reference is a positive one: The American Cancer Society stresses the protection that oral contraceptives provide against ovarian cancer.

As the millennium nears, forty years after the first Pill hit the marketplace, the pharmaceutical industry and the cancer establishment continue to trivialize the risks of breast cancer posed by the Pill, as evidenced by their misinterpretation of *The Lancet* 1996 study cited at the beginning of this chapter. Proclaiming that the results of this latest meta-analysis of fifty-four epidemiological studies means that "no link between the Pill and breast cancer exists," the media and the industry failed to recognize the following:

- **Short duration of study**: The results of the studies examined in *The Lancet* article were based mostly on relatively short and inadequate follow-up periods, generally less than twenty years after women stopped using the Pill. Furthermore, the studies focused on the first-generation Pill, a form of low-potency oral contraceptive on the market only until about 1980, which women then took for relatively brief periods of time. Any studies performed on current oral contraceptives, then, would have far less than twenty years of follow-up available. The risks to most women using the Pill today, therefore, remain unknown.

- **Dismissal of high-risk subgroups**: The analysis clearly showed a much higher risk for women who started using the Pill as teenagers and who used it over a long period of time: Women who started using the Pill before the age of 17 and used it for more than a year, for instance, increased their risk by more than 80 percent within four years after they stopped using it. Among current and recent users, women who started using the Pill within five years of their menarche have the highest relative risk of breast cancer.

- **Dilution of risks**: Scientists derived the results of themeta-analysis by averaging a wide range of studies, such as women starting the Pill as teenagers in contrast to those starting later in life after having children, and thus diluting or smoothing out much higher risks found in some of the studies, particularly risks from early and prolonged use.

PERSONAL PROTECTION

As convenient as oral contraceptives may be, they represent an avoidable risk of breast cancer, especially in young women or in women who use them for more than a year. Fortunately, safer birth control methods exist.

WHAT YOU CAN DO

- Avoid using hormonal contraceptives, if possible.
- Use one of the safe and effective alternatives to the Pill, and teach sexually active adolescents about safer forms of birth control.

AVOID USING ORAL CONTRACEPTIVES IF POSSIBLE

If you are sexually active and do not wish to become pregnant, you and your partner have a decision to make about birth control. Without question, the risks associated with an unwanted pregnancy are very real, sometimes tragic, and should be prevented with the use of effective birth control. In most instances, the prevention of pregnancy by convenient hormonal contraceptives may well be more important than is any increased risk of breast cancer.

In most cases, however, the Pill is not a good first choice of birth control because its benefits do not outweigh the significant risk of breast cancer and other complications, especially with prolonged use starting at an early age. Furthermore, the Pill provides no protection against sexually transmitted diseases, which are currently reaching epidemic proportions. If you are using the Pill or another hormonal contraceptive, consider switching to a different method unless you have a compelling reason to continue. Consider discontinuing the Pill immediately if you:

- Have not yet had a full-term pregnancy

- Are under the age of 25, even more so under the age of 20

- Have a family history of breast cancer

- Have a history of benign breast disease

CHOOSE ONE OF THE SAFE, EFFECTIVE ALTERNATIVES TO THE PILL

As we head into the twenty-first century, we face many medical and social challenges, especially when it comes to issues of reproductive health. Rates of unwanted pregnancies and sexually transmitted diseases continue to soar in tandem. Yet the development of new, safer, and more effective methods of birth control appears to be a painstakingly slow process. In a December 27, 1995, article in the *New York Times*, Susan Tew, of the Guttmacher Institute, a leading reproductive research center, had discouraging words about the development of safer contraceptives for men and women:

> *There's clearly a need for better contraceptive methods, when well over half the pregnancies to U.S. women are unplanned. And we clearly need more methods that offer dual protection, from pregnancies and from sexually transmitted disease. But it doesn't look like we'll see much on the market soon.*

So far, the following methods of birth control are in widespread use. Each has its own risks and benefits, and you should discuss the matter thoroughly with your doctor and your sexual partner.

The Condom

The *male condom* has been used for centuries as a barrier method to prevent pregnancy and protect against the spread of disease. Today, lubricated latex condoms that contain a spermicide are up to 98 percent effective against pregnancy when used properly. Condoms also have the advantage of protecting against sexually transmitted diseases. No side effects exist with condom use, although some men and women complain of decreased sensitivity during the sexual act. It is important to avoid using condoms coated with talc, which has been incriminated as a cause of ovarian cancer.

The *female condom* is a rubber sheath placed in the vagina to cover the cervix. When used properly it is an effective barrier against pregnancy and sexually transmitted diseases. However, most women and men find it awkward and uncomfortable.

The Diaphragm

The most effective barrier method for women, the diaphragm, has a 98.5 percent success rate, again, when used properly and in conjunction with a spermicide. You need to see a doctor to be fitted for a diaphragm: A proper fit is crucial to its effectiveness. The side effects of diaphragm use are minimal and rare. They include cramping, infection, and inflammation. The diaphragm does not provide protection against most sexually transmitted diseases.

The Intrauterine Device

The intrauterine device, or IUD, is 95 to 98 percent effective in preventing pregnancy. The IUD is a small piece of plastic that is inserted into the uterus by a physician. The IUD prevents pregnancy by creating changes in the lining of the uterus that make it difficult for a fertilized egg to become implanted and grow. Common side effects include increased bleeding and pain during menstruation. Rarer and more serious complications include pelvic inflammatory disease and ectopic pregnancy. The IUD provides no protection against sexually transmitted diseases.

The Cervical Cap

A plastic cap designed to fit snugly over the cervix, the cervical cap is similar in design to the diaphragm and must be fitted by a physician. When used with a spermicide, the cervical cap is just as effective as a condom (98 percent) but does not provide protection against sexually transmitted diseases.

Other Products

Among the products still in the developmental stage are new vaginal sponges, cervical caps, and other barrier devices that may also have the ability to block viruses such as herpes and the human immuno-deficiency virus, or HIV. Contraceptives for men (other than the condom) appear to be several years away from being available. One method involving weekly injections of testosterone to reduce sperm count may be just as dangerous to men as hormone contraceptives are to women, because testosterone causes proliferation of the cells of the prostate and other reproductive organs.

4

Estrogen Replacement Therapy: Pros and Cons

> Estrogen replacement therapy (ERT) is an avoidable cause of breast cancer. Risks are greatest with prolonged use and high doses, and also with estrogen-progestin combinations. Safer alternatives are available.

MEDICINE FOR A GENERATION

Susan Love, M.D., stated in a *New York Times* op-ed piece on March 20, 1997:

> *Just as the baby boomers hit middle age, the pharmaceutical industry and the medical profession have discovered a new disease: menopause, or as it is called clinically, estrogen deficiency disease, [but] menopause is not a disease; it is a normal part of life. A woman's ovaries don't shut down at menopause. They continue to produce low levels of hormones well into a woman's 80s. Synthetic hormones don't replace something that is missing when women reach menopause. They add something that is not naturally there. . . . Women must redefine menopause as something natural.*

Susan Love's editorial marks a late entry into a three-decade-long debate on the safety and necessity of estrogen replacement therapy

(ERT). Her approach represents a distinct departure from the prevailing attitude about menopause, one that relegates menopause to a disease that should be treated with ERT in every woman. This view of menopause as a disease has deep roots and gained widespread popularity with the 1966 publication of Dr. Robert Wilson's bestseller, *Feminine Forever*. In it he wrote:

> *The unpalatable truth must be faced that all post-menopausal women are castrates. . . . Our streets abound with them—walking stiffly in twos and threes, seeing little and observing less. It is not unusual to see an erect man of 75 vigorously striding along on a golf course, but never a woman of this age. . . . Now, for the first time in history, women may share the promise of tomorrow as biological equals of men. Thanks to hormone therapy, they can be feminine forever.*

In *Feminine Forever*, one of the top-selling books of 1966, New York City obstetrician-gynecologist Robert Wilson offered women (and the men in their lives) estrogen as a kind of "miracle cure" for the perceived loss of sexuality and vitality associated with aging. Wilson first insulted older women, then promised them eternal youth and sexual equality—as long as they took estrogen. Wilson's book sold more than 100,000 copies in its first seven months of publication, and its subject—estrogen replacement therapy—soon became one of the hottest topics in both medicine and the media. Robert Greenblatt, then the chairman of the Department of Endocrinology at the Medical College of Georgia, wrote that Wilson "sounds the clarion call, awakening a slumbering profession to a woman's needs." Articles about ERT appeared in the *New Republic*, *Vogue*, and *Time*, among many other publications.

Within 10 years, estrogen had become the fifth most commonly prescribed drug in the United States, and since then the popularity of ERT has only grown. Today, doctors dispense ERT in the form of pills, patches, and creams to more than 25 percent of menopausal women, making it one of the top-selling prescription drugs in the country. The media continues to extol its virtues as well: "Estrogen Replacement: More Important than Ever," read a 1995 headline in *Consumer Reports on Health*. A 1995 *Reader's Digest* cover story called ERT "The Pill that Keeps Women Young." What the media continues to ignore, however, are the serious risks of breast cancer and other health risks posed by ERT.

As the baby boomer generation begins to cross the threshold of middle age in greater numbers every year, the issues surrounding menopause become ever more urgent. Indeed, by the year 2010, more than fifty million American women will be at or through the passage from fertility to late life. Today, the fastest growing segment of the population consists of men and women over the age of 85.

Estrogen replacement therapy is an entrenched industry that exploits the protective power of hormones. As we age, our bodies stop or slow production of a variety of different hormones, including the primary sex hormones. Some scientists believe that replacing these hormones as they diminish may help the body stay young and vital far longer than the present seventy years or so, and the media has taken up this cry of "forever young" with enthusiasm. At the same time, many physicians have cautioned against taking hormones of any kind. Hormones are very powerful substances that have the potential to affect every organ and system in the body. We have only to look at our experience with ERT, in use by many millions since the 1960s, to see the potential dangers involved.

We take a position somewhere in between Dr. Love's almost blanket condemnation of ERT and Dr. Wilson's uncritical if not reckless promotion of hormone replacement. Indeed, ERT has its benefits; however, it also has its risks, some of which are quite serious, such as that of breast cancer. ERT is *not* a cure for aging, nor is it the only option for women who want to protect their health and vitality after menopause. In this chapter, we define these risks and benefits of ERT so that you can make an informed decision for yourself.

THE RISKS AND BENEFITS OF ESTROGEN REPLACEMENT THERAPY	
Benefits	Risks
Reduces	*Increases*
Heart disease and stroke	Breast cancer
Osteoporosis	Uterine cancer
Colon cancer	Ovarian cancer
Alzheimer's disease	Blood clotting
Urinary incontinence	Benign breast disease
Vaginal atrophy	Uterine fibroids
Menopausal symptoms: hot flashes, night sweats; mood swings	Premenstrual syndrome symptoms
	Weight gain
Thinning skin	Gall stones
	Aggravation of asthma

UNDERSTANDING ESTROGEN REPLACEMENT THERAPY

The uses of ERT and its risks in regard to breast cancer and other side effects remain the subject of considerable controversy, cover-up, and contention among the medical establishment, physicians and their patients, and the media, especially when it comes to breast cancer. In 1993, at the very same time that the *New York Times* declared that "The pendulum . . . is now clearly on the side of women taking [estrogen supplements], at least for most women," the large-scale Harvard Nurses' Health Study published in the *New England Journal of Medicine* found that women who use ERT increase their risk of breast cancer by 30 to 70 percent.

Clearly, many pros and cons exist regarding the use of ERT during and after menopause. How long, how much, and what type of ERT you take, as well as your risks of heart disease and osteoporosis are among the important issues you and your doctor must discuss before you decide whether to use these powerful drugs or choose one of the many safer alternatives available.

Types of Estrogen Replacement Therapy

Estrogen is the term used to describe a broad range of related female sex hormones. In humans, there are three principal natural estrogens: estradiol, estrone, and estriol, with estradiol being the most potent and active form. ERT preparations consist of varying amounts of these estrogens, alone or in combination, and of either natural or synthetic formulas. Produced in the laboratory from animal sources, the natural estrogens are almost identical to those found naturally in the body. In contrast, synthetic estrogens are more potent than are the natural hormones. In fact, synthetic estrogens are used chiefly to make birth control pills, which require higher doses in order to suppress ovulation. Almost all women taking ERT to relieve menopausal symptoms, however, take natural estrogen (along with progesterone, discussed later in this section).

Of the dozen or so natural estrogen preparations, the most commonly prescribed brand is a conjugated equine estrogen known as Premarin, which is manufactured by Wyeth-Ayerst Laboratories. Conjugated estrogen is a mixture of some ten naturally occurring estrogens derived from the urine of pregnant mares, hence its name *pre* (for pregnant) *mar* (for mare) *in* (for urine). Another common ERT preparation consists of estrone, a weaker form of estrogen produced both by the ovaries and through the conversion of androgens (male hormones) by fat cells. Estradiol a more potent estrogen, is the main constituent of the pills marketed under the brand name Estrace (estradiol, micronized) manufactured by Bristol-Myers Squibb.

Most women take estrogen in pill form; however, ERT also exists in cream and patch forms. Women can apply estrogen creams directly to vaginal tissue to help alleviate localized symptoms of menopause, including dryness, itchiness, and urinary tract infections. Although some of the hormone is absorbed into the body (including breast tissue), it tends to be less effective for other common symptoms and side effects of menopause, including hot flashes, osteoporosis, and heart disease. The most recently developed form of ERT is the transdermal patch. Once applied to the skin (usually on the hip, thigh, or abdomen), the patch dispenses estrogen directly into the bloodstream in a steady dosage. As do ERT creams, the patch bypasses the liver but also offers some protection against osteoporosis and heart disease. The risk of breast cancer from creams and patches depends on the type and concentration of estrogen and their duration of use; there is minimal information on long-term effects of these products.

Adding Progesterone

Most women who use estrogen also take progesterone, which is the hormone that becomes active in the second half of the menstrual cycle. Progesterone inhibits cell division in the uterus and breast, and so is thought to counteract the stimulation of cell growth caused by estrogen. As with estrogen, progestins are either derived from natural animal sources or produced synthetically; synthetic progestins tend to be stronger than natural progestins and are used most often as a component of oral contraceptives. Several different types of progestins are used as part of menopausal therapy. Medroxyprogesterone acetate, known by the brand names Provera, Amen, and Curretab, manufactured by Upjohn, Carnrick, and Solray, respectively, is the most commonly prescribed progestin.

Unfortunately, in its synthetic form, progesterone actually increases the risk of breast cancer.

Adding Testosterone

A relatively new and disturbing trend among physicians treating menopausal women is to add testosterone to the ERT mix in order to "perk up" libido and increase the sex drive. Although many women find it helpful and physicians extol the virtues of testosterone, scientists have conducted very few long-term studies on the risks to women of taking this powerful male hormone. The problem is that a woman's body fat converts testosterone to estrogen, and therefore the addition of testosterone almost always results in higher levels of estrogen and in estrogen stimulation, especially in overweight women. One of the few studies performed on testosterone in women, published in a 1996 issue of the *Journal of the National Cancer Institute*, showed that this increase in estrogen levels elevates the breast cancer risk. Clearly, more research is needed to assess the long-term risk factors of testosterone before doctors prescribe it to women, or women take it on a regular basis.

THE ESTROGEN REPLACEMENT THERAPY REGIMEN

Most doctors prescribe ERT so that it will mimic a woman's menstrual cycle. For most women, ERT means taking oral estrogen for about twelve days, then oral estrogen and progestin together for about thirteen days. At about twenty-five days, both pills are discontinued and withdrawal bleeding occurs, although not as heavily as during a normal period. Dosages for the patch and for creams vary.

Estrogen replacement therapy has both positive and negative effects on your body, and you must keep in mind that taking ERT is likely to have long-term implications for your health, including increasing your risk of breast cancer. Nevertheless, ERT does offer some major benefits that you should consider.

THE BENEFITS OF ESTROGEN REPLACEMENT THERAPY

For women, the transition into late life begins to occur at an average age of 51 (women can enter menopause anytime between the ages 45 and 58), when the ovaries decrease their production of estrogen, or earlier following surgical removal of the ovaries. Although the ovaries and adrenal glands still secrete small amounts of estrogen, the dramatic decline in estrogen triggers many changes in the body, including and primarily, the loss of fertility. The effects of estrogen however, extend far beyond the reproductive system into the cardio-vascular, musculoskeletal, gastrointestinal, and nervous systems. When a woman loses estrogen, her bones may become weaker, her heart and blood vessels more vulnerable, her skin less supple and moist, and her sex drive diminished.

Right from the start, it is important for you to realize that there may be good reasons to take ERT. For many women, the risks associated with the loss of estrogen far outweigh the risks of replacing it with ERT. The two most documented risks related to estrogen loss are heart disease and osteoporosis.

HEART DISEASE

Although we tend to think of cardiovascular disease—specifically coronary artery disease and stroke—as a "male problem," women, especially postmenopausal women, indeed are at risk. According to the American Cancer Society, three times as many women (95,819) aged 35 to 74 died of heart disease in 1996 compared with women of the same age who died of breast cancer (28,216).

Although it is true that women suffer from less cardiovascular disease than do men (before the age of 50, a man is six times more likely to die from a heart attack than is a woman of the same age) that picture dramatically changes after menopause. Within ten years after menopause, women lose their "female" advantage against heart attacks, and women's rates of the disease soon match the rates of men.

It is unclear exactly why this marked disparity exits; however, researchers believe that both estrogen and progesterone play an important role in protecting women from the ravages of athero-sclerosis, otherwise known as hardening of the arteries. The connection appears to be the way in which female sex hormones affect cholesterol levels in the blood. Cholesterol is a natural chemical that travels through the bloodstream by combining with lipids (fatty chemicals) and certain proteins. When combined, these substances are called lipoproteins. It is the relationship between different kinds of lipoproteins that determines the type of cholesterol in the blood. Low-density lipoproteins (LDLs)— "bad" cholesterol—carry about two-thirds of circulating cholesterol *to* the cells: It is this fat that we often speak of when referring to the plaque that builds up and causes atherosclerosis. High-density lipoproteins (HDLs)—"good" cholesterol—carry cholesterol *away* from the cells and blood vessel walls to the liver, which eliminates the cholesterol from the body.

Estrogen appears to help maintain a healthier balance between LDL and HDL levels during a woman's fertile years. The exact mechanism by which estrogen does this is still unclear; however, several studies show that when estrogen is withdrawn, through natural menopause or hysterectomy, the amount of "bad" cholesterol dramatically increases.

However, there are many other ways to reduce your risk of cardiovascular disease that do not involve taking hormones or other drugs. Changing your diet, improving exercise habits, and better controlling conditions known to exacerbate heart disease, such as diabetes and hypertension, are among the safest and most effective ways to protect your cardiovascular system.

OSTEOPOROSIS

The term *osteoporosis* comes from the Greek *osteo* (bone) and *porus* (pore or passage). Osteoporosis refers to a disease that affects mostly older women whose bones become brittle and weak. This disease has now reached epidemic proportions, affecting fifteen to twenty million American women annually. Every year, more than one million fractures occur because of osteoporosis, including 250,000 hip fractures. About 50,000 elderly women die every year from complications of hip and other fractures. Taking ERT usually helps prevent the process of osteoporosis from taking hold.

Although we tend to think of bone as solid material, it is actually living tissue enriched by blood vessels that travel through it. Bone consists of two major layers of cells: the smooth outer surface tissue, known as cortical bone; and a spongy inner meshlike material made up mostly of collagen, the protein-based connective tissue that also is a major component of skin tissue. When hardened by the metallic mineral calcium, collagen forms a network of solid tissue called trabeculae. Calcium gives bones their strength and density. Calcium also helps other parts of the body to function properly, including muscles, nerves, the endocrine glands, and blood cells.

For women, one major element in maintaining a healthy musculoskeletal system is estrogen. Estrogen helps protect bones from being "robbed" of calcium by other parts of the body. It also stimulates the production of another hormone called calcitonin, which helps the bones take up calcium from the bloodstream. Finally, estrogen helps to produce and maintain collagen, an important component of bone that also decreases in direct relationship to the decrease in estrogen during menopause.

Whether ERT provides efficient and sufficient protection against osteoporosis is the subject of some debate. One study in the *New England Journal of Medicine* found that for ERT to protect against osteoporosis, women must take the drug for many years:

> *For long-term preservation of bone mineral density, women should take estrogen for at least seven years after menopause. Even this duration of therapy may have little residual effect on bone density among women 75 years and older, who have the highest risk of fracture. . . . Among women older than 75 or 80, the protective effect of estrogen (usually taken earlier in life) is negligible.*

A study on 875 women aged 45 to 64, however, reached a different conclusion. The study known as the Postmenopausal Estrogen/ Progestin Intervention (PEPI) and sponsored by the National Heart, Lung, and Blood Institute, showed that women first starting ERT in their 60s (not immediately following menopause) not only slowed bone loss, but actually increased bone mass within three years. Another study, called the Study of Osteoporotic Fractures, showed that estrogen alone was less effective than estrogen/progestin combinations. It also reported that women with the greatest bone density had more than double the risk of breast cancer than women with the least bone density.

Other recent studies, such as the 1997 Rancho Bernardo Study, indicate that it is the *current* use of estrogen that provides the most benefits: Women over the age of 60 currently using estrogen had 60 percent fewer wrist fractures and 40 percent fewer hip fractures than did women who had never taken estrogen. Unfortunately, women who had taken estrogen and then stopped, even if they had taken it for ten years or more, had no decrease in their risk of fractures. At the same time, it appears that it is possible to attain almost the same protective benefits by taking estrogen starting at the age of 60, rather than at 52, or when menopause first begins.

Balanced against the increased risk of breast and other reproductive cancers, as well as blood clots, weight gain, and other common side effects, taking ERT for thirty years or more to prevent osteoporosis may not be the best alternative for you. We will show you a host of other ways to protect yourself from developing this debilitating disease after menopause, including taking ERT only when a bone density scan shows that your bones are beginning to thin, which may be a decade or more after menopause.

OTHER BENEFITS

In addition to heart disease and osteoporosis, ERT may protect against several other diseases, conditions, and symptoms frequently experienced during menopause, which we consider next.

Colon Cancer

Recent studies, including one in a 1995 issue of the *Journal of the National Cancer Institute*, show that ERT may reduce the risk of colon cancer by as much as half. This reduction is maintained for about ten years after a woman has stopped taking ERT.

Alzheimer's Disease

According to government-sponsored estimates, about 2 to 4 percent of individuals over the age of 65, particularly those with a family history, suffer from the chronic, degenerative brain disease known as Alzheimer's disease, and approximately 100,000 elderly men and women die from it every year. Alzheimer's disease affects the cerebral cortex, the cap of the deeply grooved tissue considered the seat of the brain's higher powers. As the disease takes hold, short-term memory falters and the ability to perform routine tasks begins to deteriorate. As Alzheimer's disease spreads through the cortex, it also begins to destroy language ability and long-term memory. Although the cause or causes of this disease remain a mystery, scientists believe that a virus, a genetic defect in certain brain cells either inherited or triggered by exposure to environmental toxins, or (most likely) a combination of several factors may contribute to the progressive brain degeneration in a given individual.

To date, scientists have found neither a cure nor a sure way to prevent Alzheimer's disease. However, in late 1993, a study reported in the *Medical Tribune* revealed a remarkable connection between ERT and Alzheimer's disease. Researchers followed 9,000 women living in a southern California retirement community and found that those who took ERT had only a 7 percent incidence of Alzheimer's disease, whereas those who did not take ERT suffered an 18 percent incidence of the disease. More recently, *The Lancet* published a study showing that just 6 percent of postmenopausal women who took estrogen developed Alzheimer's disease compared with 16 percent who did not take it. Women who took the hormone for longer than one year had an even greater reduction in risk. A study by the Baltimore Longitudinal Study on Aging published in *Neurology* in June 1997 showed that estrogen reduced the risk of developing the disease by more than 50 percent in a group of 472 women observed over sixteen years.

How does estrogen affect brain cells? Both human and animal studies support the theory that certain neurons contain estrogen receptors on their surfaces and these same neurons also have receptors for a substance called *nerve growth factor*. Scientists believe that nerve growth factor and estrogen somehow work together to protect brain cells from degenerating. Apart from boosting nerve growth factor, estrogen also appears to protect brain cells from various toxins such as amyloid, the protein that accumulates in the brain of Alzheimer's disease patients. Some consider amyloid to be the cause of the disease. Evidence from studies on female rats and monkeys and healthy women in their thirties suggests that estrogen also improves mental function and memory. Although more studies are needed, there is now growing evidence that ERT may be important in protecting against Alzheimer's disease. A large-scale, long-term study by the Women's Health Initiative of the National Institutions of Health is now underway; its results, however, will not be known for about another decade.

Urinary Tract Problems

Another set of troublesome and very common side effects of menopause is urinary tract problems, including incontinence and infections. Urinary tract problems occur more often as estrogen is lost because it plays such an important role in maintaining the health of body tissue. As estrogen levels decrease, the outer membranes of the urethra (the tube that carries urine from the bladder to the outside) and bladder become thin, weak, and more prone to infections and dysfunction. Taking ERT appears to help many women avoid these problems. In 1995, a pooled analysis of twenty-three earlier studies found that ERT does, in fact, ease urinary tract dysfunction related to menopause, a condition affecting up to 35 percent of women over 60.

Skin Changes

The skin is your largest organ, and it changes as you age, as do all other parts of your body. The skin has three major layers: the epidermis, the skin's surface layer; the dermis, the middle layer; and the bottom layer, which is made up of fatty tissue and muscle. Age and lack of estrogen affect each layer in a slightly different way. Estrogen helps the epider-

mis stay moist and supple by stimulating water retention and oil lubrication, and therefore as estrogen becomes less abundant, the skin
tends to dry out. Without estrogen, collagen breaks down far more
quickly than it would normally. Finally, estrogen provides most
women with an extra layer of fatty tissue throughout the body. When
the levels of this fatty tissue begin to decline, this extra fat layer begins
to shrink and pucker, causing the skin to wrinkle.

Vaginal Changes

Just as does your skin, the vagina changes in many ways with age and
loss of estrogen. In fact, vaginal tissue is more dependent on estrogen than is any other part of the body. The vagina is made up of
three layers: an internal mucous membrane lining responsible for
providing lubrication and elasticity; a layer of connective tissue filled
with tiny veins that fill with blood during sexual arousal; and a mus-
cular layer that expands and contracts.

As estrogen levels decrease, the mucous membrane tends to become
thinner and less supple. This thinning may cause irritation, itchiness,
and even bleeding that can lead to recurrent vaginal infections. After
menopause, a measurable decrease in the quantity and quality of vaginal secretions also occurs. Not only does the vagina become drier, but
the lubrication secreted tends to be less acidic, which leaves the vagina open to yeast and bacteria that would have been neutralized by the
previously high acid content of the secretions. The size of the vagina
decreases as well, becoming shorter and narrower. Muscle tone also
lessens, leaving the vaginal passage feeling slack and loose. Many
women find that ERT helps diminish these troubling side effects.

Menopausal Symptoms

Hot flashes, night sweats, sleep disturbances, and mood swings are
among the most common symptoms of estrogen withdrawal at
menopause. All of these symptoms are related to the widespread
hormonal changes that take place at menopause. In most cases, the
symptoms decrease in severity and frequency within just a few
months, with or without ERT.

THE RISKS OF ESTROGEN REPLACEMENT THERAPY

Thus far, we have outlined a fairly strong case in support of taking ERT after menopause. By replacing estrogen you can help reduce your risk of serious diseases, such as heart disease, osteoporosis, and colon cancer, and diminish the troublesome side effects of menopause, such as skin, vaginal, and urinary tract changes. However, we have also stressed that you would do so at the price of putting yourself at increased risk for other serious diseases and the uncomfortable side effects of ERT.

Estrogen both positively and negatively affects the way many different organs function, including the liver, heart, uterus, ovaries, and breasts. Therefore, at the same time that ERT may alleviate some medical problems, it may exacerbate others. As Dr. Graham Colditz of Harvard University asked at the 1994 meeting of the American Association for the Advancement of Science, "Should . . . cancer be the price we pay for reduced risk of heart disease and fractures? . . . . Alternative approaches to preventing heart disease are available, but this is not so for breast cancer."

Unfortunately, the cancer establishment has made little effort to publicize this information. Instead, ERT remains one of the most commonly prescribed drugs in the United States today. Most gynecologists routinely prescribed ERT for recently menopausal women; most of these women (about 80 percent) fill those prescriptions and of that number about 70 percent take ERT for more than nine months, while 50 percent take ERT for five years or more.

We are only now beginning to see more negative than positive results from the widespread use of a powerful hormone. As early as 1977, Barbara Seaman wrote in her groundbreaking text, *Women and the Crisis in Sex Hormones*, that "the estrogenization of American women is a major factor in our rising rates of female cancers." In addition to breast, endometrial, liver, and ovarian cancers, ERT also promotes the development of other conditions, including benign breast disease, uterine fibroids (leiomyomas), blood clots, and gallstones. There are also several other trouble-some side effects of ERT, including weight gain and premenstrual symptoms such as cramping and mood changes. Let us consider these risks one by one.

BREAST CANCER

In 1991, the *American Journal of Epidemiology* published an article revealing a shocking statistic based on reviews pooling earlier stud-ies: ERT is responsible for up to 8 percent of all postmenopausal breast cancers in the United States—15,000 cases with 4,000 deaths annually. A series of well-controlled human studies and reviews conducted over the last two decades clearly shows that extended use and high dosages of estrogen increase the risk of breast cancer by about 30 to 70 percent. This statistic means that a 70-year-old woman on ERT may increase her chances of breast cancer from one in fourteen to up to one in five, and even higher still if she has a fam-ily history of breast cancer. Another pooled analysis found that women who had used estrogen for at least eight years had at least a 25 to 30 percent increased risk. In 1995, the Harvard Nurses' Health Study confirmed these statistics, adding that prolonged use (over five years) has a particularly significant impact on risk.

Despite this persuasive evidence, the cancer establishment and ERT industry continue to promote ERT without informing women of the potential risk. The FDA–approved package insert for Premarin pills, for instance, states that the "majority of studies . . . have not shown an association [with breast cancer] with the usual doses for estrogen replacement." Bristol-Myers Squibb, the manufacturer of the popular estradiol tablet called Estrace, concurs: "The majority of studies have not shown an increased risk of breast cancer in women who have ever used estrogen replacement therapy." Even the National Alliance of Breast Cancer Organizations (NABCO), an extensive net-work of breast cancer organizations, trivializes evidence of the risk for breast cancer with ERT, concluding that "more data [are] needed."

Estrogen Replacement Therapy and Breast Cancer: The Studies

■ In 1991, an *American Journal of Epidemiology* article cited eight major studies demonstrating increased risks of breast cancer, ranging from 20 percent up to 80 percent, among women using ERT for extended periods.

■ In 1991, pooled results from sixteen previous studies published in the *Journal of the American Medical Association* found that women who used estrogen for fifteen years increased their risk of breast cancer by 30 percent. Tenfold higher risks were reported among women with a family history of breast cancer.

■ A follow-up to this review concluded that the risk of breast cancer after ten years of estrogen use increased "by at least 15 percent and up to 29 percent."

■ Another pooled analysis similarly found that women who had used estrogen for at least eight years had a 25 to 30 percent increased risk.

■ In 1995, the Harvard Nurses' Health Study confirmed an increased risk of 30 to 70 percent for women on ERT. This risk increased with cumulative risk, especially after five years.

■ A large-scale study, based on 60,000 postmenopausal women and published in the June 1997 *New England Journal of Medicine*, showed that the use of ERT for more than 10 years increased breast cancer deaths by 43 percent. An accompanying editorial emphasized that the benefits of ERT may not outweigh the risks of breast cancer, especially for women at low risk of heart disease.

The addition of progestins, testosterone, or both to the ERT mix only makes matters worse. Scientists have known since at least 1979—when the World Health Organization published statistics—that synthetic progestins enhance the carcinogenic effect of estrogen and increase a woman's risk of breast cancer. In 1989, a joint study by the United States and Sweden reported in the *New England Journal of Medicine* that taking progesterone as part of ERT increased the risk by more than 400 percent, while a 1995 study in the same journal showed a smaller but still significant 40 percent increase in risk. This study also showed the danger of "perking up" libido with testosterone: Testosterone added to the ERT regimen increases breast cancer risk by about 60 percent.

Another important factor to consider is the risk that alcohol consumption poses to women on ERT. Recent studies indicate that having just one or two drinks a day significantly increases estrogen levels in women taking hormones. The level of circulating estrogen skyrockets by 300 percent in women on ERT who drink 4 to 6 ounces of alcohol a day. These effects can be measured within one hour of taking the drink and last for up to five hours.

OTHER CANCERS

Endometrial cancer ranks among the most common cancers in women, with an estimated annual incidence of between 39,000 and 42,000 new cases. About 3,000 women die every year from this cancer. As for ovarian cancer, approximately 27,000 new cases are diagnosed every year, accounting for about 4 percent of all cancers among women. About 15,000 women die of ovarian cancer annually, making it the most deadly cancer of the female reproductive system.

Risks for both types of these cancers, as well as for breast cancer, include having a family history of the disease, going into early menarche or late menopause, never having had a child, being overweight, smoking, and using ERT after menopause for a prolonged time.

Indeed, taking ERT sharply increases a woman's risk for developing these cancers. According to a study by Richard Theriault and his colleagues, cited in the 1995 book *Reducing Breast Cancer Risk*, the long-term risks of uterine cancer increased more than fifteenfold with estrogen use, while a 1995 study in the *American Journal of Epidemiology* showed that ovarian cancer rates increased by 40 percent after six years of ERT and by 70 percent after eleven years or more. The reason is that the cells of both the uterine lining and the ovaries (as well as the cells of the breast) are loaded with estrogen receptors and thus proliferate when estrogen is present. Estrogen may accelerate the growth of a cancer already present in these organs as well as make the cells more vulnerable to environmental carcinogens. In addition, the risk of liver cancer appears to be slightly elevated in women who take ERT.

BENIGN BREAST DISEASE AND UTERINE FIBROIDS

Benign breast disease, also known as fibrocystic disease or chronic mastitis, is a common condition affecting millions of women, mostly between 25 and 50 years of age when high levels of estrogen are circulating in breast tissue. In these women, estrogen may promote the development of fibrocystic disease, which can be painful and uncomfortable. Many women with benign breast disease who take ERT find that the disease continues to trouble them throughout and even after menopause, at a time when their peers who do not take ERT experience relief from this disease. An associated problem is that ERT tends to make breast tissue denser, which makes obtaining an accurate mammogram more difficult. Thus, a woman taking ERT is more likely to obtain a false-negative test result on mammography—and hence have a breast cancer that goes undetected—than would a woman who passes through menopause without replacing estrogen.

Fibroids that develop within the uterine wall or are attached to it are also very common in the same age group and for the same reason. Estrogen also causes uterine muscle and connective cells to divide more rapidly than normal, resulting in a condition known as endometrial hyperplasia.

BLOOD CLOTS

Otherwise known as thrombi, blood clots are a major cause of heart attacks and strokes. In high doses, estrogen may stimulate the production of some clotting factors produced by the liver. A woman with a history of thromboembolic disease or high blood pressure runs an increased risk for developing clots if she takes ERT.

GALLSTONES

The gallbladder is the sac located beneath the liver that stores the bile produced by the liver; bile is used to help enzymes digest fatty substances after they enter the small intestine. Gallstones—hard, crystalline structures that form in the gall bladder—are a common problem among Americans: An estimated one million new cases are diagnosed every year. Most gallstones (about 80 percent) are composed primarily of cholesterol; the remaining 20 percent contain mostly calcium salts of bile pigment. Normally, the acids in bile keep cholesterol from becoming too concentrated. However, when the amount of cholesterol in the bile increases beyond the ability of bile acids to maintain the balance, the cholesterol crystallizes and, in some persons, a stone forms.

Estrogen has a tendency to increase the cholesterol fraction of the bile. The incidence of gallstones in postmenopausal women using ERT is about 2.5 times greater than it is in women not using ERT. Gallstones may be painful and may require surgery for removal.

WEIGHT GAIN AND OTHER SIDE EFFECTS

Extra weight, breast tenderness, breakthrough bleeding, nausea, aggravation of diabetes, and depression are just a few of the common side effects of estrogen therapy. Many women experience one or more of these side effects so severely that they stop taking ERT. According to a recent survey, about 50 percent of women stopped taking ERT after a year because of the adverse effects.

PERSONAL PROTECTION

As you can see, ERT has many risks and benefits that you must carefully weigh for yourself before deciding whether to take it. Every woman has a different set of risk factors and concerns: You may have such a strong family history of heart disease and osteoporosis, for instance, that the benefits of ERT may outweigh its risks for you. However, keep in mind that there are several safe, effective diet and lifestyle changes you can make to help you through the passage into later life and keep you healthy and vital during the second half of your life—even if your doctor may fail to mention them unless directly asked.

In 1995, the Physicians' Committee for Responsible Medicine stated:

> *It is patronizing to assume that every postmenopausal woman is too wedded to her current diet and lifestyle to listen to competent advice. The real problem is, she is not likely to find such advice. Most doctors know little about how diet affects health, even when a mountain of research has already been done [and] is gathering dust in medical libraries. They rely instead on knee-jerk prescribing [ERT], which is continually encouraged by drug manufacturers' aggressive promotion. When doctors learn how to use all the tools their medical bags could really offer—including prescriptions for diet and lifestyle changes—their patients will be much better off.*

In chapters 9 and 10, we will describe in detail the connection between cancer and what you eat, drink, and inhale, how much you exercise, and how much stress you endure. Meanwhile, here are some safe and effective ways to protect yourself against the sometimes unpleasant and potentially dangerous problems that result from the loss of estrogen at menopause—without taking ERT and increasing your risk of breast cancer, other cancers, and other complications.

WHAT YOU CAN DO

- Avoid using ERT, or use it only in low doses for short periods of time.

- Avoid alcohol if you use ERT.

- Maintain your health during menopause *without* ERT

  - Stop smoking, eat a healthful diet, exercise, and maintain a normal weight.

- Take advantage of nonhormonal solutions.

AVOID ESTROGEN REPLACEMENT THERAPY OR USE IN LOW DOSES FOR A SHORT TIME

As we have discussed, the risks of breast cancer increase considerably with the use of ERT over long periods of time. Many women pass through menopause without experiencing serious menopausal symptoms or developing osteoporosis or heart disease, especially if they eat a healthful diet and exercise regularly. However, if you suffer from uncomfortable hot flashes, mood swings, or other symptoms, you may decide that taking a short course of ERT will help you through the most difficult months of menopause without putting you at a much higher risk for developing breast cancer.

Another reason to consider taking ERT is to prevent osteoporosis. If you have a family history of osteoporosis or you are otherwise at high risk for this bone-thinning disease, talk to your doctor about taking ERT starting at the age of 65 or so, when fractures related to the disease usually begin to occur. Recent evidence published in the February 1997 *Journal of the American Medical Association* shows that women who put off using estrogen for ten years or more after menopause still receive "nearly equal bone-conserving benefits as women who began in their late 40s or early 50s."

Avoid Alcohol

Studies show that alcohol consumption—even only four drinks a week—significantly increases the levels of estrogen (and thus the risk of breast cancer) in women who take ERT. When taking ERT it is best to eliminate or at least severely restrict your intake of alcohol.

Maintain Your Health During Menopause without Estrogen Replacement Therapy

By changing your lifestyle, or reinforcing healthful habits, you can avoid many of the conditions that tend to develop in women after menopause, including cardiovascular disease and osteoporosis.

Stop Smoking

According to the United States Surgeon General, cigarette smoking is the single most preventable cause of heart disease and is responsible for at least 30 percent of all deaths related to heart disease annually. The Framingham Heart Study found that the mortality rate of women smokers is fivefold over that of women nonsmokers. The dangers from cigarette smoke start with just one cigarette a day and increase with every cigarette smoked: Smoking one to ten cigarettes per day doubles the mortality rate from heart disease. Smoking ten to twenty cigarettes per day increases the mortality another 25 percent. Altogether, smokers have a stunning 70 percent higher rate of death from heart disease than do nonsmokers.

Cigarette smoking also has an impact on the development of osteoporosis because it inhibits bone repair and depletes valuable nutrients. Women who smoke lose bone mass more quickly and the loss is much more severe than in those who do not smoke, largely because smoking affects both estrogen production and the way in which the body metabolizes estrogen. (We will discuss smoking in further detail in chapter 10.)

Design a Healthful Diet

The cliché, "You are what you eat" is apt when it comes to your health. Scientists have discovered many important links between what we eat and both cardiovascular disease and osteoporosis. We recommend four dietary guidelines for menopausal women:

1. **Lower your fat intake:** Cutting down on fatty meat and dairy products may be the most important step you can take in creating a healthful diet for yourself. Leading heart disease specialist Dean Ornish, M.D., demonstrated that a nearly vegetarian diet—one that contains little or no fat— can dramatically lower heart disease risk and even reverse existing damage to the cardiovascular system. Replacing meat and dairy products as sources of protein with complex carbohydrates, such as grains, beans, and soy products, will help lower cholesterol levels and reduce caloric intake.

2. **Add complex carbohydrates to your diet:** The United States Department of Agriculture recommends that you eat from six to eleven servings of cereals and grains, three to five servings of vegetables, and two to four servings of fruits per day. Most complex carbohydrates also contain high amounts of fiber, which lowers cholesterol by helping the body excrete fat more quickly and thus reduce its absorption into the bloodstream. Fresh fruits and vegetables, especially dark green, leafy vegetables, tend to be rich in folic acid and other B vitamins that help reduce levels of the toxic amino acid called homocysteine. According to a January 3, 1996 article in the *New York Times*, "just a small decline in homocysteine levels could save 35,000 lives a year in this country."

3. **Add antioxidants to your diet:** Fruits and vegetables also contain high amounts of nutrients known as antioxidants, including the vitamins C, E, beta carotene (a precursor of vitamin A), and the minerals magnesium, zinc,

and selenium. These nutrients have the ability to destroy certain harmful molecules in the body called free radicals. Free radicals are unstable molecules that may damage both cell membranes and internal cells structures, including DNA. Scientists have linked free radicals to the development of several diseases and conditions, including heart disease, osteoporosis, and several types of cancer. (We will discuss free radicals and breast cancer in more detail in chapter 9.)

4. **Increase your intake of bone-strengthening and heart-healthy nutrients:** When it comes to osteoporosis, the most important vitamins and minerals are calcium, magnesium, and vitamins C and E. Found in grains, vegetables, fruits, and dairy products, these nutrients help bone tissue maintain its strength and resiliency, even as the effects of aging progress. Listed here are the vitamins and minerals you need every day to keep your heart and musculoskeletal system healthy:

    ▪ **Calcium:** Approximately 80 percent of women eat less than the recommended daily allowance of 800 milligrams of calcium. Not only is calcium essential to the health of your bones, it also helps to lower blood lipids and make other blood components less sticky, thereby helping to prevent cardiovascular disease. Food sources rich in calcium include green leafy vegetables, sardines, salmon, soybeans, and dairy products such as milk, yogurt, and cheese. Most doctors recommend that postmenopausal women consume about 1,000 to 1,500 milligrams of calcium per day.

    ▪ **Magnesium:** Magnesium is a mineral that works in tandem with calcium to help keep both the musculoskeletal and cardiovascular systems healthy. A recent Israeli study published in the *Medical World News*, for instance, showed that women who take supplemental magnesium can increase their bone density up to 8 percent, whereas those who did not take extra magnesium lost bone density. Although magnesium is found in a wide variety of foods, including wheat bran, raw leafy vegetables, nuts, and bananas, few women obtain enough magnesium from their diets. If you decide to take magnesium, you should balance the amount you take one for one with calcium. You can safely take about 600 to 800 milligrams of magnesium daily.

- **Vitamin B3 (niacin)**: Niacin is often prescribed to lower blood lipids and increase HDL cholesterol and homocysteine. However, because use of niacin may result in serious side effects, you should take supplements only under the care of an experienced health care provider. Always use free-form niacin, avoiding time-release forms that tend to cause the most serious side effects.

- **Vitamin C**: Vitamin C is both an important antioxidant that protects against cardiovascular disease and an essential component of bone metabolism. Foods rich in vitamin C include citrus fruits, green leafy vegetables, and tomatoes, among many others. You can safely take anywhere from 250 to 3,000 milligrams of vitamin C per day (the official recommended daily allowance is about 60 milligrams). Older women who smoke require more vitamin C, because cigarettes sap the body of its vitamin C supply. Please note, however, that the more vitamin C you take, the more likely you are to suffer from the common side effect of stomach irritation.

- **Vitamin D**: In order for your bones to absorb enough calcium, your body needs enough vitamin D. Found in fish and fortified milk, vitamin D is also produced in the body in response to sunlight. You need about 400 IU (international units) of vitamin D per day.

- **Vitamin E:** According to several recent large-scale studies, vitamin E provides excellent protection against heart disease in postmenopausal women. The Harvard Nurses' Health Study, for instance, reported that nurses who took vitamin E supplements had only two-thirds the heart disease risk compared with nurses who did not take supplements. Women who took vitamin E for more than two years cut their risk in half. A study in the *American Journal of Epidemiology* reported that women with the highest intake of vitamin E lowered their risk by 65 percent compared with women with the lowest intake.

  Vitamin E is also known to help relieve menopausal symptoms such as hot flashes and night sweats. Back in 1950, a study published in the *Annals of Western Medicine and Surgery* showed that "vitamin E is undoubtedly effective in treating [menopause] and some associated symptoms." Vitamin E also helps alleviate benign breast disease in many women.

- **Phytoestrogens:** As we will discuss in greater detail in chapter 9, certain plants contain estrogen-like substances. Found primarily in soy products such as tofu and soybeans, phytoestrogens help protect against bone loss. Indeed, several studies that show osteoporosis is very uncommon in countries in which soy consumption is highest, such as China and Japan. You can also reduce your risk for heart disease by consuming more soy: One study published in *The New England Journal of Medicine* in 1995, found that eating about 47 grams of soy protein (the amount found in three-quarters of a pound of tofu) per day lowers cholesterol levels up to 20 percent in persons with high cholesterol. It also showed that phytoestrogens found in soy also appear to increase protective HDLs while lowering total cholesterol. In chapter 9, we will discuss the importance of these key chemicals to the prevention of breast cancer.

Maintain a Healthy Weight

According to a 1990 report by the Framingham Heart Study group, obesity is a major cardiovascular risk factor, especially for women after menopause. Even ten extra pounds puts a heavy burden on the heart and blood vessels; for each pound of excess weight, the heart is forced to pump blood through an additional several hundred extra miles of blood vessels a day. Even a 10 percent reduction in weight is more likely than an exercise program to improve blood pressure readings, cholesterol levels, and the ability of the body to process blood sugar, all of which influence coronary disease risks. Being overweight also places more stress on bones that may become more brittle as you age, thus increasing your risk of osteoporosis process. As you will see in chapter 9, obesity also plays a major role in the development of breast cancer.

Exercise Regularly

Without question, for a woman entering or past the age of menopause, exercise may be the single best thing she can do for her emotional and physical health. Exercise mitigates three of her most pressing health problems: cardiovascular disease, osteoporosis, and weight gain. Aerobic exercise helps keep the heart pumping and blood vessels clear, while weight-bearing exercise helps strengthen bones and muscles. Just 30 minutes of aerobic exercise three times a week helps prevent cardiovascular disease in older women. Many women also find that exercise alleviates other menopausal symptoms, including annoying hot flashes. A recent study among women at Wayne State University showed that more than 50 percent of those who suffered from hot flashes decreased the frequency and severity of their episodes by exercising regularly. A menopausal women who exercises may also notice that her skin looks and feels younger as more blood is pumped into the tiny capillaries that feed the dermis. Improved circulation will also help her digestive system stay healthy and her immune system stay strong. Exercise has a positive effect on her brain and her emotions as well. Like skin, brain tissue is fed by thousands of tiny capillaries, and the more blood coursing through them, the more mentally alert and emotionally satisfied a woman will feel. Part of the reason is that certain body chemicals called endorphins, known to dull pain and produce mild euphoria, are released during vigorous exercise. Finally, exercise helps prevent breast cancer, a matter we will take up in more detail in chapter 10.

TAKE ADVANTAGE OF NONHORMONAL SOLUTIONS

If you are like most women, stopping smoking, eating right, and exercising regularly will help you stay healthy and feeling vital and vigorous throughout menopause. However, if you remain plagued by menopausal symptoms or side effects, there are several herbal and nonhormonal remedies available to you:

- **For skin changes**: Avoiding the sun and using sunscreen are the very best ways to protect your skin from age-related changes, including increased dryness and wrinkling.

- **For vaginal dryness**: Several safe and effective lubricants are available over the counter, including almond, coconut, or vitamin E oil. Water-soluble products, such as Astroglide, glycerin, and K-Y Jelly, are also helpful.

- **For preventing heart disease**: Several recent studies show that, at least among men, taking one aspirin a day can help prevent heart disease. As yet, no such information is available for women, however. Several medications are also available that help lower high blood pressure and reduce serum cholesterol. All drugs, including aspirin, however, have their own side effects and associated risks that you must be aware of before you take them.

■ **For preventing or treating osteoporosis:** In addition to eating a diet rich in calcium, magnesium, and vitamin D, and exercising regularly, you can also take one of several different medications developed to treat osteoporosis. Fosamax (alendronate)—manufactured by Merck and Company, Incorporated—and Miacalcin (calcitonin)—manufactured by Sandoz—may help keep bones strong after menopause; however, both have side effects and their long-term effects are unknown. Fluoride by prescription too, has side effects.

Discuss the matter thoroughly with your doctor. It is also important that you avoid or restrict taking prescription and over-the-counter medications that increase bone loss. Indomethacin, ibuprofen, and other non-steroidal anti-inflammatory drugs (NSAIDs), anticonvulsant medications, some cholesterol-lowering drugs, corticosteroids, and the antibiotic tetracycline are some of the most common culprits. Antacids containing aluminum may also interfere with the ability of the body to use other bone-building materials and thus should be avoided. Again, talk to your doctor for more information.

■ **For preventing colon cancer:** The Harvard Nurses' Health Study showed that women who took two or more aspirin weekly for more than twenty years had a dramatic 44 percent reduction in colon cancer. Taking four to six aspirin per week gave the greatest protection. See your doctor before you begin taking aspirin, however, because aspirin has side effects of its own, including exacerbating osteoporosis and causing stomach irritation.

■ **For preventing Alzheimer's disease:** Studies released in a 1997 issue of the *Journal of Neurology* indicate that ibuprofen, an inexpensive over-the-counter anti-inflammatory drug, may reduce the risk of Alzheimer's disease by as much as 60 percent. Although the findings are preliminary, and you should not take ibuprofen for this reason alone, if you are already taking it for arthritis or another inflammatory condition you can take heart in knowing that you may be protecting yourself against Alzheimer's disease at the same time.

5

The Case Against Mammography

Mammography, long hailed as the most effective "prevention" method for breast cancer, is overrated as a screening method. Its risks to premenopausal women especially—false alarms, missed cancers, the spread of early undiagnosed cancer caused by breast compression, and radiation to the breast—far outweigh its negligible benefits. Safer alternatives are available, particularly self- and clinical examination.

"My breast cancer was diagnosed at 45 with a mammogram. I'm sure I'm alive today because I was screened."

"I faithfully received annual mammograms but found my own cancer by breast self-exam five months after the last mammogram. It's growing and spreading so fast, I'm not sure I'll survive. And I'm only 49."

"I wonder now, at age 63 and with breast cancer, if the radiation I've received over the last 20 years from yearly mammograms has anything to do with the development of my cancer. I mean, radiation does cause cancer, doesn't it?"

These three sentiments sum up very succinctly the pressing issues surrounding mammography. These sentiments also reflect the profound confusion about the issue that decades of misinformation, reversals of opinions, and conflicting interpretations of studies by the cancer establishment have caused among health professionals and the public alike. Indeed, the debate leaves millions of women wondering if mammography offers the benefits touted by the American Cancer Society's well-known slogan, "The best protection is early detection"; offers no benefits at all; or actually puts them at increased risk for misdiagnosis or even for developing breast cancer and other complications.

Mammography Debate Time Line

Whereas most experts agree that postmenopausal mammography is a useful screening tool, the debate over *premenopausal* mammography has been one of the longest and most bitter in modern medicine. In 1997, when the National Cancer Institute (NCI) broke ranks with the American Cancer Society (ACS) and declined to recommend the procedure to women under the age of 50, its decision was met with outrage. Dr. Leon Gordis, chairman of the expert panel that made the recommendation, stated that, "The arguments have gotten so one-sided [in favor of mammograms] that people are unwilling to listen."

Before 1977 No specific guidelines.

1977 The NCI and ACS recommend that women aged 40 to 49 have mammograms only if they or their mothers, aunts, or sisters have had breast cancer.

1980 The ACS recommends one-time mammograms for women aged 35 to 40 to establish a future baseline and advises women under 50 to consult their doctors about their individual needs for mammograms.

1983 The ACS recommends that symptom-free women aged 40 to 49 have mammograms every one or two years.

1987 The NCI adopts working guidelines: Begin screening by the age of 40, with mammography every one to two years; the ACS also adopts this guideline.

1989 The 1987 guidelines are officially adopted by a conference of leading cancer organizations.

1993	The NCI changes its recommendation, saying "Experts do not agree on the value of routine screening mammography for women aged 40 to 49." ACS and other organizations disagree.
January 1997	The National Institutes of Health (NIH) consensus conference says not enough evidence exists to support a recommendation that all women aged 40 to 49 receive mammograms. The ACS says it is "disappointed" by the decision.
March 1997	The ACS advises women aged 40 to 49 to have a mammogram every year. Days later, the NCI reverses its position and recommends that women aged 40 to 49 have a mammogram every one to two years "if they are at average risk of breast cancer."

In this chapter we outline the risks of mammography for both premenopausal and postmenopausal women. Although we believe that mammography has limited benefits and carries potential risks for women at any age, we stress that premenopausal screening poses the least benefit and the most danger—and it is just that group of women, those between the ages of 40 and 49, that the cancer establishment and the mammography industries now target with the most vigor. Indeed, at this writing (July 1997), the latest round in the debate has just ended with both the ACS and the NCI issuing strong statements in favor of premenopausal mammography.

For the ACS, on the one hand, this recommendation represented a reaffirmation of its long-held policy in favor of mammography. The NCI, on the other hand, reached this decision with some difficulty and with some vocal dissension among its staff. One panelist, Dr. Donald H. Bening of Duke University, said that—at most—1.5 percent of women in their forties who have annual mammograms receive any benefits. Dr. Otis Brawley, the director of special populations at the NCI, went even further in his disapproval, remarking, "I've always believed in telling people what you know and then letting them decide for themselves. To say what some people are saying, that obviously mammography is saving lives of women in their forties, is lying to the American people."

UNDERSTANDING MAMMOGRAPHY

In the United States, mammography is the only procedure involving radiation for which women require no medical prescription. All a woman need do is visit a mammography center to receive this highly questionable and potentially dangerous treatment. And she does so believing what the cancer establishment tells her: Mammography is a preventive tool, one that is very safe and effective. Nothing could be further from the truth. First, the reality is that *90 percent of all breast cancers are found by women during their monthly breast self-examination*—not by mammography. Second, mammography does nothing to prevent a woman from developing breast cancer.

WHAT IS MAMMOGRAPHY?

Mammography is an imaging technique designed for two distinct purposes: To diagnose suspicious lumps or nodules, and to screen for early cancers in apparently normal breasts. The purpose of screening mammography is to identify breast cancer as early as possible in order to treat it most effectively. The question remains whether mammography is the safest and most effective tool for this purpose.

There are two different types of screening procedures in current use. Film mammography prints the X-ray image of breast tissue on photographic paper, and xeromammography prints the X-ray image on regular paper. Film mammography involves exposure to more radiation, especially when combined with grid-type devices, but tends to produce clearer images. Both procedures use the same basic method: A technician places one breast between two X-ray plates, then compresses the plates together, squeezing the breast as flat as possible, so that the X-ray beam penetrates the thinnest possible layer of tissue.

Whether a woman is pre- or postmenopausal influences the effectiveness of a mammogram. Before menopause, the dense, highly glandular structure of the breast is maintained by relatively high levels of estrogen production. This density tends to mask small early tumors and shield them from X rays. After menopause, the progressive reduction of glandular tissue makes the detection of early tumors much easier.

Recent developments, including techniques based on digitized mammography and computer enhancement, provide better images, especially of the dense premenopausal breast. Digitized mammography, a computerized technique, displays images using an infinite scale of gray tones that enhances the quality of the mammographic image and magnifies the view of specific areas of the breast. This technology is expected to improve the sensitivity of mammography and to decrease the radiation dose used with each mammogram.

Another specialized technique is displacement mammography, which is used as a screening method for women with silicone implants. Technicians position breast tissue away from the chest wall, while moving the implant in the opposite direction. This allows the breast to be compressed more effectively and prevents tissue from being shadowed by the implant.

MAMMOGRAPHY AND RADIATION

Although most of us tend to forget this fact, to obtain all X-ray films, including mammograms, radiation is used. Mammography narrowly focuses X rays (electromagnetic radiation capable of penetrating solid material) on the breasts. Radiation exposure is measured in rads, or radiation absorbed dose (a millirad is one-thousandth of a rad).

In the past, mammography exposed women to up to 50 rads during a single mammogram. During the early 1970s, women who underwent mammography under the joint NCI/ACS Breast Cancer Demonstration and Detection Project typically received 2 to 3 rads of exposure to each breast every year for five years. Other women received far higher dosages. A 1977 study published in *Cancer* showed that the average single-exposure dose in some seventy Pennsylvania clinics was about 8 rads, with some reaching as high as

47 rads. High dosages, up to and exceeding 3 rads, continued through the 1980s.

Current procedures expose the breast to much less radiation than did past procedures. Still, current exposures are unacceptably high, despite the reassurances of radiologists to the contrary. A common analogy touted by radiologists and doctors alike is that the dosage from a single mammogram is just a small fraction of what the average woman would receive from simply spending a week in Denver, Colorado, having a chest X-ray film, or flying on a jet to Europe.

Many studies have proved this analogy to be misleading (Table 5.1). For example, a woman who spends a week in Denver, a city whose elevation involves relatively high exposure to cosmic radiation, would receive less than 1 millirad. Flying to Europe would expose her to just a fraction more. And exposure in either of these instances would be to the whole body, whereas mammography focuses radiation on just one highly sensitive organ.

TABLE 5.1: COMPARISON OF RADIATION EXPOSURES	
Comparative Doses to the Breast	Millirads
Average dose to each breast from mammography	340
One week in Denver	less than 1
Chest X-ray film	1
Jet flight from the United States to Europe	5

From Mammography Screening: A Decision-Making Guide. *New York: Center for Medical Consumers, 1990.*

Today, most film mammograms result in less than 300 millirads of exposure with every shot taken of the breast, clearly a vast improvement over past exposures. However, because it may take several films to examine the whole breast, the total breast exposure may be much higher. And the larger and denser the breast, the higher the exposure.

Technicians in most major centers take at least two films of each breast. When the X-ray film shows a suspicious or unclear lesion, the radiologist may take ten films or more, resulting in exposures over 3,000 millirads. For women with implants, the American College of Radiology routinely recommends an additional two views. You can see that many women today are receiving much more than the 300 millirads misleadingly cited by radiologists and the mammography industry as the exposure that occurs in "usual practice."

Furthermore, American radiologists screen too frequently. A Swedish study showed that screening with a single view every two to three years achieved a 34 percent reduction in postmenopausal breast cancer mortality, a result similar to that achieved with American procedures using two or more views per breast every year. Similarly, a study performed in the Netherlands reported a 50 percent reduction in mortality in postmenopausal women using just a single view at two-year intervals. To date, there is no evidence that "more views at more frequent intervals," as conducted in the United States, reduces mortality compared with the more restrained European use of mammography.

Indeed, techniques, dosages, and screening in the United States are quite different from those practiced in Europe. One expert referred to the American approach to mammography as "overkill." In the Boston's Women's Community Cancer Project's May 1992 newsletter, director Kate Dempsey summed up the unnecessarily high exposures to which American women were and still are subjected:

> Exam for exam, women in the U.S. may be receiving twice the dose of radiation necessary to accomplish the same reduction in mortality. . . . This suggests that women in the U.S. are not only unnecessarily exposed to radiation exam for exam in comparison to their European counterparts, but that they are also unnecessarily exposed year after year. . . . There is solid evi-

dence that mammography can be effective at reducing mortality with a great deal less radiation exposure overall.

In addition to the unnecessary exposures taken, the safety of the equipment used for mammograms is questionable. In fact, owing to a troubling variability of radiation exposure from mammograms in the 1970s and 1980s, the American College of Radiology attempted to standardize techniques and dosages in the early 1990s. It established a voluntary certification program that required mammography facilities to meet machine calibration and performance standards.

Because of the failure of voluntary certification, erratic compliance, and reports that more than half of the current facilities and technologists failed to meet minimal quality assurance standards, Congress passed the 1992 National Mammography Standards Quality Assurance Act. Congress intended this legislation to ensure that all radiologists are qualified to perform mammograms, equipment is specifically designed for mammography, centers have systems for reviewing results and performance, and facilities are regularly inspected.

In 1997, the United States General Accounting Office published a detailed analysis of the federal compliance program as mandated by the 1992 legislation. The report noted that "the first time these facilities were evaluated, more than ¼ had significant violations." Moreover, there were significant differences in the way inspections were conducted that could lead to "inconsistent reporting of violations, thereby limiting the FDA's ability to determine the full effect of the inspection process." The report also noted that the FDA's inspection procedures were "inadequate" and that the agency lacked procedures that would guarantee that all violations of standards were promptly and adequately corrected.

Even the Division of Mammography Quality and Radiation Programs of the FDA still admits not knowing what percentage of mammograms are of acceptable quality. Furthermore, while the regulations set a maximum dose of 300 millirads per film, they did not set a maximum number of films a radiologist could take of each breast. Therefore, women at some centers receive doses as high as 2 or 3 rads each time they have mammography performed—doses that put them at increased risk for developing breast cancer.

MAMMOGRAPHY: THE RISKS OF BREAST CANCER

M. Maureen Roberts, a medical doctor and former clinical director of the Edinburgh Breast Screening Project, made the following statement in a 1989 *British Medical Journal* article and she did so knowing she was dying of breast cancer:

> *Screening is always a second best, an admission of failure of prevention or treatment. . . . There is . . . an air of evangelism [about the benefits of mammography], few people question what is actually being done. Are we brainwashing ourselves into thinking that we are making a dramatic impact on a serious disease before we brainwash the public?*

Dr. Roberts' words echo as more and more evidence mounts against the widespread and indiscriminate use of mammography, and for two reasons. First, the cancer establishment hails mammography as a *preventive* tool, giving women false confidence that this procedure somehow protects them against developing breast cancer. In fact, by the time a mammogram can detect a cancer, the cancer can be up to nine or ten years old, can reach about 1 centimeter in diameter, and may have spread to distant sites in the body, especially in premenopausal women. At that stage, women can often detect the cancer using self-examination.

Second, radiation from mammography may trigger the very cancer it is meant to detect. The cancer establishment, radiologists, and manufacturers of mammography film and machines dismiss these serious problems and, instead, further encourage routine large-scale mammography. And they have succeeded in their efforts: From 1987 to 1992 the percentage of all American women who ever had a mammogram increased from 38 to 68 percent. Over the same five-year period, the percentage of premenopausal women submitting to mammography rose from 22 to 39 percent. Since then, their numbers have only increased. A 1993 survey published in the *Journal of the National Cancer Institute* showed that 75 percent of women aged 40 to 49 followed ACS guidelines recommending a baseline mammogram at the age of 35 and an annual screening over the age of 40. Today, however, fewer postmenopausal women submit to mammograms, with figures decreasing from 47 percent in the late 1980s to 33 percent in the late 1990s. How the latest recommendations will affect the number of premenopausal women who submit to mammography remains to be seen.

RADIATION AND BREAST CANCER

The link between radiation and breast cancer is a strong one. As radiation expert Rosalie Bertell, Ph.D., pointed out in a 1992 article in *Mothering*, a review of several previous studies, showed that women who lived through the aftermath of the atomic bombs at Nagasaki and Hiroshima suffer rates of breast cancer. Interestingly, rates are highest (a 39 percent increase for every 1 rad exposure) among those survivors who were ten years old or younger at the time of the bomb compared to less than 1 percent for older women. The two-decade lag time between exposure and cancer is only to be expected, because breast cancer usually takes a long time to develop.

Other evidence of the link between radiation and breast cancer involves the use of radiation in medicine. In the past, doctors and radiologists used radiation to diagnose and treat various diseases, with tragic results because of ignorance or reckless disregard for the risks of cancer. Until recently, doctors prescribed radiation therapy to treat crippling spinal curvature (a disease called ankylosing spondylitis), postchildbirth mastitis (infection of the nipples and breast), enlarged thymus glands in children, acne, fungal scalp infections, and cancer.

Radiation and Breast Cancer: The Studies

- In 1965, a study in the *British Journal of Cancer* found increased cancer rates after repeated and prolonged exposure to X rays (during fluoroscopy) taken to monitor the progress of tuberculosis treatment. Each examination exposed the breast to up to 8 rads, and patients typically received 100 examinations or more.

- In 1971, the *Journal of the American Medical Association* reported excess breast cancers in adults who as children had received irradiation to the thymus gland. From the 1920s until 1955, doctors routinely used chest X-ray films to diagnose an allegedly abnormal enlargement of the gland in young children.

- Reports published in the *Canadian Medical Association Journal, Radiology,* and the *Journal of the National Cancer Institute* in 1973 to 1975 and 1977 confirmed excess adult breast cancers among women with past history of fluoroscopy.

- In 1989, a small study published in the *Journal of the National Cancer Institute* found excess breast cancers among women who had been treated with X rays for spinal curvature (scoliosis) as children. These women had received an average breast dose of 13 rads at an average age of 12.

- Another 1989 study in *The Lancet* found excess breast cancer rates in women whose doctors treated fungal infections of their scalps with radiation and whose breasts were exposed to under 2 rads.

- In 1996, the *New England Journal of Medicine* published a study showing that the breast cancer risk is much higher than normal among women treated with radiation for childhood Hodgkin's disease.

- Based on a detailed review of these and a wide range of other such studies, Dr. John Gofman, a leading international authority on medical radiation, recently published his analysis in a startling book, *Preventing Breast Cancer.* Gofman claims that past medical radiation is probably the single most important cause of the modern breast cancer epidemic. An editorial in the *Journal of the American Medical Association* has attacked this conclusion as "incredible," an accusation vigorously countered by Gofman in a later issue of the same journal.

Today, doctors prescribe radiation most often to treat cancer and also use radiation to diagnose a wide variety of conditions. Highest doses of diagnostic radiation result from fluoroscopy, such as barium swallows, barium enemas, and cardiac catheterization, which entail prolonged exposures to radioactive materials. Orthopedists, dentists, and pulmonologists also widely use diagnostic radiation. Even though the breast does not receive a direct hit from most of these diagnostic procedures, it may receive damaging levels of radiation. A 1994 FDA Public Health Advisory reported that patients undergoing procedures such as cardiac catheterization were developing radiation-induced skin burns because of the nearly 2,000 rads of radiation these imaging techniques entailed.

In addition to the dangers average women face from radiation exposure involved in mammography, there are groups of women who face even higher risks, which we discuss next.

Genetic Risks

A relatively uncommon genetic disease, ataxia-telongiectasia (A-T) causes skin lesions and progressive neurological disease. People who carry the gene are highly sensitive to the carcinogenic effects of radiation. Most individuals who inherit the disorder first display symptoms in childhood. However, many can carry the gene without ever developing symptoms and, until a screening test is available, may not know they are at risk for A-T. About 1 to 2 percent of American women carry the gene and thus are highly susceptible to breast cancer, running a fivefold higher risk than women without the gene. In fact, some researchers claim that women carrying the A-T gene exposed to radiation may account for up to 20 percent of breast cancer cases annually in the United States.

Women with the A-T gene, and indeed other women already at high familial risk for developing breast cancer, find themselves caught in a vicious cycle: Because they are deemed "high risk," their doctors recommend that they have regular mammograms from a young, premenopausal age. Yet such procedures expose these women to radiation that is likely to further increase their risk of cancer. What is even more tragic is that a June 1995 article in the

American Journal of Public Health reports "There is no evidence that screening [high familial risk women] is more efficacious in reducing [their] mortality . . . than in other women in their 40s."

Hormonal Risks

Studies show that women who have higher levels of total estrogen because they have never had children or because they had children late in life are more susceptible to the carcinogenic effects of mammographic radiation. Additionally, experimental studies confirm that radiation enhances the carcinogenic effects of estrogen in rodent breasts. On the basis of these results, it is reasonable to assume that radiation will exacerbate cancer risks from hormonal contraceptives, estrogen replacement therapy, and eating beef contaminated with estrogen and pseudoestrogens.

THE VARIABLES OF RISK

As discussed, there appears to be little question that postmenopausal women benefit from mammography. However, if you are premenopausal, there is little or no evidence that you will benefit from mammography in any way. The primary reason for the special problems with premenopausal screening is that the premenopausal breast is naturally "lumpy" and dense with tissue, making it difficult to identify tumors with accuracy by mammography. Premenopausal mammograms, therefore, are likely to either miss cancers (false-negative results) or identify lumps as tumors that are merely benign tissues (false-positive results). As women pass through menopause and their hormone levels decrease, however, their breasts tend to become less dense, making tumors easier to locate.

Indeed, studies recently examined by the NCI panel showed that somewhere between none and ten women out of 10,000 in their forties would prolong their lives—but not save their lives—by receiving mammograms. Some of these studies found no effect of having regular mammograms for this age group, others found a few small benefits, and at least one study showed an increase in breast cancer.

Another important variable relates to the ability of mammograms to detect different types of breast cancer. Scientists are just now beginning to understand that breast cancer is not just one disease but many. At a recent meeting at the National Institutes of Health, several speakers described three separate diseases, with somewhat indistinct boundaries between them, that fall under the general heading of "breast cancer." Understanding these differences will help us see how limited the use of mammograms in premenopausal women may be:

- **Aggressive cancers that tend to spread and kill whether or not they are found by mammography.** These cancers account for about 13 to 17 percent of all breast cancers, and may first be discovered in the time between annual mammograms (interval cancers). Annual mammograms, then, would serve little purpose in finding these tumors.

- **Cancers that develop and spread over a period of five to ten years and account for about 50 to 70 percent of all breast cancers, primarily in postmenopausal women.**

- **Ductal carcinoma *in situ*, or preinvasive milk duct cancers, which are relatively benign even if left untreated for years, even until a woman can feel the lump herself.** This type of cancer accounts for about 10 to 15 percent of all breast cancers but 40 percent of all tumors detected in younger women.

These statistics show that about from 50 to 60 percent of premenopausal women with breast cancer are unlikely to benefit from mammography: Either they have virulent cancers that grow and spread too quickly to benefit from early detection, or they have cancers that will remain relatively harmless until they can be felt in a self-examination or clinical examination.

In postmenopausal women, mammography may detect small tumors earlier than could self-examination or clinical examination, thus providing up to two years' lead time in diagnosis and a reduction in mortality rates. Nevertheless, the benefit of this earlier diagnosis may not outweigh the risks of mammography.

IS SCREENING SAFE AND EFFECTIVE FOR PREMENOPAUSAL WOMEN?

The premenopausal breast is one of the most radiosensitive organs. In 1971, the prestigious National Academy of Sciences estimated that the overall risk of breast cancer increases by about 1 percent for every single rad exposure. Several more recent reports confirm this estimate.

Mammograms and Premenopausal Mortality

A Swedish study involving 42,000 women aged 45 to 69 showed that those under the age of 55 who received regular premenopausal mammography experienced a 29 percent greater risk of dying from breast cancer.

Another Swedish study of 60,000 women aged 40 to 64 showed a 7 percent increase in breast cancer mortality after premenopausal mammography.

A pooled analysis of six major international mammography screening programs found increases in mortality among healthy premenopausal women being screened for breast cancer.

Nevertheless, and despite warnings by its own senior staff (particularly the notable epidemiologist John Bailar, M.D.), the NCI, with the enthusiastic support of the ACS, embarked on the ill-conceived and poorly designed and conducted Breast Cancer Detection and Demonstration Project in 1972. Some 300,000 women, about half of them premenopausal, received free mammograms with assurances that they were safe, despite the high radiation exposures involved.

A confidential memo from Nathaniel Berlin, M.D., the senior NCI physician responsible for the project, may explain why women were not informed of the basic motivation for the study or its risks:

> *Both the [ACS] and the NCI will gain a great deal of publicity because they are bringing research funds to the public and applying them. This will assist in obtaining more research funds for basic research and clinical research which is sorely needed.*

Over the next two decades, questions of the safety and effectiveness of premenopausal screening came under closer scrutiny. On June 2, 1991, a front-page story in London's *Sunday Times* brought these concerns to the public under the headline "Breast Scans Boost Risk of Cancer Death." The report described interviews with Dr. Cornelia Baines (Department of Preventive Medicine and Biostatistics, University of Toronto, Toronto, Ontario, Canada) and Professor Anthony Miller (World Health Organization, Geneva, Switzerland), the senior investigators of the Canadian National Breast Screening Study. These researchers found that women aged 40 to 49 who had undergone mammography and physical examination had a higher death rate from breast cancer than did women who had undergone only a single physical breast examination.

Commenting on these findings, an editorial in *The Lancet* concluded the following:

> *The 44 deaths from breast cancer in the screened group translates into a 52 percent increase in breast cancer mortality among those screened. Although these results are the first to show a statistically significant increase in breast cancer mortality in a population who underwent screening mammography, other published studies have shown non-significant trends in the same direction, ranging from three to 29 percent with six to eight years' follow-up. There is no evidence to support introduction*

of service mammography for women under 50, and
some may argue that there should be a moratorium on
all mammography for symptom-free women in this age
group outside randomized clinical trials.

In another 1992 article in the *New Republic*, the chairman of
the United States Preventive Services Task Force was quoted as
saying that premenopausal women who enrolled in one of the
first large-scale mammography trials in the 1960s, conducted by
the Health Insurance Plan (HIP) of New York, received no benefit at all:

When you look at the data on women who enrolled in
the HIP trial in their 40s, you see that most who appear
to have profited from screening were closer to 50 than
40 at the time they started, and that their tumors were
detected not while they were still in their 40s, but when
they were in their 50s. The clear implication is that the
results would have been the same if they had waited
until 50 to start mammography.

These concerns were confirmed and extended with the 1993 publication of the results of a pooled study. Based on six well-conduct-
ed American and European clinical trials, the study showed excess
breast cancer deaths among premenopausal women who had had
regular screening with even modern "low-dose" mammography.
Within three years, breast cancer death rates were consistently higher among women who underwent premenopausal screening than
they were among those who did not. Based on the study the authors
concluded the following:

This evidence provides no basis for the promotion of
mammographic screening in women under 50 in the
general population. If mammography is to be offered to
the asymptomatic woman of that age who requests it,

> *appropriate information including the fact that there
> has been no demonstrated ultimate benefit should be
> given.*

Reluctantly bowing to the persuasive scientific evidence and a
ground swell of concern from activists and the public, the NCI convened an international workshop in 1993. Its published report concluded that the pooled results of eight major screening studies, some
dating back to the 1960s and others more recent, produced no evidence of benefit from screening under the age of 49. Having strongly recommended premenopausal screening for decades, the NCI
finally broke ranks with the American College of Radiology, the ACS
and the American Medical Association—groups that continued to
insist that the benefits of mammography outweighed the risks—and
recommended screening only for postmenopausal women. Then, in
early 1997, the NCI once again reversed its position. (Throughout
the duration of these flip-flops, the NCI consistently recommended
screening for *high-risk* premenopausal women, despite evidence that
radiation exposure is likely to further increase their risks, particularly if they carry radiation-susceptible genes.)

Both the ACS and the American College of Radiology—and now,
again, the NCI—continue aggressively to recommend mammography for premenopausal women. In recommending annual screening to all women aged 40 to 49, in March 1997, the ACS and NCI
relied on an analysis of seven studies of mammography for women
in their forties that found a 17 percent reduction in mortality.
However, even the NCI panel making the recommendation admitted that although 17 percent "appears impressive, it is actually difficult to detect with a high level of certainty," explaining that the figure was derived by combining data from studies that were not truly
comparable. Furthermore, Dr. Barbara K. Rimer, chair of the advisory group and director of the program on cancer prevention at
Duke University, reported that only two of the seven studies
involved *annual* screening. In addition, of these two studies, one

found that the death rate from breast cancer declined whereas the other found that mammography actually increased the risks of breast cancer.

Unfortunately, in recommending routine mammograms to women aged 40 to 49, the NCI and ACS relied on studies that were designed on the basis of chronological rather than menopausal age. Therefore, not only was menopausal status of women ignored, but any benefit of screening before age 50 could not be distinguished from that of screening after 50.

IS SCREENING SAFE AND EFFECTIVE FOR POSTMENOPAUSAL WOMEN?

Although less public and emotional, there is also a debate among scientists over the risks and benefits of mammography for women after menopause. In 1989, David Eddy, M.D., later key advisor on health care reform to the Clinton administration, was among the earliest experts to challenge routine screening for postmenopausal women. Basing his opinion on extensive analyses comparing the effectiveness of annual clinical examinations with a combination of clinical examination and mammography, Eddy concluded that, at best, mammography only marginally reduced mortality.

Others agreed with Eddy. In 1995, for instance, a federal panel of health experts warned physicians against mammography for women under 50 and over 70 years of age. The authors of a 1995 article in *The Lancet* concurred:

> *Little publicity has been given to the results of the four subsequent trials . . . showing no significant benefit in any age group. . . . It is disappointing that the marginal improvement in terms of reduced mortality is only perceptible in older women. . . . Since the benefit achieved is marginal, the harm caused is substantial, and the costs incurred are enormous, we suggest that public funding for breast screening in any age group is not justifiable.*

The High Price of Mammography

In strongly recommending routine annual mammography screening of women aged 40 to 49, the ACS and NCI have apparently ignored the overwhelming costs involved. The average cost of a screening mammogram in the United States is now $125. If every woman in this age range—about 20 million, according to the Census Bureau—submitted to an annual mammogram, the total annual cost would be $2.5 billion. This figure excludes substantial extra costs for further tests in the relatively high percentage of premenopausal women with mistakenly diagnosed (false-positive) breast cancers. These costs are in excess of NCI's 1997 total budget of $2.2 billion, and more than eight times the $300 million NCI budget for their breast cancer research program, only a small fraction of which do they devote to prevention. Contrasted with the minimal expense required to institute and maintain a national educational and training program for the breast self-exam—a safer and equally effective method of detecting breast cancer—the costs of mammography are clearly excessive.

We believe that older women who have received mammograms on a yearly basis—as recommended by the cancer establishment—for the last twenty or more years have by now been exposed to dangerously high levels of radiation. Based on evidence from past exposures, it is clear that some women today have received as much radiation from mammography—particularly from the misguided NCI/ACS Breast Cancer Demonstration and Detection Project—as from an atomic bomb blast (about 50 rads). And, unfortunately, the results are likely to be similar: Radiation accumulates in tissue, and therefore it does not matter if you receive a megablast from an atom bomb or smaller repeated exposures over several years. Rosalie Bertell, Ph.D., a leading expert on radiation risks, warns that "X-ray and nuclear exposures are cumulative in effect, and spreading them over time tends not to reduce the risk of developing breast cancer in later years."

MAMMOGRAPHY: THE OTHER RISKS

Besides breast cancer, mammography poses other risks, including receiving false-negative and false-positive results, interval cancers, and the spread of undiagnosed breast cancer after breast compression.

FALSE-NEGATIVE RESULTS

A false-negative result is a mistaken conclusion that a mammogram is normal when, in fact, a cancer is present. Many studies show that false-negative results are common, ranging from 7 to 70 percent of total mammograms taken in any given year. Most of the time the problem does not lie with the technique itself, or even the X-ray image, but rather with the radiologist who diagnoses an abnormality as benign rather than malignant. As Jane Brody wrote in the *New York Times* on December 2, 1994:

> A new study [in the New England Journal of Medicine] has raised serious questions about radiologists' reliability in reading mammograms and making recommendations about what to do when a suspicious lesion is found in the breast. . . . They disagreed on the diagnosis more than 20 percent of the time. . . . In addition, in some cases the radiologists disagreed [as] to which breast should be biopsied.

False-negative results tend to be particularly common among certain groups:

- **Premenopausal women:** The premenopausal breast is relatively dense due to its higher glandular structure and minimal fat content, and therefore small cancers are more likely to be missed.

- **Postmenopausal women on estrogen replacement therapy (ERT):** Because estrogen stimulates the growth of breast tissue, about 20 percent of women on ERT develop breast densities that may make their mammograms as difficult to read as are those of premenopausal women.

- **Women with breast implants:** Implants make the identification of early cancers very difficult by casting a shadow on breast tissue, compressing adjacent tissue, increasing mammographic density, and reducing contrast. Not surprisingly, women with implants who develop breast cancer tend to be diagnosed with more advanced disease and with a higher percentage of invasive lesions, and thus with a worsened prognosis.

INTERVAL CANCERS

About one-third of all cancers are diagnosed *between* annual mammograms. A study at a University of Louisville (Louisville, Kentucky) screening center showed that from 17 to 77 percent of premenopausal cancers surfaced quickly in the intervals between annual screening examinations and also were more likely to metastasize. This type of cancer tumor can double in size in one month, so that women or their doctors sometimes detect lumps by self-examination or clinical exam within just a few weeks after a negative mammography result. This problem is just another indication that premenopausal screening is of little or no benefit to women, particularly women lulled into a false sense of security by the idea that mammography offers "the best protection" and who then fail to perform their own monthly self-examinations as a result.

FALSE-POSITIVE RESULTS

For every cancer they detect by mammography, radiologists mistakenly diagnose some five to ten other lesions as cancer, resulting in unnecessary anxiety, more mammograms, biopsies, and scarring. Overall, women between the ages of 40 and 49 who have mammograms every year run a 30 percent chance of being told that an abnormality has been found, even though their breasts are normal.

According to a 1989 article in *Clinical Radiology,* some 84 to 97 of 100 "positive" mammograms are false-positive results. Breast cancer experts Devra Lee Davis, Ph.D., and Susan Love, M.D., emphasized in a 1994 article in the *Journal of the American Medical Association* that "overall [only] about one of ten biopsies recommended on the basis of mammography will be cancerous." Premenopausal women and postmenopausal women taking ERT are two groups more likely to get false-positive mammogram results.

As discussed, the most common false-positive results radiologists and surgeons identify as cancer are actually precancerous lesions called milk duct cancers (ductal carcinoma *in situ*), the incidence of which has tripled over the last few decades. Although at least 75 percent of these lesions never progress to cancer, many surgeons treat them as cancer and operate, often performing lumpectomies or total mastectomies (removal of the breast). In 1992, for instance, some 23,000 American women were diagnosed with this cancer and about half submitted to mastectomies.

On the basis of these figures, and considering the low potential for carcinomas *in situ* to become invasive cancer, it appears that for every woman who receives a life-saving mammogram, three others receive unnecessary mastectomies and an erroneous diagnosis of a fatal disease.

SPREAD OF CANCER CELLS

As early as 1928, an article in *Radiation* warned that doctors should handle cancerous breasts with care "for fear of accidentally disseminating cells" and spreading cancer. Nevertheless, today's mammogram requires very tight compression of the breast, which may lead to the rupture of blood vessels and spread of cells from as yet undetected breast cancer. In fact, recent studies show that the number of metastases can increase by up to 80 percent when a tumor is manipulated mechanically. In a Swedish study in which technicians used "as much compression as the women could tolerate," the screened group had nearly 30 percent more deaths than did the unscreened group. Unfortunately, as emphasized in a 1992 article in *The Lancet,* as yet, neither the United States nor the United Kingdom has standards for the force to be used during mammographic procedures nor "has the possible risk associated . . . ever been properly assessed."

SAFE ALTERNATIVES TO MAMMOGRAPHY

Are there safe alternatives to mammography? The short answer to this important question is yes. Several safe and more effective methods exist for women and their doctors to detect and diagnose breast cancer. Some of these methods are now readily available, others harder to find, and others are still on the drawing board. Unfortunately, the powerful cancer and mammography establishments continue to discourage—if not block—the development and large-scale application of these alternative screening methods, a subject we will discuss in depth in chapter 13.

BREAST SELF-EXAMINATION

Breast self-examination, without doubt, is far safer and at least as effective as mammography. Remember that 90 percent of all breast cancers are found by women during their monthly breast self-examinations. Even the ACS, now a fierce proponent of routine mammography, once extolled the effectiveness of self-examination:

> It is probably true that, from the point of view of the greatest possible gain in early diagnosis, teaching women how to examine their breasts is more important than teaching the technique of breast examination to physicians, for we must keep in mind the fact that at least 90 percent of the women who develop breast carcinoma discover their tumors themselves.

According to a 1985 article in *The Lancet,* breast self-examination leads to "earlier detection and improved survival." A pooled analysis of several 1993 studies published in the *Journal of the National Cancer Institute* showed that women who regularly perform breast self-examinations detect their cancers much earlier and with fewer positive nodes and smaller tumors than women who do not perform self-examinations. A 1992 study of Finnish women practicing self-examinations reported a 30 percent decrease in breast cancer mortality compared with the general population.

The key to success in almost anything is practice and proficiency, and this is also true of breast self-examination. The number of false-positive and false-negative results may be just as high with self-examination as with mammography. A study in *The Lancet* showed that there is an 80 percent chance that an abnormality detected by breast self-examination will be benign, particularly among premenopausal women. As for false-negative results, women who previously found abnormalities later proved to be benign are much more likely to dismiss future abnormalities. The same study concluded:

> *The risk here is that the patient may delay a further visit to a physician for efficacious breast screening (clinical or mammographic) or, worse, for the assessment of a malignant lump, subsequently found by the patient but thought benign because of her previous experience.*

With training, however, women can decrease the frequency of both false-positive and false-negative results. A 1980 article in the journal *Cancer* found that "training increases reported breast self-exam frequency, confidence, and the number of small tumors found."

The use of a new tool, called the Sensor Pad, further improves the reliability of self-examination. The Sensor Pad consists of two sealed plastic sheets with lubricant between them. You lay the sheets over the breast to enhance your ability to detect abnormalities in the breast. A woman who used the Pad told a *Wall Street Journal* reporter in 1994 that "There is no question that the Sensor Pad increases my tactile ability. . . . It makes it 100 percent easier." The Sensor Pad is now freely available in most countries worldwide; however, in the United States it is available only by prescription.

CLINICAL EXAMINATION

Combined with regular self-examinations, regular clinical examinations represent the most effective and important screening method now widely available. When the physician takes adequate time and is well-trained, the detection rate can be as high as 87 percent, with great success in finding even small tumors.

TRANSILLUMINATION WITH INFRARED LIGHT SCANNING

Believe it or not, a machine exists that can screen for breast cancer by shining a perfectly harmless (though intense) infrared light through the breast, then scanning the light on a closed-circuit television monitor. Because tumors absorb more infrared light than does normal tissue, they show up as distinct masses on the television screen. A recent innovation, called ballistic two-dimensional imaging, uses ultrafast shutters that limit the amount of light scattering associated with transillumination.

Although early forms of transillumination techniques were less reliable, a 1985 article in *American Surgeon* concluded that it is now a "sensitive indicator of both benign and malignant breast disease [and a] reliable predictor of clinically apparent breast lesions without the potential problems of radiation exposure." The procedure is also more effective than is mammography for women with scarring from previous biopsies, partial surgical procedures, or reconstruction, because it can distinguish the differences between these lesions and cancerous lumps. The only drawback is that cancers deep within the breast may be missed with transillumination.

Nevertheless, this screening method is a safe and effective alternative for most women. It is particularly useful for women carrying the A-T gene, who are at high risk for developing radiation-induced breast cancer, and for women who require repeated examinations. Most women who have had both mammography and light scanning clearly prefer the latter. Unfortunately, the FDA—whose expert panels are largely made up of radiologists anxious to protect their own turf—has blocked approval, seizing transillumination machines from screening centers that attempt to use them "illegally" and claiming that their safety has not been sufficiently assessed.

THERMOGRAPHY

Because breast cancers emit more heat than does normal tissue, they can be detected by a method in which an image of this heat can be translated onto a heat map. A 1980 report in *Cancer* stated that although thermography "has not proven to be of significant value in detecting early breast cancer, it can be useful . . . in reducing the number of women who should receive routine mammograms for screening purposes."

One application now under development is the use of heat-sensitive detectors in bras. Scantek's Breast Thermal Activity Indicator consists of two fiber pads, which a woman places inside her bra for about fifteen minutes. When she removes it, a color-coded system indicates an abnormality and the need for further screening. This safe and useful method is currently available by prescription only.

ULTRASONOGRAPHY

Ultrasonography exposes the breast to pulsed high-frequency sound waves. The reflected and transmitted echo patterns are then displayed as electronic images. Although ultrasonography may very well replace mammography in the future, it still has two major drawbacks as a screening tool. First, it is unreliable for detecting lesions less than 1 centimeter in diameter. Second, about 30 percent of cancers have variable ultrasound characteristics, which means that these cancers have physical characteristics that make detecting their sound patterns more difficult.

For now, ultrasonography offers women with suspicious breast abnormalities found by other screening techniques another option besides biopsy. In April 1996, the FDA approved the use of high-definition digital ultrasound for the diagnosis of suspicious lesions found in routine mammographic screening. This new and safe technique produces very sharp images and could reduce by 40 percent the 700,000 biopsies annually performed in the United States.

MAGNETIC RESONANCE IMAGING

More commonly known by its acronym MRI, magnetic resonance imaging uses magnetic fields to produce high-contrast images of breast tissue that has been injected with a dye designed to concentrate in (and thus define) cancer cells. MRI may be especially useful in detecting cancers in dense premenopausal breasts and in breasts with implants—cancers that are often missed by mammography.

Currently, MRI has three major drawbacks: First, it cannot distinguish between benign and malignant lesions. Second, it is expensive—about $800 per scan, or six to ten times more than the cost of mammography, a cost that could be sharply reduced as the procedure becomes more widely employed. Finally, MRI exposes a woman to electromagnetic radiation, which itself may trigger breast cancer development (chapter 11). At this time, the MRI is now widely used in Germany as a follow-up to abnormal mammograms, thus reducing the need for biopsies, and may soon be used the same way in the United States.

ESTROGEN TESTS

Because estrogen plays a strong role in influencing the risks of breast cancer, blood and urine tests are being developed to evaluate both overall levels of estrogen and the ratio of "good" to "bad" estrogen. Because estrogen levels are higher in urine, urine testing seems more promising at this time.

In combination with breast self-examinations, clinical examinations, and other safe screening methods, estrogen tests may be helpful in identifying women at higher risk for developing breast cancer. Once these women understand that risk, they can work to reduce any other risk factors they may have by, for example, changing their diets to avoid contaminated beef and dairy products, and exercising on a regular basis.

THE SPRINGER TEST

The Springer test is somewhat like an allergy test. A doctor injects tumor antigens into the skin and then waits to see if your body reacts quickly to the antigens. Either a rash develops in the area injected or the area becomes inflamed. When either occurs, it means that your immune system has produced antibodies to cancer cells already present in your body. Although the Springer test is nonspecific—that is, it indicates the presence of an undetected cancer somewhere in the body—it may be useful for women who have had suspicious results on mammography.

ANTIMALIGNIN ANTIBODY IN SERUM TEST (AMAS)

Another nonspecific cancer screening test, the Antimalignin Antibody in Serum test, measures serum levels of antimalignin, an antibody found in the serum at elevated concentrations in patients with cancer. In some cases, the AMAS test can detect cancer up to nineteen months before a clinical examination would find it. Reports in a 1994 issue of *Cancer Detection and Prevention* and a 1992 issue of *Oncology Times* have shown that the AMAS test has a very low incidence of false-positive and false-negative results.

A one-year follow-up study by researchers at the Baptist Hospital in Miami claimed that the AMAS test had a 96 percent sensitivity rate in patients who had previous abnormal results on mammography, and that the test detected breast cancers as small as 1 millimeter in diameter.

GENE DAMAGE SCREENING

Just now ready for clinical trials (which means the general public might not see it in use for several years), the gene damage screening test analyzes the extent to which genes have been damaged and thus become precancerous or cancerous. A surgeon performs a fine-needle biopsy (a procedure that removes cells from an abnormal mass in the breast), then submits the tissue for analysis. This test can identify precancerous changes in DNA, thereby detecting cancer long before a life-threatening tumor appears. In addition, because cells that are likely to metastasize have more DNA damage than do relatively noninvasive cancer cells, doctors could use this test to determine whether newly diagnosed breast cancers are likely to spread. By doing so, they could prevent women with cancer *in situ* from submitting to unnecessary mastectomies.

PERSONAL PROTECTION

It may be very difficult for women to ignore the panoply of voices in favor of mammography: Advertisements and pamphlets from the ACS, advice from their own doctors, and admonishments from concerned relatives. Nevertheless, as we have carefully spelled out in this chapter, for most women, most of the time, mammography offers few benefits and a great deal of risk.

WHAT YOU CAN DO

- Use mammography sparingly.
- Use safer alternatives whenever possible.
- Avoid all nonessential medical radiation.

USE MAMMOGRAPHY SPARINGLY

If you are a premenopausal woman, refuse a baseline mammogram or annual mammography screening—however strongly your gynecologist or physician recommends or insists. If breast cancer runs in your family or if you have other risk factors, be absolutely scrupulous about performing careful monthly self-examinations and receiving annual clinical examinations.

If you are postmenopausal, submit to a single-view mammogram every two years, only at a dedicated mammography center, and then only up to the age of about 70. Women at all ages with the A-T gene or family history of A-T should refuse mammography altogether.

When you choose a mammography center after menopause, look for a clinic or hospital center accredited by the American College of Radiology that fully meets the 1994 standards. The center should have a staff licensed by the state to practice mammography. Also be sure that the center performs at least ten to twenty mammograms daily, because experienced radiologists are less likely to make mistakes. Make sure that the center uses its machines only for mammography, the machines are calibrated at least annually, and the average dose per exposure is 300 millirads or less. Insist on receiving numerical information on the annual percentages of false-positive and false-negative results at the center.

USE SAFER ALTERNATIVES

Women of *all ages* should routinely practice monthly breast self-examinations and have annual clinical examinations. When it comes to maintaining breast health, the best thing you can do for yourself is to receive breast self-examination training. Mammacare, and other breast self-exam training programs, widely available throughout the United States teach women the most effective method of self-examinations and train them to work with their doctors and nurses to detect breast cancer as early as possible. When women receive training in palpation with breast models, they rapidly achieve a high level of competence.

In the meantime, these instructions show you how to perform a breast self-examination. Every month, preferably on the same day and at about the same time:

- Stand in front of a mirror with arms at your sides. Look for any changes, such as puckering or dimpling of the skin, discharge from the nipples, or a change in size of one or both breasts. Repeat the examination first with your arms overhead, and then with arms on your hip and tensing your chest muscles.

- Lift one arm behind your head. Take the other hand and massage the entire breast with your fingertips. Move counterclockwise and from the outer portion of the breast inward toward the nipple. Feel for any lumps, thick patches, or tenderness. Repeat this process on the other breast.

- Lie down and place one arm under your head. Using the fingertips of your other hand, once again examine the portion of the breast inward toward the nipple. Squeeze the nipple gently and note any discharge. Repeat this process on the other breast. If you feel an abnormality, do not panic. More than 90 percent of all lumps discovered by breast self-examination (or mammography for that matter) are benign. Breasts are extremely sensitive to hormonal changes; a lumpy, tender breast at any age could be due to natural stimulation by estrogen or other hormones. Nevertheless, it is important for you to see your doctor for further evaluation.

To make the self-examination even easier and more accurate, ask your doctor to prescribe the Sensor Pad for you. As you reach menopause, seek safer alternatives to mammography, such as thermography or the AMAS test.

AVOID ALL NONESSENTIAL MEDICAL IRRADIATION

Always keep in mind that "routine" or "safe" medical irradiation does not exist: Every exposure carries with it some risk. Whenever possible, avoid having any X-ray films taken for any reason, including as part of "routine" dental examinations, even though you are likely to be assured of their safety by your physician, radiologist, or dentist.

6

Breast Implants: The Whole Story

In addition to causing serious complications including rupture, pain, and autoimmune disease, silicone gel implants, particularly those wrapped in polyurethane, pose clear risks for breast cancer. The cancer establishment, plastic surgeons, and the breast implant industry have known about and ignored these risks for decades. Safer alternatives are available.

Female breasts: Objects of desire and sexuality, icons of motherhood and nurturing, ideals of aesthetic beauty for painters and sculptors throughout the centuries. Today, thanks largely to an unrealistic ideal of large-breasted, tiny-waisted women made popular by the Barbie doll, *Playboy* magazine, and myriad television and advertising images, we have a booming plastic surgery industry ready to exploit women eager to meet that ideal—no matter the cost to their health and safety. As we will discuss in this chapter, we also have a cancer establishment and breast implant industry unwilling to recognize or publicize the serious risks implants pose for breast cancer.

To date, over one million American women have had breast implants, about 80 percent for cosmetic reasons and about 20 percent for reconstruction after mastectomy. (Although the Food and Drug Administration (FDA) estimates that closer to two million women have had implants, Dow Corning, a major manufacturer of breast implants, puts the figure closer to one million.) "While there is no direct proof that silicone causes cancers in humans," reads a 1987 FDA task force report prepared by scientists who were then summarily reassigned, "there is considerable reason to suspect that it can do so." Because breast cancer usually takes many years—if not decades—to develop, the fate of these women remains in grave question.

THE HISTORY OF BREAST IMPLANTS

The history of cosmetic breast implants began during the occupation of Japan by the United States after World War II. Asian prostitutes, eager to satisfy the United States servicemen's preference for large breasts, began asking their doctors to augment their breasts with injections of silicone or paraffin. Two decades later, when technology improved and with social changes brought on by the sexual revolution, the practice of breast augmentation caught on in the United States.

Until the early 1960s, plastic surgeons enlarged women's breasts by injecting liquid silicone directly into the breast—an extremely dangerous practice that frequently resulted in infection, poisoning, and the early development of cancer. Developed in the late 1960s and 1970s, modern breast augmentation generally involved implanting a pouch filled with silicone gel or, less often and more recently, with saline (saltwater) solution. Saline implants involve surgically implanting a pouch then injecting saline into the pouch through a valve; leakage and deflation of the implant are the chief disadvantages.

Silicone gel implants come in two forms: 1) wrapped in a seamless silicone outer envelope, and 2) in an envelope wrapped in polyurethane foam (PUF). The PUF implants, marketed under brand names such as Meme, Natural Y, and Replicon, have been in widespread use since the mid-1980s. Until recently, seven major United States companies, including Dow Corning and Bristol-Myers Squibb, manufactured about 40 types of implants. Of the women who received silicone implants since the early 1960s, about 300,000 have implants made with polyurethane foam.

Safety issues have surrounded the implants since their inception. By the early 1980s, unpublished industry studies showed that the silicone gel used in implants caused cancer in rats; however, the market for implants continued to grow. It wasn't until September of 1991 that the manufacturers "voluntarily" withdrew polyurethane foam implants after adverse publicity about their cancer risks—risks that the manufacturers continue to trivialize. In 1992, the FDA banned all silicone gel implants, allowing only women taking part in controlled, clinical trials to receive them for reconstructive purposes. Saline-filled breast implants, however, continue to be freely available both for the purpose of reconstruction and augmentation.

Health Complications of Implants

Quite apart from increasing your risk of breast cancer, breast implants result in other serious complications:

- **Rupture of implants:** The most common complication is rupture of the implant, which causes the silicone contents of the implant to leak into the body. If rupture or leakage of a saline implant occurs, the saline itself is naturally absorbed; however, the empty silicone envelope must then be surgically removed. If rupture or leakage of a silicone gel implant occurs, the more viscous gel may ooze out so slowly that the woman is unaware of the problem.

  In fact, even intact silicone gel implants leak microscopic particles of the gel into surrounding breast tissue: A study by Boston's Massachusetts General Hospital found that patients with implants had five times the blood levels of silica or silicon as did patients who had never had implants—and this was true whether or not the implants had ruptured. Once inside breast tissue, these particles can then be carried to distant sites in the body by the lymph and blood systems. Specialized microscopic and chemical tests have also identified silica in such distant sites as joint lining tissue, lung cells, and skin, as well as in inflamed tissue surrounding the implants.

  The toxic gel can thus be in contact with body tissue for many years—causing chronic inflammation in the breast or anywhere

(continued)

else the silicone settles as well as the development of autoimmune disease (see below)—before surgery, X-ray film, or magnetic resonance imaging identifies the rupture.

- **Hardening:** Both gel and saline implants can develop surface hardening, which occurs when breast tissue interacts with the silicone envelope, causing an inflammatory reaction called *capsular contraction*. The contraction can be painful and cause the implants to harden and occasionally crack with minimal trauma. When cracking occurs, the implants rupture and leak. Polyurethane implants were originally introduced in attempts, which proved unsuccessful, to reduce the chances of this complication.

- **Autoimmune disease:** Breast implants may cause the body to produce abnormal antibodies, which are immune system cells that attack foreign invaders (such as viruses and bacteria) they perceive as "nonself" or harmful. In the case of autoimmune diseases, however, the immune system generates autoantibodies that attack normal body cells. According to a 1993 study in the *Archives of Internal Medicine*, 35 percent of women with implants may develop autoantibodies. These autoantibodies can cause rheumatoid arthritis, systemic lupus erythematosus, and scleroderma, three diseases, that affect the connective tissue (joints, muscles, and tendons) and skin. A wide range of other studies published in prestigious journals fully confirm these findings.

The 1992 FDA restriction on silicone gel implants has met and continues to meet stiff resistance from the ACS's American Society of Plastic and Reconstructive Surgery, American College of Radiology, American Medical Association, and some major women's groups, including the National Alliance of Breast Cancer Organizations (NABCO) and its subset, Y-ME, which is funded by the implant industry. All of these groups continue to insist that the benefits to women (particularly women who want implants as reconstruction after breast cancer surgery) outweigh the risks. In September of 1996, Nevada Congresswoman Barbara Vucanovich—supported by the ACS, the American Society of Clinical Oncology, and NABCO—filed a citizen's petition asking the FDA to ease current restrictions on the use of silicone gel implants in patients who have had mastectomies for breast cancer.

At the same time, since 1992 more than 18,000 lawsuits have been filed against manufacturers of breast implants. Three of those manufacturers agreed to a global settlement of $4.2 billion to compensate women with implants who had developed complications. However, neither the lawsuit nor the ban on silicone implants considered any cancer risk (they did not even mention such a possibility). Instead, the global settlement concentrated on other serious side effects, including implant rupture, leakage of silicone gel through the capsule (gel bleed), and atypical autoimmune and rheumatoid diseases.

IMPLANTS AND BREAST CANCER RISK

Participants in Congressional hearings on implants and their risks— including women with implants, plastic surgeons, internists, and industry representatives—consistently fail to mention breast cancer. Nevertheless, substantial scientific animal and human evidence clearly demonstrates the significant risk of breast cancer to women with silicone gel implants, especially those wrapped in polyurethane foam.

THE RISKS OF SILICONE GEL

By the early 1980s, studies sponsored by Dow Corning showed that silicone gels used in breast implants were carcinogenic in rats. However, Dow Corning buried the data, which still remains unpublished. It was only in the course of a routine 1987 inspection that the FDA discovered another unpublished report of a particularly damning two-year Dow Corning study on rats. The report showed that silicone gel injected under the skin of rats induced "pronounced increases in the incidence" of malignant tumors at the implant site. Moreover, these tumors were highly invasive and rapidly lethal.

On the basis of this information, an FDA senior staff scientist urged the agency to immediately inform women. "A medical alert should be issued," the message read, "to warn the public of the possibility of malignancy development in humans following long-term implant of silicone breast prostheses." The FDA ignored the warning and, as did Dow Corning, buried this information in its own confidential files. In 1990, after Ralph Nader's Health Research Group obtained the report from the FDA under the Freedom of Information Act, it finally emerged in an issue of the *Federal Register*. Even then, Dow Corning attempted to explain away these findings on a variety of grounds including that the cancers were nonspecific or of no relevence to human risk.

Women with implants and women who wanted implants remained unaware of these dangers, even as evidence continued to mount: A 1994 study in the *Journal of the National Cancer Institute* showed that injections of silicone gel into the abdominal cavities of mice induced a high incidence of plasma cell tumors; these tumors are closely related to multiple myeloma, a rare and fatal human bone marrow cancer, generally not seen except in the elderly. Of still further concern is a evidence that silicone degrades in the body to crystalline silica, a known potent carcinogen in both animals and humans.

Not only is silicone gel carcinogenic in animals, it also acts like estrogen in rodents, as clearly demonstrated by a series of studies by Dow Corning published in 1972. Additionally, an unpublished FDA report emphasized that the gel binds to and concentrates estrogen and progesterone. The FDA report stated, "Possible uptake of high concentrations of hormones at the implant site was postulated to be the cause of the increased cancer incidence found in animal studies."

THE RISKS OF POLYURETHANE FOAM

The polyurethane foam used to cover some silicone gel implants is even more carcinogenic than is the gel itself. Polyurethane foam is an industrial wrapping and insulation material manufactured from the carcinogen 2, 4-toluene diisocyanate (TDI) that persists as a contaminant in the foam implants. Once in the breast, the foam gradually infiltrates local tissues and degrades while releasing more TDI that, in turn, is converted into another carcinogen, 2,4-diamino-toluene (TDA). TDA is the same carcinogenic chemical used in dark hair dyes that made them so dangerous the cosmetic industry was forced to "voluntarily" remove it in 1972, after studies had shown it induced liver cancer in rats (chapter 10). Nevertheless, the implant industry had no qualms about bathing sensitive breast tissue of unsuspecting women with this carcinogen.

As early as the 1960s, a series of scientific publications reported that polyurethane foam rapidly degrades in the body and induces highly malignant cancers when implanted under the skin or in the abdomens of rodents. Wilhelm Hueper, then embattled head of the Environmental Cancer Division of the National Cancer Institute and a leading international expert in carcinogenesis and cancer prevention, emphatically warned that:

> Since polyurethane plastics have been used in cosmetic and orthopedic surgery during recent years, these observations are of distinct significance and practical importance . . . (and) should caution [the industry] against the indiscriminate use of polyurethane plastics in medical practice.

By the early 1980s, a series of other studies confirmed that both TDI and TDA induce breast and other cancers in rodents. In 1986, the Environmental Protection Agency stated in an internal report that TDA was "probably carcinogenic to man," which the Federal National Toxicology Program confirmed in 1991, and more recently in 1994, with particular reference to the carcinogenic effects of TDA in the breasts.

Further proof of the dangers of breast implants comes from the fact that free TDA has been found in the urine and breast milk of women with PUF implants. In 1991, the FDA requested Bristol-Myers Squibb to conduct tests to determine the amount of this carcinogen in the urine, blood, and breast milk of women with implants. While complying with the requests, Bristol-Myers launched a vigorous damage-control counteroffensive. Key to this was their claim that implants do not pose a significant risk of cancer, because the levels of the TDA in human urine "were extremely low" compared with the higher levels required to induce breast cancer in rodent feeding tests. This comparison is extremely misleading: The level of carcinogen reaching rodent breasts from feeding tests is clearly much lower than the levels of carcinogen directly contaminating breast cells of women with implants. Striking support for this conclusion is provided by recent findings of very high concentrations of TDA in breast tissue surrounding PUF implants.

A June 28, 1995, FDA press release claimed that a Bristol-Myers Squibb study demonstrated "very small amounts" of TDA in 80 percent of women with implants and in only 13 percent of women without implants. Both the FDA and Bristol-Myers claimed that the risk was "negligible," but the study remains unpublished.

ETHYLENE OXIDE

Routinely used to sterilize both silicone gel and foam implants, ethylene oxide persists on the surface of implants after surgeons insert them into breasts. Several studies, reviewed in 1987 by the International Agency for Research on Cancer, showed that this sterilant induces breast and other cancers in rodents.

THE IMPLANT INDUSTRY'S DENIAL

More than 60 case reports dating back to the 1960s have been published on breast cancer occurrences after silicone injection and silicone gel and foam implants. Both the National Cancer Institute (NCI) and the FDA have recognized the significance of the reports, as evidenced by a June 1995 press release in which the FDA stated, "These case reports all have in common a long latency period . . . associated with complications related to silicone migration." In addition, because implants make it difficult for both mammograms and self-examinations to pick up signs of early cancer (chapter 5), it is quite possible that many more women with implants have undiagnosed breast cancer.

Nevertheless, the breast implant industry continues to claim that no evidence exists of increased breast cancer risks among women with implants. A 1986 industry-funded study published in *Plastic and Reconstructive Surgery*, for example, claimed that there were actually *lower* than expected breast cancer rates in premenopausal women with breast implants. A close look at the study reveals its flaws:

- **Duration of study:** The study followed women for only six years, much too short a time for cancers to develop. Still, even this report concluded that older women who have had implants for a longer time experienced a "slight excess of breast cancer." A 1992 update of this study again claimed that the breast cancer rates were lower among pre-menopausal women with implants; however, the follow-up period averaged only about ten years, with increasing rates again noted among women with a longer follow-up. In addition, the study admitted that women with implants suffered an increase in lung, vulva, and cervical cancers, clearly showing the carcinogenic nature of the implants in other sites in addition to the breast.

- **Dismissal of risk factors and high-risk groups:** The authors also admitted that they failed to consider various breast cancer risk factors, and recognized that the relatively low cancer rate in young women with implants could be due to the fact that it is unlikely that women with a family history of breast cancer would ever be given implants. In addition, the authors ignored the fact that most women who get implants for cosmetic reasons do so because they have smaller-than-average breasts, which puts them at less risk than their larger-breasted peers, and thus should be expected to have lower rates of breast cancer.

Another study, this one done in 1992, also showed lower rates of breast cancer among Canadian women with implants; however, again, its conclusions were skewed. The average follow-up time was only about ten years, and the authors acknowledged that they could not exclude "the possibility that implants increase the risk of breast cancer" because the women in this study, too, had smaller-than-average breast size. The follow-up report to this study, released in 1995, once more showed increasing numbers of breast cancers, further demonstrating how long it takes for breast cancer to develop.

The industry tried hard to use these studies to give breast implants a clean bill of health. However, the NCI, responding to a congressional demand for a report on the risks of implants, admitted in an article in the *Journal of Clinical Epidemiology*:

> *Only a few epidemiologic studies on long-term effects have been published, and all have had methodologic limitations, including the possibility of inappropriate comparison rates, limited and/or incomplete follow-up, absence of information on patients' characteristics, and lack of specific information on types of implanted material.*

MULTIPLE MYELOMA AND BREAST IMPLANTS

An uncommon cancer usually occurring only in the elderly, multiple myeloma is a cancer of the bone marrow that affects the blood plasma cells. The FDA has received reports of about 20 cases of multiple myeloma in relatively young women after breast implantation. Combined with the animal studies that showed an increase in a related cancer (plasma cell tumors) in mice, these reports persuaded both the FDA and the NCI to establish poorly organized and poorly publicized breast implant/multiple myeloma registries in 1995—but without telling the women who participate the reasons the registries had been set up in the first place. To date, twenty-six women between the ages of 35 and 79 who have multiple myeloma have been registered with the NCI by a few surgical centers, nearly half of them under the age of 50—a remarkable finding considering the rarity of this cancer in this age group.

UNCOVERING INDUSTRY AND FOOD AND DRUG ADMINISTRATION COVER-UPS

By 1992, articles in the *Medical Tribune, New York Times,* and other publications exposed shocking evidence that the implant industry had longstanding secret knowledge that implants posed cancer risks to women and withheld this information from the public while aggressively marketing their products. A 1995 publication in the *International Journal of Occupational Medicine and Toxicology* documented this evidence—some of it obtained through the Freedom of Information Act and through confidential sources. The study made it clear that plastic surgeons also joined in this self-interested conspiracy of silence—a conspiracy in existence for more than two decades:

- In 1971, industry sources admitted in internal memos that the experimental evidence of carcinogenicity of polyurethane foam was relevant and "significant in those applications . . . for use inside the body."

- In 1985, Medical Engineering Corp., a Bristol-Myers Squibb subsidiary, frankly stated in a memo, "Polyurethanes have no real history of implantation without deterioration and we know deterioration products of polyurethanes are toxic and in some cases carcinogenic. . . . Whether they are released in such low levels as to be no threat to the human body, time will tell."

- In 1985, another industry official warned in a memo, "The breakdown products of the fuzzy implant material may well be carcinogenic. How would anyone defend himself in a malpractice suit if a patient developed a breast malignancy?"

- In 1985, at an industry-sponsored meeting, a leading plastic surgeon and co-author of the 1986 industry-funded epidemiological publication cautioned that "foam could be a time bomb . . . [in view of its] carcinogenic potential. Surgeons should not go on implanting."

- In an October 26, 1988, "Confidential, Destroy" memorandum, Batelle Laboratories in Columbus, Ohio, under contract to the breast implant industry, noted that polyurethane foam contaminants were detectable in implants and admitted their carcinogenicity in rats and mice.

- In 1989, a Surgitek consultant noted in a private memorandum, "I am at this point concerned about the amounts of TDI and [TDA] products detected in the 'clean' PUF presented to us for evaluation. Our initial methods of development were directed towards detection of ppb [parts per billion] levels; what we are detecting is parts per thousand which is significantly more concentrated than expected."

- In 1990, a Bristol-Myers Squibb memorandum revealed, "There is pretty solid evidence that [diaminotoluene] is a carcinogen to humans. The question is does PUF foam, used as we do, release [diaminotoluene] in the human breast to an extent that causes an unacceptable risk of cancer?"

- In 1991, a Surgitek consultant protested that while his prior negative findings on TDA in the urine of women had "previously been accepted as reliable by Surgitek," his more recent findings on high levels of contaminants in urine were rejected as being unreliable.

- In the latest effort to cover up the dangers of implants, Dr. James Rosenbaum, an implant industry consultant from Oregon Health Services University in Portland, published an article in *Science* that brazenly called for "Activism by Scientists" to organize opposition to any claims that breast implants posed any health risks. Dr. Rosenbaum's ignorance of the scientific literature is illustrated by his insistence that "epidemiologic studies have failed to show an association between silicone breast implants and various diseases [including] breast cancer."

With the breast implant industry and the FDA ignoring or trivializing the breast cancer risk of long-term implantation, women still have not received any information or warning about such risks. An immediate medical alert warning of breast cancer risks should be sent to all women with implants, especially those with PUF implants. A national surveillance program, funded by industry, should also be implemented, and women should be offered financial assistance for removal of their implants.

PERSONAL PROTECTION

WHAT YOU CAN DO

- Have a surgeon remove your implants as soon as possible.

- Choose a safer alternative to implants.

- Ask for special screening if you have implants and need a mammogram.

HAVE A SURGEON REMOVE YOUR IMPLANTS

Increasing numbers of women across the country are now visiting plastic surgeons—not to receive breast implants, but to have them removed. Most do so because they suffer from scleroderma or other autoimmune diseases, or because they have heard the increasingly alarming stories about implants splitting apart and causing breast deformities. In 1994, nearly 29,000 women had their implants removed, compared with just 18,000 in 1992. If you currently have implants, we strongly urge you to join these women, especially because of the very real breast and other cancer risks they pose. It may be a difficult decision to make, particularly if you worry that the surgery to remove the implants might disfigure you. It should reassure you to know that, in most cases, the surgery usually leaves minimal scars and that the breasts usually return to their normal, healthy, pre-implant shapes within a few months.

You may also be worried about the financial cost of such a decision, and for good reason. Even if you have insurance, you may find it difficult to convince your insurer to pay for the removal of implants—unless you can persuade the company that you have suffered some implant-related complications with the aid of documentation from your doctor. According to a 1992 article in the *Wall Street Journal*, many insurance companies assert that the procedure is unnecessary. If your insurance will not pay, you may find the price tag of the surgery $5,000 or higher too big a burden.

If you are among the 3,000 or so women whose breast implants have ruptured or begun to leak, you may be eligible to have them removed at the expense of the manufacturer. Representative James A. Traficant, Jr., of Ohio, recently introduced the "Breast Implant Accountability Act" (H.R. 2796), requiring breast implant manufacturers to notify women that funds will be provided for the voluntary surgical removal of breast implant surgery performed before January 1, 1994. (The recent declaration of bankruptcy by Dow Corning, however, limits the amount of money available to women in need.) Similar bills have been introduced at the state level. Making such initiatives difficult is the poorly informed but enthusiastic endorsement of the value and safety of silicone gel implants by the mainstream National Alliance of Breast Cancer Organizations (NABCO).

You may also find it difficult to find a plastic surgeon to perform the procedure. Many doctors fear that performing the procedure will expose them to future malpractice suits; others resist because they do not want to admit the risks of implants, because they fear malpractice suits, or because they are simply unaware of the facts that implants pose health risks to women. Keep trying, though, for your future health is well worth the inconvenience and expense.

Choose Safer Alternatives to Implants

Despite the controversy over breast implants, thousands of women still seek breast augmentation—7,000 more women received implants in 1994 than did in 1992. If you have been thinking about obtaining breast implants, read about these safer alternatives before you visit a plastic surgeon:

- **Implants:** A relatively new type of implant uses peanut oil instead of saline or silicone gel. It has a nonsilicone shell and, because the body will readily absorb this food material, any rupture of the implant would be unlikely to cause any serious effects. Saline and soybean oil implants are safer than are silicone gel implants; however, because they have silicone shells, they still pose a risk. At all costs, avoid any silicone gel implants.

- **Transplantation:** A procedure that involves transplanting tissue from other parts of the body (usually the abdomen or back) into the breast, this method of breast reconstruction is a safer alternative to implants, according to an article in a 1995 issue of *Plastic and Reconstructive Surgery*. In this procedure, the surgeon creates a breast from a flap of skin, muscle, and fat taken from another part of the body. However, the surgery is not an easy one. It is complex, costly, and requires a long recovery period. You will want to research this procedure and discuss it thoroughly with your doctor before you decide.

Request Specialized Screening When You Need a Mammogram

As discussed in chapter 5, standard mammography is unreliable for women with implants. If you have implants and need a mammogram, make sure your doctor is aware of your condition. Insist on a displacement mammogram, during which the technician moves the tissue of your breast away from the implant before taking the image. Another possibility is for you to have a magnetic resonance imaging (chapter 5), a sophisticated procedure that can penetrate silicon implants to view the breast thoroughly. Currently, these tests are extremely expensive—about $800 or more—and your insurance company probably will not pay for this procedure.

7

The Case Against Chemoprevention

Chemoprevention is the use of nutrients or synthetic drugs in attempts to prevent breast cancer in healthy women. Tamoxifen is a synthetic hormonal drug now being tested in clinical trials because some scientists believe that it could reduce risks of breast cancer. However, there is little evidence of any such effect. Moreover, treatment of healthy women with this drug poses serious, even life-threatening, risks. There are safer and much more effective ways of reducing breast cancer risk.

E strogen is the common link between most breast cancer risk factors—genetic, reproductive, dietary, lifestyle, and environmental. It both stimulates the division of breast cells (healthy as well as cancerous) and, especially in its "bad" form, increases the risk of breast cancer. Thus, hormonal drugs such as tamoxifen that block the effects of estrogen on the breast might be expected to reduce the risk of breast cancer developing in healthy women.

THE TRUTH ABOUT TAMOXIFEN

About twenty years ago the pharmaceutical industry developed a drug called tamoxifen. Tamoxifen is the first generation of a group of drugs, now known as "Selective Estrogen-Receptor-Modulators (SERMs), which have both antiestrogenic and estrogenic effects.

Tamoxifen is antiestrogenic to the breast, and estrogenic to the uterus and, to a lessor extent, the heart, blood vessels, and bone. Tamoxifen is currently sold under the brand name Nolvadex by Zeneca Pharmaceuticals, an American spin-off of the British Imperial Chemical Industries, one of the world's largest manufacturers of industrial chemicals and pesticides; Zeneca is now the world's largest cancer drug company, second only to Bristol-Myers Squibb.

Animal studies show that tamoxifen prevents estrogen from binding to receptor sites on breast cells. Tamoxifen also reduces the incidence of breast cancer in rodents after administration of a breast carcinogen.

Starting in the late 1970s, oncologists began using tamoxifen to treat women with breast cancer, often in combination with other drugs, radiation, or surgery, such as lumpectomy and mastectomy—and with modest success. Today, doctors are treating about one million American breast cancer patients with tamoxifen, about 20 percent of them for more than five years. As studies published in the *New England Journal of Medicine* in 1989 and the *Journal of the National Cancer Institute* in 1991 show, women with breast cancer who take tamoxifen reduce their chances of developing cancer in the other breast (called *contralateral cancer*) by about one-third.

Based far more on wishful thinking than on science, the National Cancer Institute leapt to the conclusion that tamoxifen's antiestrogenic effects in relation to breast cancer treatment means that the drug will prevent breast cancer from developing in healthy women. The NCI also claimed that tamoxifen reduces the risks of osteoporosis and heart disease because—paradoxically enough—tamoxifen has estrogenic and thus protective effects on bone, blood cholesterol, and the heart.

As a result, in April 1992, the NCI launched a $60 million breast cancer prevention trial, aiming to recruit 16,000 healthy women in about 270 centers in the United States and Canada. Still ongoing, the trial now involves 13,000 healthy women over the age of 35 considered at high risk for breast cancer because of a strong family history of the disease or suspicious breast lumps (atypical hyperplasia), as well as women over 60 with or without risk factors. For five years, half the women receive tamoxifen and half receive a placebo. The drug is supplied free by manufacturer, Zeneca Pharmaceuticals. Results of the trial are expected by 1999.

Unfortunately, this misguided and dangerous approach to prevention stems from the entrenched fixation of the NCI on the use of chemical drugs to prevent cancer which may have been induced by chemical pollutants, medical technology (such as radiation from X rays), and carcinogenic/estrogenic drugs in the first place. Instead of attempting to reduce the carcinogenic chemical burden under which we struggle to maintain our health, the NCI believes that the solution is to add more chemicals to the mix. Their approach prompted Dr. Susan Love to protest, "It is a sad state of affairs when we have to add yet more chemicals to counteract the effects of other chemicals."

This attitude extends to the way the NCI treats the women in the trial. They are given no guidance on alternative protective measures, such as increasing exercise, maintaining a healthy weight, eating a protective diet, and avoiding exposures to environmental carcinogens, let alone being fully informed about the serious risks of taximofen.

Apart from this fundamental problem, the NCI's logic about the tamoxifen trial is flawed in other essential ways:

- A 1992 report in the *New England Journal of Medicine* emphasized that no basis exists for any comparison between the breasts of healthy women and the unaffected breast of women with cancer in the opposite breast.

- The same report showed that tamoxifen may reduce the incidence of contralateral cancer, but only in premenopausal women and then in only three of eight trials.

- In another 1992 study in *Acta Oncologica*, tamoxifen not only failed to reduce contralateral cancers in premenopausal women, it actually increased their incidence.

- On the basis of an audit of long-term clinical trials, the NCI reported in a December 1995 letter to physicians that tamoxifen provides "no advantage" for preventing contralateral breast cancer in women treated with tamoxifen for more than five years. The NCI further admitted "a troublesome possibility . . . that tamoxifen might actually be detrimental." In other words, even by NCI's own admission, tamoxifen *does not* provide long-term protection against contralateral breast cancer, which was the original basis for the prevention trial. Nevertheless, the NCI persists with the trial.

- Several trials with tamoxifen failed to show that tamoxifen has any effect on bone density, and thus on the prevention of osteoporosis. In three other trials, bone density increased slightly in lower spinal vertebrae, but not in longer bones or in hip bones, those particularly susceptible to fractures and potentially fatal complications.

- Regarding its effects on heart disease, tamoxifen does appear to reduce total cholesterol levels. Its effect on the levels of "good cholesterol," and thus on the buildup of arterial blockages and clots, however, is less certain. A detailed review of the drug's alleged protective cardiovascular effects prompted the National Heart, Lung, and Blood Institute—a once strong proponent and funder of the trial—to sharply reduce its support because the evidence of benefit proved so inadequate.

Clearly, the cancer establishment has exaggerated the benefits of tamoxifen as a preventive tool for breast cancer, osteoporosis, and heart disease. In addition, tamoxifen poses risks of serious side effects in the healthy women who are induced to take it, leading them to take these risks with little to no chance of reaping any benefits.

THE RISKS OF TAMOXIFEN

Among the well-documented complications of tamoxifen are premature menopausal symptoms, eye damage, blood clots, hepatitis, and liver, uterine, and other cancers. A woman taking tamoxifen to fight against life-threatening breast cancer may consider these risks acceptable; however, no healthy cancer-free woman would, or should, feel the same.

- **Menopausal symptoms:** Tamoxifen often induces menopausal symptoms in young women, ranging from hot flashes to vaginal discharge, vaginal atrophy, and other debilitating changes.

- **Eye damage:** According to a 1978 study in *Cancer Treatment Reports* and another in *Cancer* in 1992, about 6 percent of women taking tamoxifen suffer damage to the retina, corneal opacities, and decreased visual acuity.

- **Blood clots:** Several studies, including one reported to the FDA Oncological Drugs Advisory Committee by the National Surgical Adjuvant Breast and Bowel Project in 1991, show that the risk for developing life-threatening blood clots increases about seven times in women taking tamoxifen.

- **Hepatitis, liver, uterine, and other cancers:** Tamoxifen is toxic to the liver, and there have been reports of acute hepatitis in patients treated with tamoxifen. Furthermore, animal studies show that, according to Gary Williams, medical director of the American Heart Foundation, tamoxifen is also a "rip-roaring" liver carcinogen, inducing highly aggressive cancers in about 12 percent of rats at dosages equivalent to those used in the prevention trial. The incidence was much higher at twice this dose and in rats primed by prior exposure to other chemical carcinogens. Even Zeneca, the manufacturer of tamoxifen, admits that it is a liver carcinogen, while nevertheless aggressively promoting its use in prevention trials.

Laboratory studies show how tamoxifen acts as a carcinogen. It binds tightly and irreversibly to DNA, the genetic blueprint of a cell, causing a cancerous mutation to take place. Even the conservative British Medical Research Council warns that no amount of tamoxifen is safe when it comes to carcinogenic effects.

When cancer develops in the other breast of patients treated with tamoxifen, the cancer tends to be highly aggressive and rapidly fatal. Should tamoxifen have a similar effect in healthy women in the trial, the results would be disastrous. Furthermore, patients with breast cancer treated with tamoxifen run a 50 percent increase in risk for developing other cancers, particularly of the digestive tract.

Risks of aggressive uterine cancers are sharply increased by tamoxifen, a not surprising finding in view of its estrogenic effects on this organ. A 1992 article in *The Lancet* quoted a leading proponent of the trial as admitting this risk, but dismissing it as "no big deal," easily treated by hysterectomy—an appalling example of medical sexism.

TAMOXIFEN LOBBY

On the basis of a detailed review of the studies cited above (and many others), an eight-member Carcinogen Identification Committee, appointed by the state of California in 1995 and chaired by Dr. Thomas Mack of the University of Southern California, unanimously concluded, as reported in *Science,* that tamoxifen is unequivocally carcinogenic. The Committee emphasized that both Swedish and American trials found a sixfold increase in uterine cancer in patients treated with tamoxifen. A report by the California Environmental Protection Agency stated:

> *Evidence from case-control and cross-sectional studies support the conclusion that tamoxifen causes endometrial cancer in women. Supporting evidence is also provided by numerous reports of endometrial and other gynecological changes associated with tamoxifen treatment. Tamoxifen has been clearly shown to cause cancer in humans and animals.*

Only intervention by California Governor Pete Wilson and aggressive lobbying by Zeneca prevented the state of California from immediately placing tamoxifen on its list of carcinogens. In fact, California's 1986 Proposition 65 requiring prominent labeling and warning of exposure to a known carcinogen, obligated the state to do so. Had the state so defined tamoxifen as carcinogenic the NCI might well have been forced to discontinue its tamoxifen trial.

Instead, the state's Environmental Protection Agency received a letter from Dr. Leslie Ford, a senior NCI staffer, challenging the carcinogenicity of tamoxifen. She dismissed the strong evidence associating tamoxifen with increased uterine cancer as "premature," claiming that carcinogenic effects in rats were seen only at high doses. In fact, the doses the rats received were equivalent to the doses women typically receive in the trial. Ford also dismissed tamoxifen's potential to cause liver cancer, simply because women in the trial had not yet developed the disease. Because liver and other cancers may take ten years or more to develop—and very few women have been taking tamoxifen for more than about seven years—Ford's logic is flawed at its base. In fact, the same logic would strike many carcinogens off the state's list of carcinogens, including asbestos, benzene, and vinyl chloride. Nevertheless, California still has not added tamoxifen to the Proposition 65 list.

In late 1995, the International Agency for Research on Cancer of the World Health Organization announced the creation of a seventeen-member task force to review information on the carcinogenicity of tamoxifen for publication in its monograph series. The unequivocal evidence before it persuaded the agency formally to confirm carcinogenicity of the tamoxifen in February 1996.

Nevertheless, the chemoprevention trial goes on and continues to enlist more women without warning them of the serious risks of tamoxifen. Its consent form, which it claims to be "one of the most comprehensive informed-consent forms" in medicine, is misleading in the extreme. It exaggerates the highly questionable benefits of tamoxifen and trivializes its very dangerous risks. The form's waiver of compensation for illness and injury is unlikely to protect the NCI, its investigators, or the hundreds of centers involved from a future flood of malpractice and punitive claims for cancer and other complications. Informed consent exists only when all the risks and benefits are clearly and completely spelled out by the prescribing doctors. The NCI clearly fails to do so in its patient consent forms.

THE NEXT GENERATION

It should be noted that a second generation of related SERM estrogen/antiestrogen drugs is now under active development. These drugs are antiestrogenic to the breast, where they bind to alpha estrogen receptors, while estrogenic to the heart, blood vessels, and bones, where they bind to beta receptors. Leading the SERM race is Eli Lilly's raloxifene, which experts estimate may be on the market within about a year. Raloxifene appears to be more protective than tamoxifen against heart disease and osteoporosis and—unlike tamoxifen—does not seem to pose risks of uterine cancer. Nevertheless, there are unresolved concerns with regard to other health risks, notably liver cancer. Moreover, the long-term effects of large-scale hormonal manipulation of healthy women, a population eagerly pursued by the pharmaceutical industry, is extremely problematic. Safer and more effective methods of breast cancer prevention are readily available for most women.

PERSONAL PROTECTION

By its very nature, treatment of a serious disease like breast cancer entails risks. However, the risks of prescribing tamoxifen to healthy women—in an ill-conceived effort to reduce their risks of developing breast cancer in the future—far outweigh any potential benefits. We strongly urge you to avoid this and related drugs for preventive purposes.

What You Can Do

- Say no to tamoxifen for prevention of breast cancer.
- Use safer and more effective methods of preventing breast cancer.

SAY NO TO TAMOXIFEN FOR PREVENTION

Healthy women should *never* use tamoxifen. Do not enter the NCI tamoxifen prevention trials. If you are currently taking part in the tamoxifen trial, withdraw immediately and insist that the center give you regular physical examinations on a long-term basis to prevent or treat delayed drug-related complications—and at its own expense. Keep in mind that you may have grounds to sue your doctors for medical malpractice because they did not inform you of the drug's risks for serious and potentially fatal complications.

USE SAFER ALTERNATIVES TO PREVENT BREAST CANCER

Fortunately, there are far safer ways to protect yourself against breast cancer than submitting to dangerous hormonal therapy:

- **Lifestyle changes:** Improving your diet by increasing foods that protect against breast cancer and losing weight if you need to (chapter 9), exercising on a regular basis, and consuming minimal amounts of alcohol (chapter 10) will help you reduce your risks of breast cancer—and a host of other conditions—with virtually no risk.

- **Nonhormonal drugs:** Believe it or not, common anti-inflammatory drugs, including aspirin and ibuprofen, reduce breast cancer risk more safely and effectively than does tamoxifen. A 1996 study showed that women who took aspirin three times a week for five years reduced their breast cancer risk by as much as 30 percent. In other words, the average 40-year-old woman, who normally has a one in 217 lifetime chance for developing breast cancer, can reduce her risk to 1 in 154—just by taking aspirin on a regular basis. This finding confirms at least five earlier studies, published in *Epidemiology, Journal of the National Cancer Institute,* and *Cancer Research.* The lead researcher in a 1996 study explained the potential benefits of aspirin in an issue of *Science News*:

> *These results indicate that nonsteroidal anti-inflam-matory drugs [such as aspirin] may have chemopreventive potential against the development of breast cancer. . . . I'm very excited about this. I think it's a promising lead in the prevention of these types of malignancies.*

The fact that such a simple and inexpensive class of drugs has such protective effects is probably one that the monopolistic cancer drug industry would rather you did not know. We strongly urge the further testing of aspirin's potential for preventing breast cancer, with NCI taxpayer-supported funds.

8

Common Medications and Your Risks

Common prescription drugs may trigger or exacerbate the development of breast cancer. They include medication used to treat hypertension, bacterial infections, psychiatric disorders (such as anxiety, depression, and psychosis), cancer, high cholesterol, and indigestion and ulcers. Safer alternatives exist, and women should ask their doctors for them whenever possible.

Medical advances, made with speed and ingenuity during the twentieth century, continue to save countless lives. Indeed, drugs that lower blood pressure and antibiotics that cure once-fatal infections are among the remarkable achievements contributing to a more than 50 percent increase in life span in under 100 years (from about the age of 49 in 1900 to nearly 75 as we reach the millennium). That said, clear evidence exists that medical technology has outpaced our ability to recognize and control its side effects. For instance, diethylstilbestrol (DES), a synthetic hormone designed to prevent miscarriage and prescribed with impunity to millions of young pregnant women despite long-standing and well-documented evidence of its carcinogenicity in rodents, increased women's risks of breast cancer, caused birth defects in their infants, and caused rare vaginal cancers in their daughters.

In this chapter, we provide information about certain medications that may have dangerous and generally unrecognized side effects, particularly increasing risks of breast cancer or spread of existing cancers. As you read about these medications, keep in mind what drugs really are: Potent chemicals designed profoundly to affect bodily processes. As such, then, it is not hard to imagine that along with their intended effects, they may also cause unintended but serious side effects. You should take all medications with care.

ANTIHYPERTENSIVES

High blood pressure is the most common chronic illness in the United States today. The American Heart Association estimates that more than sixty-two million Americans suffer from high blood pressure, and only a minority has it under control. Pharmaceutical industry scientists have developed several types of antihypertensive medications, four of which may increase breast cancer risks: reserpine, hydralazine, spironolactone, and atenolol.

SERPASIL (RESERPINE)

Derived from the rauwolfia plant, reserpine is one of the oldest and still most widely prescribed antihypertensives. A 1980 article in the *Journal of the American Medical Association* described reserpine as the "treatment regimen of choice" for 25 percent of persons with hypertension. Reserpine is one of a class of drugs (peripheral adrenergic antagonists) that lowers blood pressure by inhibiting the release of norepinephrine, an adrenal hormone that constricts blood vessels. The most common brand of reserpine prescribed today is Serpasil, manufactured by Cibageneva Pharmaceuticals. In another brand, sold under the name Ser-Ap-Es, reserpine is combined with two other drugs, another adrenergic antagon-ist called hydralazine hydrochloride and the diuretic drug hydrochlorothiazide.

In the early 1970s, several studies from the United States, the United Kingdom, and Finland established links between reserpine and breast cancer, showing that long-term reserpine treatment resulted in a tripling of breast cancer risks. One of these studies, published in *The Lancet* in 1974, showed that women who used the drug for more than ten years had up to a fivefold greater risk. Another, in a 1978 issue of the *Journal of the National Cancer Institute*, similarly reported "a significant but low-level association . . . between the occurrence of breast cancer and the use of rauwolfia derivatives for five or more years." Despite this and other evidence, a 1979 Food and Drug Administration (FDA) advisory panel recommended that the drug remain on the market, claiming that human studies were inconclusive. Since then, further studies—in both humans and animals—have confirmed the earlier findings.

The problem with reserpine is that it increases the blood concentration of prolactin, a pituitary hormone involved in the growth of both normal and breast cancer cells. According to several studies, published during the early 1970s in prestigious journals such as the *New England Journal of Medicine*, *International Journal of Cancer*, and *Medical Journal of Australia*, about one-third of human breast cancers depend on the presence of prolactin to grow and develop. Thus, drugs that increase prolactin levels are also likely to increase breast cancer risks.

In 1984, a study published in *Cancer Research* showed that women who had taken reserpine for five or more years had substantially elevated blood levels of prolactin. The study also reported that elevated prolactin levels persist for weeks after a woman stops taking the drug.

There is also experimental evidence of risks of breast cancer from reserpine. A 1980 National Toxicology Program study reported that the drug induced breast and other cancers in mice and rats. The result of this study is frankly admitted in the 1996 edition of the *Physician's Desk Reference*, which also notes that "The[se] breast neoplasms [cancers] are thought to be related to reserpine's prolactin-elevating effect. Several other prolactin-elevating drugs have also been associated with an increased incidence of mammary neoplasms in rodents."

APRESOLINE (HYDRALAZINE)

Sold by Cibageneva under the trade name Apresoline, hydralazine is a *vasodilator*—a drug that lowers blood pressure by dilating arteries—often prescribed to patients who fail to respond to reserpine. The results of a 1978 study published in the *Journal of the National Cancer Institute* showed that women taking the drug for more than five years doubled their risk of breast cancer. Although a 1987 study in the *Journal of the National Cancer Institute* found no evidence of increased risk among short-term users, its authors admitted that the long-term risks of breast cancer have not been adequately evaluated. In rodents, the drug induces lung but not breast tumors.

ALDACTONE (SPIRONOLACTONE)

Spironolactone is a *diuretic*, which means it lowers blood pressure by increasing excretion of body fluids in urine. Long known to cause breast enlargement (gynecomastia) in men, spironolactone also induces a statistically significant incidence of breast cancers in rodents and precancerous changes in monkey breasts.

To date, human studies have found only a modest link between Aldactone and breast cancer risk. However, the fact that the manufacturer of the drug, G.D. Searle & Co., falsified results of its carcinogenicity tests in 1975 (an action Senator Edward M. Kennedy characterized as an "exceedingly grave development") raises serious questions about the reliability of their data. In addition, the 1996 edition of the *Physicians' Desk Reference* warns patients and physicians that "carcinoma of the breast has been reported in patients taking spironolactone." Nevertheless, the FDA still allows unrestricted use of Aldactone.

TENORMIN (ATENOLOL)

Sold under the brand name Tenormin, atenolol belongs to a class of drugs known as *beta blockers* that reduces blood pressure by reducing the output of blood by the heart and reducing the heart rate. The 1996 *Physicians' Desk Reference* cites one rodent study in which atenolol caused breast and pituitary cancers, suggesting that women should avoid this drug.

ANTIBIOTICS

Antibiotics fight bacterial infections. Since scientists developed the first effective antibiotic—penicillin—before World War II, more than one hundred different antibiotics have been developed to ward off a full spectrum of bacterial diseases. Two types of antibiotics appear to increase breast cancer risk: metronidazole and nitrofurazone.

FLAGYL (METRONIDAZOLE)

One of the most widely prescribed antibiotic drugs, Flagyl, kills trichomonas, the yeast that causes vaginal yeast infections. Millions of women have used Flagyl since G.D. Searle first introduced it in the 1970s. In fact, by the mid-1970s alone, doctors wrote more than two million prescriptions for Flagyl each year.

Although two inadequate short-term human studies found no excess of breast cancer after the use of Flagyl, animal studies raise a clear warning. Several studies published in the 1970s and early 1980s showed a connection between Flagyl and breast cancer risk. The *Journal of the National Cancer Institute* published a study showing "noteworthy excesses of breast cancer in male rodents" after dosing with Flagyl, causing researchers to characterize the drug as having "considerable carcinogenic potential." A subsequent animal study also reported "significant" excesses of breast cancer.

FURACIN AND FUROXONE (NITROFURAZONE)

Used for treating wounds, burns, and skin infections, these closely related drugs are available in many forms: pills, creams, ointments, powders, solutions, sprays, suppositories, and surgical dressings. Many doctors now prescribe Furoxone to treat gastric ulcers caused by bacteria called *Helicobacter pylori*. Two studies, one reported in *Cancer Research* in 1970 and the other by the National Toxicology Program in 1988, showed that Furacin significantly increases breast cancer in rodents. Despite these findings, no epidemiological data are available about how these drugs may affect breast cancer risk in humans.

PSYCHOTHERAPEUTICS

Used to treat emotional and psychological problems ranging from anxiety and sleep disorders to depression and psychosis, psychotherapeutic drugs are prescribed to millions of women in the United States and around the world. Some 40 percent of American women and 25 percent of Canadian women, for instance, have taken an antianxiety medication such as Valium (diazepam) at some point in their lives. Unfortunately, some studies show that these drugs may pose hazards to breast tissue.

TRANQUILIZERS

Valium (diazepam) and the related benzodiazepine, Xanax, appear to increase blood levels of prolactin, a hormone known to stimulate the growth and development of invasive breast cancer, particularly among premenopausal women. The link between benzodiazepines and breast cancer has been a matter of concern and controversy since the late 1970s.

In 1976, for example, studies showed tranquilizer use was more common among women with invasive, rather than noninvasive, breast cancer, particularly among those developing recurrences within twelve months of surgery. This result suggested that Valium may increase invasiveness of early undiagnosed cancers. Animal studies in the late 1970s showed that Valium accelerated the growth of transplanted breast tumors in rats. Of particular concern, was the finding that even a low dose "only 2-3 times the usual daily dose," tripled the weight of the tumors within one month. The authors of one 1981 study, reviewed in the *New Scientist*, issued this warning:

> *If formal, rigorous studies are finally initiated, and if the connection of diazepam and cancer is confirmed, then the implications are horrendous . . . they suggest that a treatment almost universally offered to cancer patients—tranquilizers, which seemingly must be offered to curb anxiety—actually accelerates the disease in the people they are meant to help.*

ANTIDEPRESSANTS

Depression affects more than twenty million Americans every year, some two-thirds of them women. Elavil (amitryptiline hydrochloride) and Prozac (fluoxetine hydrochloride) are the most widely prescribed drugs for depression and other psychiatric conditions, including obsessive-compulsive disorder and panic attacks. According to a 1992 study in *Cancer Research*, both drugs promote the growth of breast cancer in rodents after administration of a chemical carcinogen.

ANTIPSYCHOTICS

Used to treat psychotic disorders such as schizophrenia and to control tics and the unintended explosive utterances that mark Tourette's syndrome, Haldol (haloperidol) triggers the release of the cancer-promoting hormone prolactin and induces significant increases of breast cancer in rodents.

CANCER DRUGS

It is not generally recognized that almost all cancer drugs, while effective in treating a particular cancer, may also be responsible for the induction of other future cancers, because paradoxically they themselves are actually carcinogenic. According to the National Cancer Institute (NCI), women prescribed nitrogen mustard, vincristine, procarbazine, and prednisone (a steroid) for treatment of Hodgkin's disease and other cancers are at significantly higher risk for developing breast cancer fifteen or more years later. In addition, several studies show that procarbazine induces breast and other cancers in rats.

CHOLESTEROL-LOWERING DRUGS

An industry-funded study of Pravachol (pravastatin) reported a rate of breast cancer twelve times higher among women taking this drug, designed to lower blood cholesterol, than among women not using the drug. Bristol-Myers Squibb, the manufacturer of the drug, labeled this result a "statistical fluke." However, a recent report in the *Journal of the American Medical Association* concluded that commonly used cholesterol-lowering drugs—fibrates and statins—cause breast and other cancers in rodents and that their use "should be avoided." With a new emphasis on preventing heart disease among women, the implication of this study should be explored in more depth.

ANTACIDS

Tagamet, until recently a prescription drug, is now available over the counter to treat indigestion and ulcers. Although it is not a carcinogen, Tagamet appears to alter the body's metabolism of estrogen, decreasing the levels of "good" estrogen and increasing the levels of "bad" estrogen. These estrogenic effects explain the higher rates of gynecomastia (breast enlargement) in men, as well as a report of breast cancer in a man treated with Tagamet. "After being on the drug for eight months," a 1981 article in *The Lancet* revealed, "he was found to have a hard malignant mass replacing his right breast."

Clearly, studies in humans on this drug are overdue, especially since millions of women (and men) use it.

PERSONAL PROTECTION

When you become ill with a condition that warrants taking a prescription drug, it may be difficult to think beyond just getting better—or feeling better—as quickly as possible. However, you must keep in mind that any drug you take may have unwanted and undisclosed side effects, including increasing your risk of breast cancer.

WHAT YOU CAN DO

- Avoid using drugs that may increase your risk of breast cancer.
- Use safer alternatives.

AVOID USING DRUGS THAT MAY INCREASE YOUR RISK OF BREAST CANCER

We have said it before: Knowledge is power. Before you take any medication, it is up to you to learn all you can about its intended effects and known or suspected side effects. Not only should you ask your physician about any drug he or she prescribes for you, but you should also read patient package inserts very carefully. Ask your pharmacist for an insert for each drug you take. Another way to stay informed is to purchase a *Physician's Desk Reference* (PDR), which is published by Medical Economics Data Production Company. Available for about $60 at most large bookstores, the PDR is easy to read and has several indexes enabling you to look up a drug by its generic name, its brand name, or its intended use. The information the PDR provides covers how the drug is supposed to work, the illnesses it is used to treat, its success rate, and its acute and chronic side effects, including cancer.

USE SAFER ALTERNATIVES

Armed with knowledge about the drugs you take, you can work with your doctor to find safer alternatives. In some cases, you might be able to adopt dietary and lifestyle changes that eventually decrease or even eliminate your need to take medication. However, do not under any circumstances stop taking medication without first discussing the matter with your physician. By doing so, you could seriously risk your health.

High Blood Pressure

One of the safer blood pressure medications is a drug called Esidrix (hydroclorothiazide), also sold under the brand name HydroDIURIL. Ask your doctor if this drug—which poses no risk of breast cancer—might work as well for you.

Lifestyle changes, including eating a diet low in sodium and animal fat and high in fiber, can reverse some cases of hypertension. You should avoid salt, which can exacerbate hypertension, while increasing your intake of calcium, magnesium, and potassium, which protect the cardiovascular system and help reduce blood pressure. Apricots, bananas, dates, broccoli, canned salmon with bones, dandelion greens, spinach, and nonfat yogurt are just some of the most healthful, vitamin-rich foods people wishing to reduce their blood pressure should include in their diet. In addition to improving your diet, you should lose weight if you need to, exercise regularly, and above all, stop smoking.

Antibiotics for Yeast Infections

If you use Flagyl to treat vaginal yeast infections, take the drug for just one day per infection. To relieve symptoms of a yeast infection (and to reduce the chances of reinfection), take a tub bath twice a day, wear cotton underwear, and avoid wearing pantyhose or tight pants.

Antibiotics for Ulcers

Many natural remedies for ulcers are available. Several studies in such journals as *Clinical Trials Journal, Gut,* and *The Lancet* during the early 1970s show that deglycyrrhizinated licorice (licorice with the chemical glycyrrhizin, which gives it its flavor, removed) performed as well as many typically prescribed drugs. Raw cabbage juice is another good remedy. Cabbage contains a natural chemical called glutamine, which scientists believe stimulates the regeneration of the protective mucus lining of the stomach. Ulcer sufferers should avoid aspirin unless it is enteric-coated, stop smoking, and reduce consumption of dairy products, caffeinated beverages, and wine.

Drugs for Psychological or Psychiatric Disturbances

At this time, most individuals with psychotic diseases such as schizophrenia require treatment with Haldol or related drugs, despite the risk they pose for breast cancer. To date, no effective alternatives exist. Severe cases of depression and anxiety also frequently require drug therapy. However, women with breast cancer or those at high risk should try not to rely on Valium, Prozac, or related drugs to relieve mild or moderate stress or depression. In less severe cases, counseling and behavioral modification may be all you need, because they actually produce the same kind of biochemical changes triggered by psychotherapeutic drugs. A February 15, 1996, *New York Times* article explained:

> *Psychotherapy can produce changes in brain function similar to those seen with psychiatric medication. . . . This tells us that effective behavioral treatments can have biological effects, not just psychological ones. So you can think of these therapies as ways you can change your own biology.*

Alternative medical practitioners have developed a number of nutritional and plant-based strategies for treating minor sleeplessness, anxiety, and depression. However, their usefulness and safety have not been critically evaluated.

Antacids for Indigestion and Ulcers

Among the over-the-counter alternatives to Tagamet are Phillips' Milk of Magnesia and Alka-Seltzer, at least on a short-term basis. Dietary supplements such as deglycyrrhizinated licorice and cabbage juice are also effective.

PART III

Dietary and Environmental Breast Cancer Risks

9

Eating for Health and Longevity

A diet high in calories and animal fat represents two major risk factors for breast cancer: Obesity, and exposure to carcinogenic and estrogenic industrial chemicals in animal fat. A low-calorie, low animal fat diet rich in fiber, vitamins, minerals, and antioxidants offers the best protection against these diet-related risks.

A lthough "you are what you eat" may be a cliché, it is apt when discussing your risks of breast cancer. The food you eat affects your risks in two basic and related ways: First, if you consume more calories than you burn as energy, you will gain weight, which puts you at greater risk for breast cancer and a host of other medical problems. Second, carcinogenic pesticides and other industrial pollutants contaminate many of the foods you eat. Foods containing animal and dairy fat are particularly vulnerable to this type of contamination, but fish, fruit, vegetables, and even your drinking water may also contain toxic and cancer-causing pollutants.

The cancer establishment has long minimized between the typical American diet and health. Focusing on just one small part of the dietary puzzle—the amount of fat we eat—the establishment ignores the larger issues of food contaminants and the danger they pose to our health. In this way, it protects the interests of the prime polluters of the planet—the petrochemical, pesticide, and pharmaceutical industries, and the powerful cattle lobby—whose representatives sit on its boards and provide funding for its programs. At the same time, the cancer establishment persistently fosters a "blame the victim" mentality: If your diet is putting you at higher risk, all you have to do is lower fat intake to reduce your risk. It is your fault if you fail to do so and then get cancer.

Although it is true that maintaining a healthy weight by eating less animal and dairy fat reduces breast cancer risk, an equally if not more crucial aspect of dietary risk is the amount of carcinogenic hormones, pesticides, and other industrial pollutants that contaminate many of the foods you eat. Fortunately, you can address both issues by creating an eating plan featuring healthy foods that are low in animal fat and also contain low levels of contaminants. At the end of the chapter, we will show you how to do just that.

In the meantime, we will first discuss the connection between obesity—probably the number one health problem in America— and breast cancer. Then we will describe those toxic food contaminants known to increase your risk for developing breast cancer.

OBESITY AND BREAST CANCER RISK

It is a fact: The United States is rapidly becoming a nation of the overweight. Today, more than 33 percent of American men and women are obese (commonly defined as being 20 percent or more over their ideal or optimal body weight), a full 8 percent more than were obese fifteen years ago. This growing tendency toward obesity appears to be a distinctly American phenomenon (only 6 percent of French people are overweight, for instance), and it is a problem that starts in our youth.

The proportion of overweight American children has more than doubled over the last three decades—nearly five million children aged 5 to 16 are now overweight—and that number, too, seems to be increasing. Statistics also show that overweight children tend to become overweight adults, who then must struggle with a myriad of weight-related health problems, including breast cancer. If a woman is 10 pounds overweight at the age of 30 and continues to be overweight, for instance, she increases her risk of postmenopausal breast cancer by about 25 percent; gaining an extra 15 pounds further increases her risk by 37 percent.

Several factors have combined during the last several decades to create this widespread problem. First, Americans have made fast foods and processed foods—which are traditionally filled with fat, calories, and preservative chemicals—staples of their daily diets. Second, television produces generation after generation of "couch potatoes" who also become consumers of the high-fat, nutritionally empty foods advertised on the screen. Indeed, a headline of an American Medical Association press release announced that "Kid Couch Potatoes More Likely to Become Obese," and cited a 1996 study showing that children who watched more than five hours of television daily were more likely to be overweight than those who watched two hours or less. Finally, the world of modern technology, filled with televisions, computers, automobiles, and automated appliances, now keeps us more sedentary than ever before. This lack of activity allows the food we eat to collect in our tissues rather than get used up as energy. As we will discuss further in chapter 10, lack of exercise itself is an important risk factor for breast cancer at every age.

OBESITY AND YOUR HEALTH

The health consequences of the "fattening of America" are dire. Indeed, obesity ranks as an important risk factor—along with a sedentary lifestyle—in decreased longevity and the development of most common and debilitating modern diseases, such as hypertension, heart disease, diabetes, and several types of cancer, including colorectal, endometrial, ovarian, and, particularly, breast cancer.

Statistics from studies collected over the past several decades show that obesity increases a woman's risk for developing postmenopausal breast cancer by 50 to 100 percent; this percentage increases the older she gets and the longer she stays heavy. If she also has other risk factors for breast cancer, such as a family history or late age at first pregnancy, her risk increases up to 600 percent, a study in the *New*

England Journal of Medicine shows. An obese woman of 60 with other risk factors, then, raises her chances of getting breast cancer from one in twenty-four to one in two. To make matters worse, not only are overweight women more likely to get breast cancer, they are also more likely to die from it.

Obesity and Breast Cancer: The Studies

- A 1977 study in *Preventive Medicine* found that breast cancer risk in obese postmenopausal women was about 50 percent greater than in the nonobese.

- A 1977 Netherlands report in *Cancer* showed that the overall risk of postmenopausal women increased in proportion to their weight. Furthermore, the more overweight the women, the more serious the course of cancer.

- In 1978, a report in *Preventive Medicine* revealed that Japanese women over 50 and at least 5 percent above the national average weight were at significantly increased risk.

- A 1978 Canadian study in the *American Journal of Epidemiology* found an excess breast cancer rate among heavier menopausal women.

- A large-scale 1979 ACS study in the *Journal of Chronic Disease* reported that breast cancer mortality was 50 percent greater in very obese women compared with those carrying less excess weight.

- A 1979 study in the *Journal of the National Cancer Institute* confirmed that breast cancer risks increased progressively with weight.

- A 1980 study in the *American Journal of Epidemiology* found that the heaviest women had an almost 40 percent increased risk compared with the lightest.

- A 1983 study in the *American Journal of Epidemiology* showed that any degree of obesity was associated with a 50 percent increase in risk.

- A 1988 study of Chinese women found that "high average body weight" was associated with breast cancer risk, especially among women over age 60, as reported in *Cancer Research.*

- A 1994 Netherlands study in the *British Journal of Cancer* found that risk of breast cancer increased 90 percent among the heaviest women.

- A 1996 study of Asian-Americans in the *Journal of the National Cancer Institute* found twice the risk among the heaviest rather than the lightest women. "Women in their 50s . . . with a recent gain of more than 10 pounds," the study confirmed, "had three times the risk."

THE OBESITY/ESTROGEN CONNECTION

Estrogen is produced not only by the ovaries and adrenal glands, but also by abdominal fat cells that convert other hormones (particularly testosterone) into estrogen. The more weight a woman carries, particularly around the abdomen, the more estrogen circulates in her body and the higher her risk of breast cancer. Several recent studies, including a 1990 study in the *Journal of American Epidemiology,* proved this point: It followed 40,000 postmenopausal women and found that those who subsequently developed breast cancer had a higher waist-to-hip ratio than their healthier counterparts.

Obesity affects a woman's risk of breast cancer risk in different ways and at different ages. In premenopausal women, obesity appears to offer about a 10 to 20 percent decrease in breast cancer risk. Obesity in young women is associated with lower overall estrogen levels (which results in irregular menstruation and ovulation) and higher levels of estrogen-binding proteins that reduce free estrogens. However, against such decreases in risk must be counted the negative effects of obesity-related health problems, such as heart disease and diabetes. In addition, most women tend to gain weight as they get older, and thus a woman who is obese before menopause is likely to be obese later in life.

Obesity in postmenopausal women, on the other hand, has just the opposite effect. The fat in the buttocks, thighs, and breasts contains an enzyme (aromatase) that can convert testosterone and other steroid hormones into estrogen. After menopause the activity of aromatase increases, which means that heavy women secrete more estrogen into the bloodstream and breast tissues. In addition to higher overall estrogen levels, postmenopausal obese women have a higher proportion of "bad" estrogen and lower levels of estrogen-binding protein.

Obesity also keeps the "estrogen window" open significantly longer than usual: Being obese lowers the age at which a young girl first menstruates and then raises the age at which a woman enters menopause. The estrogen window opens sooner than usual after breastfeeding, too, if a woman is obese; she misses fewer periods and starts ovulating sooner when breast feeding than do her leaner counterparts. Finally, at every age, obesity almost always coexists with inactivity, itself a risk factor for breast cancer.

Obesity Opens the Estrogen Window

Being more than 20 percent above your ideal body weight increases your risk of postmenopausal breast cancer by:

- Hastening menarche
- Hastening ovulation after breast-feeding
- Delaying menopause
- Increasing total estrogen levels postmenopausally
- Increasing levels of "bad" estrogen postmenopausally
- Decreasing estrogen binding postmenopausally

If you or your daughters are overweight, now is the time to address the problem. At the end of the chapter, we will show you safe and effective ways to lose weight while eating healthy, nutritious, and delicious food. In the meantime, it is important to understand what has become a subject of great controversy in the breast cancer debate: The relationship between the fat in our diets, the fat in our bodies, and breast cancer risk.

Dietary Fat and Breast Cancer: The Whole Story

Although many complicated cultural, social, genetic, and psychological factors influence how much you weigh, the physiological equation for weight gain is rather simple: If you eat more calories than you burn off, you'll gain weight. And it is easy to eat too many calories when food is filled with fat because, ounce for ounce, fat contains twice the calories of protein or carbohydrates. Thus, all other factors being equal, most overweight individuals tend to eat more fat than their thinner counterparts.

Scientists have long believed that the underlying cause of obesity-related breast cancer might be the higher levels of dietary fat most heavy women consume. As early as 1917, it was known that feeding laboratory animals high amounts of fat increased their breast cancer rates. Studies performed in the 1970s reinforced this hypothesis by showing that breast cancer rates of immigrants from Japan, where fat consumption is very low, quickly increase when they are exposed to the high-fat American diet.

However, more recent studies successfully challenged that assumption. The Harvard Nurses' Health Study examined the dietary habits of nearly 90,000 women and found no difference in the rates of breast cancer between those who consumed diets containing less than 25 percent of fat and those with diets containing more than 49 percent fat. In 1993, *Science* magazine confirmed what many scientists felt this and other similar studies showed, namely that "The popular theory among cancer epidemiologists in the 1980s—that eating fatty foods during adulthood greatly increases breast cancer risk—seems to have bombed out."

Prodded by the cancer establishment to bolster the fat-breast cancer link, scientists conducted several studies in the early 1990s. These studies, analyzed in a 1996 article in the *New England Journal of Medicine*, found no evidence that diets containing under 20 percent fat reduced breast cancer risk. Unfortunately, the conclusions of this study—that further investigation of a fatty diet as a cause of breast cancer is a "dead end and ultimately a distraction"—fail to consider several important links between dietary fat and breast cancer.

First, as we have discussed, fatty diets often lead to obesity, which itself is a risk factor for breast cancer. Second, there is suggestive evidence that consuming a low-fat, high-carbohydrate diet reduces breast density, a known risk factor for breast cancer. Finally, none of the multimillion-dollar diet studies generously funded by the cancer establishment over the last four decades even considered, let alone investigated, the role of food contaminants, many of which accumulate and concentrate in dietary and body fat. Indeed, converging lines of evidence involving animal studies, wildlife reports, test-tube experiments, and human studies make one fact clear: *It's not the fat itself that increases risk, it's what's in the fat.*

What the cancer establishment still isn't telling you is that dietary fat contains a wide range of contaminants—pesticides, other industrial pollutants, and sex hormones known to cause breast cancer and/or to have estrogenlike effects (pseudoestrogens). Other foods may also contain lower levels of these toxic substances. Once in the body, these contaminants tend to accumulate and concentrate in body and breast fat at levels thousands of times greater than in food, thus putting the breast at special risk.

Fortunately, women are finally learning how important a pure and unadulterated food supply is to their health. Nancy Evans, a breast cancer survivor and founder of Breast Cancer Action in San Francisco, recalls growing up on her Midwest farm:

> *We sprayed DDT constantly. The pesticide probably got into our food supply. We always had cows we butchered and a smokehouse where we smoked hams and bacon. We always had beef and chicken. We thought we were having a wonderful diet because we could afford meat. I ate this kind of a diet until I was about forty.*

Now Evans realizes that, although breast cancer is a disease that often has many causes, her diet certainly may have been a contributor. She hopes that by publicizing her story, and by urging women and men to pressure the food industry to make changes in the way it prepares and markets food, she may help to reduce the risks of breast and other cancers. For Earth First! activist Judi Bari, however, the change will come too late. Before her death from breast cancer in March 1997, she told friends that she attributed her breast cancer to hormone-laden foods and other toxins produced by the industrialized society she lived in.

UNDERSTANDING DIETARY CONTAMINANTS

Abundance, choice, and convenience: Our grocery stores' shelves, lined as they are with thousands of fresh, frozen, canned, and packaged products, are living testaments to these apparent mottos of the American food industry. No other country in the world offers as much to so many.

Unfortunately, this ostensible bounty comes at a high price. First, we have to wonder just how much truly valuable nutrition these modern products actually contain considering the depleting effect of the packaging and shipping process. More importantly, the food industry has developed and continues to use potent and potentially toxic chemicals to grow and market enormous quantities of agricultural and other products and sell them at a huge profit. The most important of such chemicals are: pesticides that kill crop pests as inexpensively as possible, but then leave residues that pose hazards to consumers; sex and growth hormones that bolster meat and dairy production; plastic wrapping and packaging products; food coloring dyes; and radioactive pollutants from nuclear plants (Table 9.1).

Dietary contaminants affect breast tissue in two different though related ways. They may be *carcinogenic* to the breast and other organs in experimental animals, which means that they trigger healthy cells to become cancer cells by deranging their DNA. Or they may be *pseudoestrogenic*, which means that they act like female sex hormones although they are structurally very different (chapter 2). Several contaminants, including the pesticide atrazine, have both carcinogenic and estrogenic effects, which makes them particularly dangerous.

TABLE 9.1: DIETARY CONTAMINANTS AND THEIR EFFECTS

Chemical	Estrogenic	Breast Carcinogen	Food
Pesticides			
Atrazine	+	+	Water, radishes, carrots
Benzene hexachloride	+	+	Beef, lamb, chicken, freshwater fish, limited saltwater fish
Chlordane	+	+	Beef, lamb, chicken, freshwater fish, limited saltwater fish
Chlordecone	+	–	Freshwater fish from limited areas of Virginia
Cyanazine	+	+	Water
DDT	+	–	Beef, lamb, chicken, freshwater fish, limited saltwater fish
1,2-dibromo -3-chloropropane	–	+	Water
1,2-dibromoethane	–	+	Water

Chemical	Estrogenic	Breast Carcinogen	Food
1,2-dichloroethane	–	+	Water
1,3-dichloropropene	–	+	Water
Dichlorvos	–	+	Wine
Dicofol	+	–	Fruits (apples and raisins) and fruit juices (apple and orange)
Dieldrin	+	+	Beef, lamb, chicken, freshwater fish, limited saltwater fish
Endosulfan	+	–	Fruits, vegetables
Ethafluralin	–	+	Water
Ethylene oxide	–	+	Spices
Etridiazole	–	+	Water
Heptachlor	+	+	Beef, lamb, chicken, freshwater fish, limited saltwater fish

(continued)

Chemical	Estrogenic	Breast Carcinogen	Food
Lindane	+	–	Beef, pork, lamb, chicken, fresh-water fish, limited saltwater fish
Methoxychlor	+	–	Fruits, vegetables, grains
Mirex	+	–	Great Lakes fish
Oryzalin	–	+	Grapes, wine, water
Prometon	–	+	Water
Propazine	–	+	Carrots, celery, fennel, water
Simazine	+	+	Water
Sulfallate	–	+	Water
Terbuthylazine	–	+	Water
Terbutryn	–	+	Water
Toxaphene	+	–	Freshwater fish; peanuts, peanut butter
Tribenutron methyl	–	+	Water

Chemical	Estrogenic	Breast Carcinogen	Food
Industrial Pollutants			
Methylene chloride	–	+	Decaffeinated coffee
Polychlorinated biphenyls (PCBs)	+	–	Freshwater/saltwater fish from inland waterways, bays, estuaries, harbors, marinas, other enclosed waterways; Eastern European meat
Polycyclic aromatic hydrocarbons (PAHs)	+	+	Seafood from bays, estuaries, harbors, marinas, and other enclosed waterways; heavy charcoal grilling of meats and seafood
Animal Drugs			
Growth-stimulating sex hormones	+	+	Beef, lamb

(continued)

Chemical	Estrogenic	Breast Carcinogen	Food
Bovine growth hormone (BGH)	−	±	Dairy
Nitrofurazone	−	+	Beef, lamb, poultry
Food Coloring and Packaging Materials			
Bisphenol A	+	−	Plastic food packaging and in lining of food cans
Nonylphenol	+	−	Plastic food packaging and in lining of food cans
Polystyrene	+	−	Plastic food packaging and in lining of food cans
Red Dye No. 3	+	±	Processed foods (cereals, artifically colored drinks)
Nuclear Fission Products			
Iodine-131 and other short-lived isotopes	−	±	Beef and dairy in proximity to nuclear facilites

+ = *causal relation;* ± = *suggestive relation;* − = *no relation*

A series of studies dating back to the 1960s demonstrate that consuming these dietary contaminants indeed increased breast cancer risk. These studies fall into three different categories: those that show some of these contaminants, particularly pesticides, induce breast cancer in rodents; those that show that dietary contaminants selectively concentrate in the cancerous human breast; and those that show higher concentrations of contaminants in the blood of breast cancer patients.

CARCINOGENS

The major categories of carcinogens in the food supply consist of pesticides, industrial pollutants, and sex hormones. Scientists have known of the existence of these dietary contaminants for decades, yet the cancer establishment continues to deny that they raise risks of breast cancer. Both animal studies from the 1960s and studies in humans from the 1970s confirm the fact that these dietary contaminants cause cancer. Some studies show that carcinogens concentrate in human breast tissue, while other studies prove the point in a different way by showing higher concentrations of these carcinogens in the blood of breast cancer patients.

Pesticides pose special dangers to the food supply. They enter your body primarily through contaminated food, but also by inhalation and or absorption through the skin. Pesticides are sprayed, powdered, or dropped as pellets in and around places where the general public may walk or engage in recreational activities. In fact, a wide range of pesticide residues is commonly found in the fatty tissue of almost everyone in the United States and, as a study published in a 1985 issue of *The Lancet* showed, in human breast milk and cow milk.

In 1993, another well-controlled study showed a strong association between high blood concentrations of DDE (a breakdown product of the pesticide DDT) and breast cancer compared with women without cancer. In fact, the risk was four times greater for

Pesticides and Breast Cancer: The Studies

- A 1976 World Health Organization study of Brazilian women found that the industrial pollutant polychlorinated biphenyls (PCBs) and the pesticide DDT selectively concentrate in breast cancer in contrast with nearby noncancerous tissues. Other pesticides, either carcinogenic and/or estrogenic to the breast (benzene hexachloride, dieldrin, and heptachlor epoxide) demonstrated "more or less the same tendency."

- A small 1982 study found high concentrations of DDT and benzene hexachloride in breast cancers compared to adjacent normal breast tissue.

- Higher levels of benzene hexachloride were found in breast cancers compared to normal breast tissues in a well-controlled 1990 study. Women with the highest levels were at a nearly eleven times greater risk of breast cancer.

- A 1992 study found that concentrations of PCBs and dichlorodiphenyldichloroethylene (DDE), a breakdown product of DDT, were up to 60 percent higher in tissues of women with cancer compared to those with benign breast disease.

- In 1993, researchers found that women with the highest blood levels of DDE were at four time greater risk for breast cancer compared to those with the lowest levels.

- In 1994, Canadian researchers reported that concentrations of a wide range of carcinogenic and pseudoestrogenic pesticides and industrial pollutants were higher in the fat and blood of women with estrogen-sensitive breast cancers than in healthy women.

- A "strong, positive association between DDE and breast cancer in Caucasian and African-American [women]" was found in a 1994 study, supporting a three- to fourfold increase among Caucasians with the highest exposures.

women with the highest levels of DDE compared to those with the lowest levels. The results prompted *USA Today* to lead with the headline "Breast Cancer May Have Link to Pollutants" and a leading scienti-fic journal to remark that the study had "extraordinary global implications for the prevention of breast cancer and should serve as a wake-up call for further urgent research." Then, in a 1994 study in the *Journal of the National Cancer Institute*, Canadian researchers reported that concentrations of a wide range of carcinogenic and estrogenic pesticides and industrial pollutants were higher in the fat and blood of women with estrogen-positive breast cancers than in healthy women.

In 1997, the same research group showed that there was a strong relationship between concentrations of estrogen receptors in the breast cancers of these women and DDE levels in their breast fat. This strongly suggests that exposure to DDT-type estrogenic pesticides explains, at least in part, the increase in estrogen receptor levels in breast tumors observed during the past two decades.

Despite this evidence, the cancer establishment has not publicized the danger, advised Congress and regulatory agencies, or encouraged the food industry to change its practices. Nor has it exposed the facts about the danger of nuclear power plant emissions that may affect millions of women and their families in the United States.

THE RISKS OF NUCLEAR FISSION BY-PRODUCTS

Every day, nuclear power plants release carcinogenic by-products into the atmosphere. These by-products then contaminate grasses and water on which dairy cows feed, thus entering the marketplace—and the human body—in the form of dairy products like milk and cheese. The body stores some types of radiation in the bone, where it can damage the bone marrow tissue responsible for producing immune system cells, as well as in breast tissue.

Although both the cancer establishment and the nuclear industry deny that nuclear by-products invade the environment, there is evidence to the contrary. An alarming study of the area around the

Millstone I reactor in Waterford, Connecticut, cited in a 1993 article in the *International Journal of Health Services*, reported the "highest emissions of airborne and liquid fission products ever released from any nuclear reactor in the United States"—cumulatively fifteen times higher than emission levels that existed at Three Mile Island after the nuclear accident.

What happens to these hazardous pollutants? They mainly end up in the local dairy supply: Milk produced in Waterford in 1976 contained levels of strontium-90, a deadly radioactive isotope, that were higher than levels recorded during the height of nuclear weapons testing. Other examples of high-risk nuclear by-products involve the communities of Suffolk and Nassau counties on Long Island, New York, each of which is home to a major nuclear reactor. The milk produced in these communities contains high doses of strontium-90 and, according to claims in a 1993 study in the *International Journal of Health Services*, the risk of dying from breast cancer there has increased sharply as strontium-90 levels have risen (see chapter 11 for more information about environmental exposures).

PSEUDOESTROGENS

The Florida panther is nearing extinction because pollutants have feminized the sexual organs of males. Wild gulls of the Great Lakes are born with deformed beaks, their egg shells are abnormally thin, and same-sex nesting of female birds occurs as a result of contamination. Wildlife ecologist Theo T. Colborn summed up the situation by saying, "We have reached the point where there are measurable changes in humans and the environment from the chemical soup we carry around in us."

Pesticides and industrial pollutants that have estrogenic effects are rampant in our natural environment. And while industrial estrogenic pollutants continue to deform and kill wildlife of all types, animals are not the only victims. Serious health risks to humans from these toxic chemicals include breast and other cancers.

Many industrial dietary contaminants not only are carcinogenic, but have estrogenic effects as well. That is, despite having quite different chemical structures, they act like natural estrogen once in the body, attaching to the same receptors on cell membranes intended for natural estrogen and then inducing similar, although much weaker, hormonal responses in the body. In the breast, estrogenic chemicals cause cells to grow and divide more quickly than normal, and also promote the growth of any abnormal or premalignant cells that might be present. Scientists have documented the estrogenic effects of certain chlorinated pesticides, including DDT, and packaging materials, such as the plastic linings in canned foods. They refer to these substances as pseudoestrogens.

The carcinogenic pesticide DDT is a typical pseudoestrogen. Banned in the United States in the early 1970s but still used widely throughout the rest of the world, DDT's estrogenic effects were first noted by scientists in the late 1940s, when they saw that the sexual organs of female rats exposed to DDT began to grow rapidly and mature. By 1950, other scientists confirmed this observation when they noted that the testicles of rooster chicks exposed to DDT remained immature and then became feminized. In 1952, a DDT derivative caused female dogs to remain in heat—even after their ovaries were removed. In 1961, a related pesticide called methoxychlor increased uterine weight in mice, and another one, kepone, caused constant estrus in mice, and the development of large ovarian follicles. Studies in humans performed in the mid-1970s showed that DDT binds to human breast estrogen receptors as well. Many other studies, such as those cited in the October 1993 issue of *Environmental Health Perspectives*, confirm these earlier studies.

Pseudoestrogens influence a woman's risk of breast cancer risk in various interrelated ways:

- **High concentrations:** Although much weaker than natural estrogens, they may concentrate in a wide variety of food, and in such high levels, that their cumulative effect is substantial.

- **Persistence:** While the body eliminates natural estrogen within 24 hours, pseudoestrogens may persist in the body for decades. Pseudoestrogens are unable to bind to proteins that would eliminate them from the body, and concentrate in body and breast fat.

■ **Metabolizing estrogen into the "bad" form:** Pseudoestrogens trigger the body to metabolize more estrogen into the "bad" form, and thus increase the risk of breast cancer even further.

CONTAMINATION OF THE FOOD SUPPLY

Pesticide regulations in the United States, while more stringent than in Third World countries, are riddled with loopholes. First, United States pesticide manufacturers continue legally to export banned pesticides, including those that cause breast cancer. The food industry then imports the foreign foodstuffs grown with these pesticides and sells them back to United States consumers. We eat squash from Mexico and the Netherlands that is contaminated with an estrogenic and carcinogenic pesticide called dieldrin. Carcinogenic pesticides such as benzene hexachloride, DDT, and lindane contaminate nuts and grains are imported from India. Norwegian-raised salmon contains these same breast carcinogens. In fact, fish farming worldwide remains virtually unregulated, and the industry frequently uses fat supplements to hasten growth, as well as veterinary drugs and pesticides to combat illness and bacterial contamination due to overcrowding. Fish caught in industrialized portions of Europe's major rivers, the Rhine and the Thames, as well as inland waters and the Baltic Sea, are usually highly contaminated by pesticides and other pollutants known to cause breast cancer.

Unfortunately, the situation in North America is not much better. Every type of food you eat may be contaminated with pollutants that could significantly raise your risk of developing breast cancer. Beef and dairy products are the most contaminated foods we eat, with residues of DDT and other chlorinated pesticides, antibiotics, veterinary drugs, and growth-stimulating sex hormones.

According to USDA monitoring reports, supermarket cuts of veal are also highly contaminated with pesticides and a wide range of veterinary drugs, and lamb may also contain a wide range of pesticides, including benzene hexacloride, DDT, hexachlorobenzene, and pentachlorophenol. The concentrations of these contaminants, however, are lower in these meats than in beef.

Pork products are relatively lean meats and, as such, contain much lower levels of pesticides than beef. However, supermarket pork products such as ham and bacon contain nitrite preservatives that combine with other chemicals in the meat or in the human body to form nitrosamines, which are very potent cancer-causing chemicals. Sulfa drugs such as sulfamethazine—known to be carcinogenic to the thyroid gland—are also likely to contaminate pork products.

Pesticides can also be found in chicken, though again at much lower levels than in beef due to the lower fat content of poultry. Low levels of antibiotics, which can cause allergic reactions as well as breed super-resistant strains of bacteria, also taint chicken. Turkey, however, is the least contaminated type of meat, containing virtually no detectable pesticide residues due to its extremely low fat content. Wild venison and wild boar tend to be safe as well.

As in Europe, fish of all types in the United States may be contaminated as well. Fish from industrialized waterways, including the Mississippi and Missouri rivers, the Great Lakes, and the inland waters of New York, Ohio, and New Jersey, contain a wide range of pseudoestrogens and breast carcinogens (including benzene hexachloride, chlordane, dieldrin, endrin, heptachlor, lindane, toxaphene, and mirex). The white croaker, a popular fish caught off the coast of Los Angeles, contains DDT and other pollutants at concentrations so high that the Environmental Protection Agency posts warnings on bays and estuaries against eating it —and yet not in supermarkets.

Considering the amount of pollution in our waterways, it should come as no surprise that carcinogenic pesticides and other industrial pollutants also contaminate our supply of drinking water. When the Environmental Working Group conducted a recent sampling of water in the Midwest, Maryland, and Louisiana, they found that tap water in twenty-eight of twenty-nine cites contained atrazine, a pseudoestrogenic herbicide known to cause human ovarian cancer as well as breast cancer in rodents. About one million Californians consume water with detectable concentrations of the breast carcinogen dibromochloropropane. Several studies from the 1970s and 1980s published by the Environmental Protection Agency and elsewhere have shown associations between pesticide contamination of water and increased rates of breast cancer. Recent unpublished studies have shown a high correlation between areas of Illinois where groundwater is heavily contaminated with atrazine and clusters of high breast cancer rates. Similar excesses, and links to breast cancer development, have been reported in St. Louis Park, a suburb of Minneapolis, where the carcinogen creosote tainted the town's drinking water.

Even fruits and vegetables—also highly touted as essential to a healthy diet—may be highly contaminated. Endosulfan, a pesticide related to DDT, is found on many fruits and vegetables and represents the seventh most commonly detected pesticide residue in food. Recently, the United States Federal Insecticide, Fungicide, and Rodenticide Act gave a green light to California raisin and strawberry growers, as well as to Washington state apple growers, to use the DDT-containing pesticide dicofol on food crops.

One of the most disturbing chapters in this saga involves recent reports from the Environmental Working Group of the U.S. Department of Health and Human Services revealing that baby food is also contaminated with carcinogenic and estrogenic chemicals. A 1984 study published in *Cancer* further notes that "Numerous studies have found that there is a greater risk of developing cancer if exposure to carcinogens begins in infancy rather than later in life." Given this information, it seems reckless that the food industry continues to ignore the danger of marketing carcinogen-laced food to vulnerable consumers.

FOOD PACKAGING

It's not only the food you eat that might put you at risk for breast cancer; it's also how that food is packaged. Packaging materials such as styrene cups, trays for microwaving prepared foods, and the lining of canned foods also may contain pseudoestrogens and carcinogens. Alkylphenols, nonylphenol, and bisphenol A—all used in food packaging materials and all known pseudoestrogens—migrate into foods, particularly when stored for long periods or heated at high temperature.

FOOD DYES

The use of carcinogenic food colors, specifically Red Dye No. 3, remains widespread, and may be one reason that breast cancer rates continue to mount. A 1997 report in *Environmental Health Perspective* estimated that the diet of American women is increasingly made up of processed foods that are likely to contain food colorants, such as Red Dye No. 3, which can bind to estrogen receptors on breast cells and thus derange the cells' DNA, turning them into cancer cells. Over the last several decades about 80 percent of our food supply has been processed by the food industry, and the use of food additives in these products continues to increase at a rate of 4 to 5 percent annually.

According to the International Association of Color Manufacturers, Red Dye No. 3 is "widely used and hard to replicate." The food industry uses it to color marachino cherries, bubble gum, and a wide range of snack foods and baked products. Researchers estimated that the average woman receives a daily dose of Red Dye No. 3 about 1,000 to 2,000 times the amount that would be required to derange the cells' DNA. In 1990, the FDA discontinued the use of all "lake" forms of Red Dye No. 3—the form used to make external drugs and cosmetics—because of reports that the chemical caused thyroid cancer in rats, but still allows its use as a food "dye."

MEAT AND SEX HORMONES

At least as dangerous as pesticides and industrial pollutants, growth-stimulating sex hormones used to fatten livestock by about 10 percent before slaughter now contaminate virtually all our beef, with the exception of a small organic market.

Hormones in beef have serious estrogenic and carcinogenic effects—effects of which the cancer establishment, the FDA, and the cattle industry have been well aware for decades. Yet the real dangers they pose—especially when it comes to women and breast cancer—have remained in the shadows until the present. (Pork, veal, lamb, poultry, and other cuts of meat, although uncontaminated by sex hormones, contain pesticides and a wide range of veterinary drugs, as discussed on pages 188–189.)

The history of growth-stimulating sex hormones and the cattle industry is a long one. It begins with the use of a chemical called diethylstilbestrol (DES), a highly potent synthetic estrogenic and carcinogenic chemical. Studies since the 1940s collected in a monograph published by the International Agency for Research on Cancer proved that DES is a highly potent carcinogen and that very low concentrations induce cancers in the breast and other hormone-sensitive organs in mice, rats, hamsters, frogs, and squirrel monkeys. DES was nevertheless widely used during the 1950s in misguided and unsuccessful efforts to prevent miscarriages (chapter 3). Women prescribed DES developed increased rates of breast cancer, their daughters developed increased rates of vaginal cancers, and their sons developed increased rates of reproductive and urinary tract abnormalities.

Despite clear evidence of its carcinogenicity, the FDA approved the use of DES as a cattle growth promoter in 1947. By the 1950s, ranchers began implanting DES in the ears or muscles of cattle as a way of forcing them to gain weight in feedlots. Predictably, use of these hormones resulted in high residues in meat.

By 1971, encouraged by infrequent federal testing for residues in meat, ranchers used DES in 75 percent of cattle nationwide. Misleading assurances of safety and stonewalling by the FDA and the U.S. Department of Agriculture—including deliberate suppression of data on residues in meat—managed to delay a ban on DES until 1979, some forty years after scientists knew that it was clearly carcinogenic. Even after the FDA was forced by Congress to ban DES, its illegal use continued until 1983, when inspectors discovered DES contamination in nearly 1,500 veal calves from five farms in upstate New York. The pharmaceutical and food industries thus exposed the entire meat-eating population of the United States to DES from the 1940s to the 1980s.

Some two decades ago, Roy Hertz, former director of endocrinology at the National Cancer Institute and world authority on hormonal cancer, warned that the cattle industry's indiscriminate and unsupervised use of hormones posed a major danger to health. He dismissed self-interested industry claims that a woman would have to eat more than 500 pounds of beef per day before she increased her daily estrogen production by more than 1 percent. He warned:

> *This business [that women would have to eat] thousands of tons of beef [to be at risk] . . . has no pertinence to the physiological problem before us. . . . We're talking about the addition to an important food item of a substance at a level of concentration which is of the same order of magnitude as that which has profound physiological effects in the human body normally, in the human body affected by breast cancer.*

After the ban—and after a meat-hormone-related 1982 epidemic of premature sexual development and ovarian cysts was reported in 3,000 Puerto Rican infants and children—the U.S. meat industry switched from DES to natural sex hormones such as estradiol, progestins, and testosterone, or to their synthetic variants. Today, the FDA allows their unregulated use by implantation of pellets under the skin of the ear in virtually all cattle raised in feedlots. Hormone use is subject only to the theoretical and nonenforceable requirement that residue levels in meat should be less than 1 percent of the daily hormonal production in children. However, unlike the easily monitored residues of DES, residues of natural hormones can be detected only by highly specialized analytic methods that make routine monitoring an extremely difficult and expensive process.

The 1982 epidemic in Puerto Rico proved to be a harbinger of current trends in the United States. A large-scale national survey, published in the April 1997 issue of *Pediatrics*, revealed that 1 percent of Caucasian and 3 percent of African-American girls show signs of pubic hair and/or breast development by the age of 3. This is a remarkable statistic considering that it is abnormal for girls to show signs of sexual maturation before the age of 8. One cause of premature puberty could well be the high levels of estradiol contamination of meat. It is also possible that much less potent pseudoestrogenic pesticides and other industrial chemicals may also be implicated in this startling finding.

Not surprisingly, a random survey in 1986 found that up to half of all cattle sampled in feedlots in Kansas, Colorado, Texas, Nebraska, and Oklahoma had hormone pellets illegally implanted in muscle tissue rather than under the ear. This practice led to higher absorption of hormones from the implants and very much higher residues that even the FDA admitted could have "adverse effects":

> USDA inspectors have reported finding the pellets in the crown of the head, between the ears, in the neck, at the base of the ear, and in the brisket, or chest area, of cattle carcasses. . . . However, feedlots implanting the pellets elsewhere may be trying to give cattle additional hormone doses.

This is hardly surprising, as hormone treatment increases profits by up to $80 per animal.

In 1989, Syntex Agribusiness, Inc., a leading manufacturer of animal drugs, petitioned the FDA to allow repeated ear implants of cattle with estradiol and progesterone (a drug called Synovex-S) at the midpoint of the preslaughter period rather than using one implant at entry into the feedlots, admitting that most feedlots practiced this method anyway. A year later, the FDA ruled in favor of doubling the dose of hormones allowed in cattle. An industry insider conceded that:

> Cattle today are receiving a lot more [hormones] than ever before. Three or four years ago, they were given only one implant in one ear. But feedlots now are putting one in each ear for more bulk at a faster rate. This is because feedlots are paid by weight for their product. They want the fastest gain in the shortest period of time."

Sex Hormones in Meat and Dairy Products— from the Confidential Files of the FDA

■ An October 1983 FDA report found that Synovex-S, a product containing estradiol and a progestin, increases estradiol concentrations in cattle muscle by twelvefold, in liver by sixfold, in kidneys by ninefold, and in fat by twenty-threefold. When cattle are slaughtered shortly following implantation, levels are even higher. With multiple implants, they are higher still; with intramuscular implants, yet even higher. Another brand, Synovex-H, produces similar results.

■ A November 1991 FDA report found that the implant REVALOR, containing estradiol and a synthetic form of testosterone, caused weight gain in the uterus and ovaries and markedly stimulated division of breast cells in implanted cows. Residues in beef liver averaged as high as 50 parts per billion.

■ Melengestrol acetate, a potent progestin which stimulates estrogen production, is fed to cows in feedlots. It induces breast cancer in mice. At typical levels, for 180 days, concentrations of up to nearly 32 parts per billion were found in fat, 12 parts per billion in muscle, and 14 parts per billion in the liver.

Disturbingly, and contrary to unequivocal public assurances, the United States Department of Agriculture (USDA) does no testing at all for hormone residues. USDA stamps on meat and poultry levels proclaiming the safety of the products refer only to general health and cleanliness, not to the concentrations of carcinogenic hormone residues.

Records of hormone levels in beef, obtained under the federal Freedom of Information Act from the FDA, show that even when ranchers implant single hormone pellets beneath the ear skin under ideal laboratory test conditions, levels of estradiol and other hormones in meat and organs are more than triple the levels found in nonimplanted controls. Much higher levels, up to three-hundredfold, result from the common practice of illegal intramuscular implants.

The extent to which hormonal meat contributes to increased breast cancer rates, apart from cancer of the uterus, prostate, and testis, has been virtually ignored. Hormonal beef may also have other endocrine-disruptive effects, such as hastening menarche. While evidence on the carcinogenic and estrogenic effects of a wide range of pesticides and other industrial pollutants is disturbing, just as disturbing is evidence of the much more potent estrogen residues in meat products.

Responding to strong consumer concerns, the European Commission and European Parliament banned the sale of meat from hormone-treated cattle throughout western Europe in 1989. However, the recent opening of global markets has placed this ban under attack. In February 1997, a panel of World Trade Organization trade experts conducted closed hearings on a challenge mounted by the United States and Canada charging that the European ban is merely protectionist and is costing North America over $100 million a year in lost exports.

The challenge is based on a 1987 report issued by two United Nations bodies, the Food and Agriculture Organization and the World Health Organization, endorsing the FDA's claims for the safety of hormonal meat. However, the joint committee that prepared this report had minimal expertise in public health and cancer prevention. It was made up mainly of veterinary and food scientists, senior FDA and USDA officials, and consultants from the cattle industry. Relying heavily on unpublished and confidential cattle industry information and on scientific citations dating back to the 1970s, the committee claimed that hormone residues in legally implanted cattle are so low that eating treated meat could not possibly induce any hormonal or carcinogenic effects.

On June 30, 1997, the World Trade Organization judges issued their report ruling against the ban on hormone-treated cattle. This decision has been vigorously challenged by Europe and will be appealed. Irrespective of the future legal outcome, the European market has made it clear that it will not allow sale of hormonal meat to its consumers.

MILK AND GROWTH HORMONES

In November 1993, the FDA approved the sale of milk from cows injected with the genetically engineered (recombinant) bovine growth hormone, abbreviated rBGH, in order to increase milk production by about 10 percent. The agency did so despite evidence that the synthetic hormone poses a wide range of veterinary and public health hazards, including the following:

- Increasing fat concentrations in milk.

- Contaminating the milk with rBGH.

- Causing udder infections in cows (mastitis), which results in contamination of milk with pus and bacteria, as well as with antibiotics used for treatment; these antibiotics may be carcinogenic and allergenic and can be responsible for the spread of antibiotic-resistant infections in humans.

- Producing milk contaminated with high concentrations of a potent growth factor Insulinlike Growth Factor I (IGF-I) or hormone which regulates cell division and growth. Levels of IGF-I in milk are further increased following pasteurization. Furthermore, IGF-I resists digestion in the human gut. When it passes into the bloodstream it can produce abnormal or premature growth-promoting effects.

In fact, IGF-I is a major culprit when it comes to the dangers of milk contaminated with rBGH. Recent studies in the prestigious *International Journal of Health Services* conclude that the supercharged levels of IGF-I found in dairy products from treated cows are likely to pose risks of breast cancer by stimulating cell division and promoting malignant transformation of normal breast cells. Additionally, IGF-I helps to maintain the malignancy of breast cancers, increasing their invasiveness and spread, and helps protect cancer cells from self-destructing (a process called apoptosis) in a normal way.

As mentioned, milk containing rBGH can be particularly dangerous to infants and children, who traditionally drink a lot of milk. High levels of IGF-I in the affected milk are absorbed across the highly permeable infant intestines and readily attach to special receptor sites. Such "imprinting" of breast cells by IGF-I is likely to constitute a direct breast cancer risk factor, as well as increase the sensitivity of the breast to subsequent risk factors, including carcinogenic and estrogenic pesticide food contaminants, mammography, and ERT stimulation.

High levels of IGF-I also pose risks of colon cancer by causing the surface lining cells of the gut to grow and divide abnormally, as further noted in a number of recent reports. This risk is confirmed by reports of increased rates of colon cancer suffered by people with acromegaly, a disease associated with a pituitary gland tumor, in which the body produces high levels of IGF-I. Women with acromegaly also suffer increased rates of breast cancer.

Even the conservative American Medical Association expressed concerns over increased IGF-I levels in milk. "Further studies will be required," the AMA's Council on Scientific Affairs sternly warned, "to determine whether the ingestion of higher than normal concentrations of bovine insulin-like growth factor is safe for children, adolescents, and adults."

Unfortunately, the long-standing unresponsiveness of the FDA, the cancer establishment, and the growing biotechnology food industry subverts the process by which the media might alert and protect consumers. When the FDA first approved the use of rBGH in 1993, it issued guidelines about the labeling of milk products that not only are scientifically flawed, but also flagrantly disregard consumers' right to know. One uniquely warped directive forbade dairy producers and distributors who did not use rBGH from advertising their products as being "hormone-free." The FDA claimed, despite overwhelming evidence to the contrary, that such a label would be "false or misleading" as there is "no significant difference between milk from treated and untreated cows." Monsanto, the company that manufactures rBGH, then attempted to sue any company that attempted to use such labeling. Significantly, it was Michael Taylor, a former legal counsel to Monsanto, who became Deputy Commissioner of the FDA just in time to develop and issue those very recommendations.

Today, the marketing and sale of dairy products contaminated with hormones continue, even as Europe and Canada have effectively banned their use. Americans are thus being subjected to what amounts to an experiment involving the large-scale adulteration of a dietary staple by a poorly characterized and unlabeled product of biotechnology. This experiment poses major public health risks to all of us.

PERSONAL PROTECTION

Protecting yourself against breast cancer risks posed by the food you eat involves eating a healthful, well-balanced diet that helps you maintain a normal weight, reduces or eliminates carcinogenic and estrogenic foods, and increases the amount of protective nutrients you eat. You should be able to meet each of these goals by eating a largely vegetarian, organic diet. By doing so, you will not only reduce your risk of breast cancer, but will also enjoy a host of additional health benefits.

WHAT YOU CAN DO
- Maintain a healthy weight.
- Eliminate contaminated food.
- Incorporate healthful diets.
- Incorporate food that contains protective nutrients.

Maintain a Healthy Weight

As discussed at the beginning of the chapter, weight gain at any age—from childhood through menopause and beyond—increases your risk of postmenopausal breast cancer and other health problems, including heart disease and diabetes.

The good news is that if you lose excess pounds—also at any age, including after menopause—you can reduce your risk of breast cancer as well as other weight-related problems. However, losing weight, and then maintaining a healthy weight, requires a lifelong commitment to eating well and exercising often. Some tips to get you started follow:

- **Minimize fat intake:** Cut way back on the amount of fat you eat to under 20 percent of your daily caloric intake. (Some physicians, including Dr. Dean Ornish, recommend even more drastic cuts, to under 10 percent.) Stay away from animal fat in meat and dairy as much as possible, particularly since this fat also contains high levels of pesticides, pollutants, and hormones.

- **Emphasize grains, legumes, and fresh fruits and vegetables:** In addition to being low in fat, these foods provide nutrients that protect against breast cancer and other diseases. (We discuss those nutrients later in this chapter.)

- **Eat frequent small meals:** Studies prove that your body digests and metabolizes food better if you eat small quantities and more often.

- **Limit alcohol:** Drinking alcohol hampers your ability to lose weight because it causes the body to store, rather than burn, fat. It also causes estrogen levels to rise sharply, as we describe in chapter 9.

- **Beware of fat substitutes:** It seemed too good to be true, and alas, it was. Fat substitutes like Olestra may decrease the amount of fat your body digests, but they also rob you of

Safe Eating Checklist

Be sure to:

- Reduce animal fats such as red meat, dairy, lamb, chicken, butter, and margarine.

- Emphasize "good" fats, particularly olive oil which can be used on bread to replace butter and margarine.

- Eat more turkey and safe seafood.

- Purchase organically grown produce, meats, and dairy.

- Eat more soy-based foods such as tofu, soy nut cereals, soy cheese, and soy milks.

- Eat more crucifers such as broccoli and cauliflower.

- Avoid packaged foods such as meats wrapped in styrene and plastic; pick foods packaged in freezer wrap instead.

protective fat-soluble nutrients such as beta-carotene and other carotenoids. Side effects like diarrhea and bloating are also common.

- **Avoid over-the-counter or prescription diet pills:** Even worse for your health are diet pills containing amphetamines that attempt to decrease your appetite. Not only are amphetamine-based diet pills addictive, they often cause serious side effects, including restlessness, rapid heartbeat, confusion, and even violence and mania.

   In 1996, the FDA approved a new type of prescription diet drug called Redux, manufactured by Interneuron Pharmaceuticals. It works somewhat like Prozac, increasing levels of serotonin, a brain chemical that both influences mood and tells the brain when appetite has been satisfied. Short-term studies show that Redux helps motivated people lose a little more weight a little more quickly than they would have otherwise. Unfortunately, no long-term studies are complete, and its safety remains in question. Indeed, a health and safety panel of the FDA initially found Redux "not very effective" and "unsafe." It later approved its use by a margin of just one vote.

In addition to Redux, other appetite suppressants include fenfluramine, for which seven million prescriptions were written in 1996, and phentermine, with eleven million prescriptions in the same year. According to *The New York Times*, sales of all antiobesity drugs nearly tripled from $179 million to $526 million from 1995 to 1996. Although they have no link to breast cancer, these popular diet drugs appear to be quite dangerous in other ways. Primary pulmonary hypertension, an often lethal condition, has been reported as a rare complication of fenfluramine. An even rarer mitral valve heart disease has been reported more recently among twenty-four women taking unapproved combinations of fenfluramine and phentermine (fen-phen) for more than a year, prompting an urgent nationwide FDA warning to doctors and medical specialty organizations. This type of heart disease has been linked to very high levels of serotonin. Other prescription drugs, particularly the fat-control hormone leptin now under development, may be the only effective methods for treating the rare genetic forms of obesity.

■ **Exercise:** Exercise is critical to weight loss and, in fact, may be even more important than diet. Not only does exercise burn calories, but it also leads to a general sense of well-being and a vastly improved metabolism. In addition, individuals who exercise often find that they almost unconsciously include less fat and sugar and more fresh fruit and vegetables in their diets. Exercise is discussed further in chapter 10.

■ **Limit television viewing:** One of the reasons that so few Americans exercise—and are thus obese—is that we spend far too much time watching television.

- **Maintain a balanced, moderate approach to eating and living:** It is a shocking fact of life that millions of women of all ages suffer from eating disorders such as anorexia, bulimia, or binge eating—all of which may result in serious health problems. The reasons for this rising trend are complex, involving societal expectations, political pressures, and concerns about body image, self-esteem, and power. Needless to say, if you are not overweight, losing weight will not reduce your risks of breast cancer, but will put you at risk for other health problems.

ELIMINATE CONTAMINATED FOOD

It is difficult, but not impossible, to eliminate, or at least significantly reduce, the amount of harmful foods and contaminants in your diet. The first step is to reduce your consumption of fatty animal foods, particularly beef and dairy, which contain high levels of industrial carcinogens, pseudoestrogens, and estrogens. In other words, you should consider hamburgers, butter, and ice cream as occasional treats and not dietary staples.

In the Resources section at the end of this book, you will find a list of markets and mail order companies that sell organic foods.

- **Eat safer meat, and less of it:** If you decide to include meat as part of your diet, try turkey, rabbit, quail, pheasant, and venison—all of which contain far fewer carcinogenic and estrogenic industrial chemical, pesticide, hormone, antibiotic, and other drug residues than commercial beef. The best choices are certified organic beef and poultry, which are free of all hormones and pesticides. Make sure you trim all fat and skin from your poultry and meat before cooking. Fortunately all of these options are becoming more available in ordinary as well as upscale supermarkets.

- **Consume low-fat or nonfat (skim) organic dairy products or dairy substitutes:** Eating low-fat or, better still, nonfat organic dairy products reduces your exposure to pesticides, hormones, and other drugs, as well as infectious materials from diseased udders of the hormonally treated animals. In the Resource section, you will find a list of hormone- and pesticide-free dairy products available from nationwide distributors. You'll also reduce your exposure by consuming low- or nonfat dairy products and salad dressings. Other alternatives include milk, cheese, and other products made from organic soy, rice, almond, and other nondairy substances.

- **Choose safer seafood:** Seafood represents a major source of low-fat protein but may be as dangerous to your health as meat because of the high levels of chemical carcinogens and pseudoestrogens some species contain. Your best choices are deep-sea species like Arctic char, halibut, orange roughy, red snapper, sea bass, and tuna. Wild shrimp and lobsters from Australia, California, Mexico, and New Zealand are also safe.

  On the other hand, you should avoid several varieties of fish caught in United States waters, including bluefish, striped bass, swordfish, New England lobster, and farm-raised catfish. European fish may also be dangerous, especially if caught in European inland seas or rivers that flow upstream through industrialized areas.

- **Opt for organic fruits and vegetables whenever possible:** Unlike conventional crops, which growers may spray with fifteen or more separate applications of pesticides before sending them to supermarkets, organic produce is pesticide-free. In addition, organic produce does not contain mineral waxes, preservatives, or fungicides—which means that immediate refrigeration and careful handling are necessary to avoid spoilage and bruising.

- **Research your drinking water:** To make sure you are not exposing your body to contamination by drinking or cooking with water from your tap, request a water quality report from your municipality or local supplier. If you prefer bottled water, request a laboratory report from the bottler or contact the National Sanitation Foundation or the Quality Bottle Water Association (Appendix A: Resources).

If you find that your water is indeed contaminated, you might want to considering purchasing a treatment unit (preferably one that uses a technique called reverse osmosis) at a cost of $300 or less. You'll be able to mount it under your sink and attach it to the plumbing. Convenient personal water filters for work or travel are also available.

- **Avoid food packaging:** Whenever possible, avoid buying canned foods or foods wrapped in plastic. If you cannot do this, make sure you remove the food from the packaging as soon as possible. Use glass cookware for oven or microwave.

Safer Nonorganic Produce

If you can't find organic produce, opt for these safer choices:

- **Fruits:** Avocados, bananas, dates, figs, guava, lemons, tangerines, tangelos, and watermelon.
- **Vegetables:** Artichokes, bean curd, corn, eggplant, escarole, garbanzo beans, green beans, kidney beans, kohlrabi, lima beans, mushrooms, navy beans, okra, peas (dried), pinto beans, red beans, rhubarb, scallions (green onions), Swiss chard, turnips, watercress, and yams.

INCORPORATE HEALTHFUL DIETS

In the end, your goal is to eat a diet that both reduces your exposure to contaminants and increases your body's ability to protect itself against breast cancer and other diseases. Three types of diets—vegetarian, Mediterranean, or Asian—can help you to do just that.

Vegetarian

Low amounts of chemical contamination, less fat, and an abundance of vitamins and minerals make vegetarian diets protective against breast cancer. In 1990, researchers pooled a dozen well-controlled studies together and found a "consistent protective effect . . . for fruit and vegetable intake." Scientists confirmed these findings in 1996 when they released a study that showed a 50 percent decline in premenopausal breast cancer among women who ate a vegetarian diet. More support comes from a recent study that shows that vegetarian premenopausal women have lower serum estrogen levels than nonvegetarians—and more of the estrogen they had was "good estrogen," that is, less carcinogenic.

Mediterranean

The Mediterranean diet emphasizes whole grains, fruits, vegetables, seafood, and olive oil while minimizing meat, dairy, and saturated fats such as butter and margarine. In fact, the Mediterranean diet shows that it is not necessarily how much fat, but rather the type of fat you eat that influences breast cancer risk. Greek women, for instance, take in about 40 percent of their daily calories in the form of fat from olive oil and yet have much lower breast cancer rates than American women, who eat the same percentage of fat but mostly in the form of animal fat. Southern Italian and Spanish women appear to enjoy the same protection, and for the same reason. However, the northern European diet is much higher in contaminated animal fat, such as butter and margarine, and breast cancer rates there are correspondingly higher.

Asian

The traditional Asian diet is low in fat and largely vegetarian. It contains high levels of phytoestrogens, which appear to be highly protective against breast cancer, as evidenced by the low levels of breast cancer in Japan, China, and other Asian countries. Studies show that other traditionally Asian foods, including maitake and shiitake mushrooms and green tea, also offer protection against breast cancer.

INCORPORATE FOODS WITH PROTECTIVE NUTRIENTS

Common to the three diets just discussed—the specifics of which you can find in more detail in other books about healthy eating—and to an even more typical American diet, are certain specific nutrients that offer particular health benefits. Whenever possible, add foods that contain these nutrients to your daily diet.

Phytoestrogens

As discussed in chapter 2, phytoestrogens are substances found in plants that, once ingested, provide the raw materials intestinal bacteria uses to form estrogen. Phytoestrogen promotes the formation of good estrogen while displacing "bad" estrogen from breast cell receptors (Table 9.2).

One of the richest source of phytoestrogens is soy, which contains a particular type of phytoestrogen called isoflavones. A 1992 study showed that Japanese women who ate a low-fat diet rich in soy foods had urine concentrations of phytoestrogens up to one-thousandfold higher than American and Finnish women. However, finding the elusive estrogenic isoflavones in soy is not as simple as it might sound. Not everything with soy in its name happens to be a particularly rich source. For example, do not look for isoflavones in soy sauce, soybean oil, and foods with many other ingredients besides soy, such as soy cheese, soy hot dogs, soy bacon, and tofu yogurt. Some foods made with soy-protein concentrate, such as veggie burgers, may be devoid of significant isoflavones, too. The method of processing is the significant factor. As we write this, the soy craze has so taken hold in Americans that many companies producing soy-based foods are now having their products analyzed to see how much isoflavones they provide.

Recent evidence shows that genistein, an isoflavonoid phytoestrogen found in abundance in soy foods, competes against estradiol by binding more tightly to beta estrogen receptors. It therefore not only is effective in preventing menopausal problems, but also may play an important role in preventing breast cancer (Table 9.3).

TABLE 9.2: BREAST-PROTECTIVE PHYTOCHEMICALS

Phytochemical	How It Works	Sources
Algin	Binds metals; is probably associated with unique polysaccharides, types of complex sugar chains in the blood that stimulate immunity	Brown kelp (also known as kombu or laminaria), used as a food seasoning and wrap (e.g., sushi) in soups and salads.
Bioflavonoids	Powerful antioxidants which inhibit chemical carcinogens; often found with Vitamin C, which is an important antioxidant, too.	Fresh fruits, vegetables, and other greens, especially deeply colored produce (e.g., orange squash, blueberries)
Carotenoids (betacarotene, luetein, zeaxantyhin)	Anticancer effects	Apricots (including dried), carrots, collard greens, kale, spinach, sweet potatoes, tomatoes, pumpkin, watermelon
Fiber	Transports estrogen and chemical toxins out of the gut and prevents their uptake by the body.	All organic whole grains, fruits, vegetables

Phytochemical	How It Works	Sources
Flavonoids	Inhibit chemical carcinogens, includes some with estrogenic activity (such as isoflavones which are a subset of the flavonoid family)	Deeply colored fruits, especially blueberries, huckleberries, oranges, lemons, strawberries, green and red peppers, broccoli
Indole 3-carbinol	Stimulate body to produce good estrogen; reduces levels of bad estrogen	Crucifers such as broccoli, cabbage, cauliflower
Phytoestrogens	Stimulate body to produce higher levels of "good" estrogen; displaces more toxic forms of estrogen	Soy foods (see Table 9.3)
Selenium	Inhibits chemical carcinogens including viruses	Brewer's yest, garlic, organic whole grains, safe seafood (tuna, shellfish); supplements combining selenium with garlic work synergistically
Sulfur-rich amino acids	Inhibit chemical carcinogens	Garlic
Sulforaphane	Inhibits chemical carcinogens	Bok choy, broccoli, cauliflower

(continued)

Phytochemical	How It Works	Sources
Vitamin C	Inhibits chemical carcinogens, enhances immune function.	Broccoli, cauliflower, citrus, peppers
Tocopherols	Prevent free-radical damage to inhibit cholesterol buildup in arteries. Stabilize and protect cell membranes	Vegetable oils, almonds, soybeans, sunflower seeds, wheat germ and wheat germ oil

Buy organic soy foods whenever possible, especially if they contain vegetable proteins (sometimes called tempeh). Otherwise, they may have lower levels of phytoestrogens. Even then, however, they offer a healthy choice. Always cook soybeans before you eat them as they contain toxic chemicals that are destroyed by high heat. To garner as much protective value as do Asian women, aim to consume the equivalent of about 8 to 10 ounces of soy foods daily.

Flavonoids

Often coexisting with vitamin C in fruits and vegetables, flavonoids are a class of phytoestrogens that also act as antioxidants and help the body to optimize its use of vitamin C, and thus may protect women against breast cancer. In 1990, a study reported lower breast cancer mortality among women with the highest intake of vitamin C, while others have suggested a role for a diet rich in vitamin C and flavonoids. This led one expert to remark that the "risk . . . in the population of postmenopausal women in North America would be reduced by 16 percent" if they consumed at least 400 milligrams of vitamin C per day. Vitamin C and flavonoid-rich foods include broccoli, green and red peppers, guavas, oranges, tangerines, tangelos, strawberries, grapefruit, and other citrus fruits.

Fiber

Fiber is a type of carbohydrate present in whole grains, fruits, and vegetables. Also called roughage, fiber is not broken down by human digestive enzymes and therefore is not absorbed into the bloodstream. Although it provides no nutrients, fiber aids in digestion and helps keep the digestive tract clean and clear. Fiber also reduces estrogen levels in three ways: It binds with estrogen in the gut, preventing its absorption into the bloodstream; it increases levels of estrogen-binding proteins, thereby processing more estrogen for elimination; and it reduces the availability of cholesterol, from which the body synthesizes estrogen. In one study, 16 of 17 women eating a high-fiber diet had overall estrogen levels 30 percent lower than average, as well as higher levels of good estrogen.

TABLE 9.3: COMPARATIVE ISOFLAVONE AMOUNTS IN SOY-BASED FOODS

Food	Serving Size	Isoflavones (milligrams)	Calories	Fat (grams)
Nutlettes breakfast cereal	½ cup	122	140	1.5
Beef(Not) textured soy protein granules	¼ cup dry	62	70	1
Roasted soy nuts	¼ cup	60	195	9.5
Tempeh	½ cup	35	165	6
Low-fat tofu	½ cup	35	45–75	1.5–2.5
Regular tofu	½ cup	35	105–120	5.5–6.5
Take Care High Protein Beverage Powder	2 scoops	35	100–130	1–1.5
Regular soy milk	1 cup	30	130–150	4
Low-fat soy milk	1 cup	20	90–120	2
Roasted soy butter	2 tablespoons	17	170	11

Thanks to the ready availability of low-fiber processed foods, the average American woman today consumes less than half the fiber-rich flours and cereals that her forebears ate in 1910. To optimize your diet, you should consume from 20 to 45 grams of fiber every day. Foods rich in fiber include whole grains such as brown rice, whole wheat bread, and oatmeal; fruits such as apricots, pears, and figs; vegetables such as green peas, broccoli, and carrots; and legumes such as kidney beans, lima beans, and lentils.

Olive Oil

Olive oil is a rich source of monosaturated fat that has little or no stimulatory effect on cancer rates. It also appears to have a positive effect on cholesterol levels, raising the "good cholesterol" levels and lowering the "bad." Thus, by using olive oil instead of butter—on your bread and pasta, as well as in your cooking—you'll be reducing your risk for heart disease as well as breast cancer.

Use extra-virgin olive oil, which contains oil pressed without the use of solvents. Buy oil that comes in glass, not plastic or metal, to avoid migration of carcinogenic or estrogenic contaminants. The protective effects of olive oil may be lost if it is cooked at high heat (as in deep frying), so use uncooked oil whenever possible.

Seaweed

Several types of seaweed appear to be highly protective against breast cancer, and help to explain the relatively low rates of breast cancer in countries that consume it in quantity. Brown kelp, for instance, is rich in algin, a substance that binds heavy metals and toxins and thus prevents them from affecting cells. As researcher Jane Teas emphasizes in her book *Nutrition and Cancer*: "Based on epidemiological and biological data, *laminaria* (a brown kelp seaweed) is proposed as an important factor contributing to the relatively low breast cancer rates in Japan."

Although brown kelp is the most protective form of seaweed, nori and wakame also offer benefits. Asian cooking uses seaweed in several different ways—as a garnish, as a flour to make noodles, to flavor soups and vegetables, to make jellies and sauces, as a wrap for raw fish (sushi), even as candy. Some people even enjoy steeping sea-weed in hot water to make tea. You can buy seaweed in Asian markets and in speciality sections of grocery stores, and you can learn more about Asian cooking at your local bookstore or library.

Garlic

In recent years, the media has helped spread the word about the myriad health benefits of garlic. Loaded with sulfur-rich amino acids, garlic has been proven to reduce breast tumors in rodents. If you add selenium to the recipe, or buy selenium-enriched garlic, you may further enhance its cancer-protecting effects. A popular readily available non-odorous source is Kyolic Aged Garlic Extract (KAGE).

Crucifers

Crucifers are vegetables that contain two known cancer-fighting chemicals, indole-3-carbinol and sulforaphanes. These substances increase levels of safe estrogen while protecting cells against carcinogens. In one 1997 study, published in the *Journal of the National Cancer Institute,* women who took 500 milligrams of indole-3-carbinol showed a dramatic increase in good estrogen in just a week.

The study also provides suggestive evidence that indole-3-carbinol stimulates production of enzyme products of the normal CYP1 gene, which increases levels of the good estrogen and decreases levels of the bad.

Broccoli, cabbage, cauliflower, brussels sprouts, mustard greens, turnips, watercress, and bok choy are all cancer fighters that help to speed estrogen metabolism. Try to eat crucifers raw, or cook them only slightly, as heat destroys the crucial indole-3-carbinol.

Carotenoids

Carotenoids, the chemicals that lend a rich orange or yellow color to certain vegetables and fruits, appear to offer protection against breast and other cancers. There is some controversy about their effects, however, since two studies—one sponsored by the National Cancer Institute and the other by the Physician's Health Study—

failed to link either eating high amounts of carotenoids or taking beta-carotene (the best-known carotenoid) pills with reduced cancer levels.

Some scientists believe, however, that eating whole food containing several different types of carotenoids will indeed decrease risk. A recent study lent merit to this hypothesis when it found a 50 percent reduction in risk among women who consumed vegetables rich in the carotenoids lutein and zeaxanthin, as well as beta-carotene and others.

Foods rich in carotenoids include carrots, pumpkins, squash, sweet potatoes, broccoli, peas, collard greens, apricots, cherries, and papaya. The darker in color the food, the richer in total carotenoids it is.

Tocopherols

Tocopherols, of which vitamin E is the best known and most common, may help protect breast cell membranes from damage by unstable molecules called "free radicals," caused by a diet high in polyunsaturated fatty acids, and thus reduce the risk of breast cancer.

A recent publication in the Japanese *Journal of Cancer Research* reported a fascinating link between vitamin E and increased breast cancer risk. Researchers found that the body produces an enzyme called catalase that break down hydrogen peroxide, a substance that stimulates the body's production of destructive hydroxyl free radicals. Unfortunately, millions of people do not produce enough catalase due to genetic malfunctions or poor diet. Indeed, three million Japanese are deficient in catalase. The researchers then selected low-catalase mice and found they also had a very high rate of breast cancer. Next, they fed low-catalase mice additional vitamin E and found that breast cancer incidence was remarkably reduced. The researchers commented that vitamin E "intrinsically has a protective effect against the development of mammary tumors, and this may also apply to humans."

Very recent and preliminary animal studies published in the *Journal of the National Cancer Institute* further confirm the protective effects of vitamin E. Administration of high doses of vitamin E in rats injected with the potent breast carcinogen nitrosomethylurea was found to be very effective in protecting them against breast cancer. Although more studies will be needed to confirm its protective effect, you can start taking vitamin E now.

We do know for sure that vitamin E does help to prevent heart disease, and scientists suggest that you increase your intake by consuming more grains, nuts, soybeans, and vegetable oils, and/or by taking a supplement. The natural form of vitamin E is most potent, so look for the letter "d" on any bottle of vitamin E pills you take. The letters "dl," on the other hand, mean that the vitamin is synthetically derived.

Selenium

Selenium, which closely resembles sulfur in its physical properties, is an essential mineral found in minute amounts in the body. It is a natural antioxidant that protects against free radicals. It works closely with vitamin E in actions like the production of antibodies, the binding of toxic elements like mercury, and the promotion of normal body growth and fertility. A 1976 study showed that selenium produced a "protective effect with increasing plasma selenium levels" among postmenopausal women using supplementary selenium.

Good food sources of selenium include grains, brewer's yeast, organ meats, fish and shellfish, grains, cereals, broccoli, cabbage, garlic, onions, and radishes, among others. If you choose to increase your selenium intake by eating more grains, make sure the grains are organic: Doctor's Data, a trace mineral research laboratory, found that nonorganic grains are often selenium-deficient.

10

Lifestyle Risk Factors and Coping Strategies

The choices you make in your daily life about smoking cigarettes, drinking alcohol, exercising, and using cosmetics are likely to affect your risks for breast cancer. Do you smoke? How much alcohol do you drink? Do you dye your hair with products that contain carcinogenic chemicals? Do you exercise on a regular basis? How do you handle stress? Do you suffer from depression and anxiety when faced with challenges, or are you more of an optimistic fighter? Your answers to these questions will help you determine your risk for breast cancer, and we'll show you safe ways to reduce those risks by making better choices.

Choices: the message we've tried hardest to impart in this book is that you have the power to make choices that will directly affect your risks for breast cancer. In this chapter, you will see that the choices you make about personal habits also have a very definite impact on your risks.

TOBACCO AND BREAST CANCER

Smoking is the single largest preventable cause of premature death and disability in this country. Experts at the Mayo Clinic estimate that one in six deaths in the United States each year is associated with cigarette smoking, and the American Lung Association states that smoking kills more Americans than cocaine, heroin, alcohol abuse, auto accidents, homicide, and suicide combined. In 1994, the Surgeon General of the United States, Dr. C. Everett Koop, identified cigarette smoking as the single most preventable cause of heart disease and related it to 30 percent of the 1.5 million heart-disease-related deaths that occur each year. The connection between smoking and lung cancer is also startling: The risk of getting lung cancer is approximately ten times greater overall for cigarette smokers as it is for nonsmokers.

The risk that cigarette smoking carries for breast cancer is less well known. Tobacco smoke contains a multitude of carcinogens in the form of small particles and gasses that the particles carry deep down into the lungs. Some of these carcinogens, such as benzpyrene, dibenzanthracene, urethane, vinyl chloride, and DDT, induce cancer of the breast and other organs in rodents. In addition, cigarette smoke represents the greatest source of breast-cancer-causing radiation in consumer products. It brings toxic levels of radioactive lead and polonium into the lungs of smokers as well as secondhand smoke recipients.

A series of studies reviewed by the International Agency for Research on Cancer in 1983 failed to detect any consistent relationship between breast cancer and smoking. Although these studies were designed primarily to investigate the relationship between breast cancer and oral contraceptives, they only incidentally addressed the relationship of breast cancer to smoking and other risk factors. More recently, a series of well-controlled studies, specifically designed to investigate the effects of smoking, revealed a very different picture. Eleven studies, published in the *American Journal of Epidemiology*, the *British Journal of Cancer*, and the *Journal of the National Cancer Institute*, among others, all show varying but significant associations between breast cancer and smoking at any age.

What is most disturbing is that the risks of breast cancer are highest among those who start smoking heavily in adolescence. Three studies published in 1991 by the *American Journal of Epidemiology* concentrated on the risks associated with starting to smoke before the age of 16. One study found that very young smokers raised their lifetime risk by about 30 percent, while other studies showed a remarkable 80 percent increase, particularly among those young people who smoked heavily.

Unfortunately, this highly vulnerable age group appears to be the very one ignoring the massive media and medical blitz about the dangers of smoking. A 1995 survey conducted at the University of Michigan and publicized by *USA Today* reported that teenage smoking is on the rise again. Thirty percent more 13- and 14-year-olds were smoking in 1995 than in 1991.

And the dangers posed by tobacco smoke aren't just limited to those who choose to smoke. We know that since secondhand smoke does not get filtered, it contains up to 150 times higher levels of carcinogens than smoke directly inhaled by cigarette smokers. Even though the surrounding air dilutes the concentration of these carcinogens, there can be no doubt that secondhand smoke poses great risks, especially to infants and young children. Nevertheless, scientists have conducted only one small-scale study to investigate secondhand smoke and breast cancer risk, published in 1994 by the *British Cancer Journal*, and the results were inconclusive.

Another important side effect—or at least a common companion of cigarette smoking—is alcohol abuse, which is itself a risk factor for breast cancer. According to a 1996 article published in the *Journal of the American Medical Association*, "The prevalence of smoking among substance abusers is two to three times that of the general population and alcoholics may constitute a quarter of all smokers." Without question, smoking and drinking often go together, especially among young people who mistakenly believe they are invulnerable to death and disease. The combination of drinking and smoking at a young age is especially devastating, and leads to a dramatic increase in risks for breast cancer.

ALCOHOL AND BREAST CANCER

Drinking in moderation plays an important and pleasurable social and personal role for millions of Americans, and in many cultures, a glass or two of wine at dinner is a tradition. The good news is that as long as we drink in moderation, alcohol provides many health benefits. (The one exception to this rule is women taking estrogen replacement therapy (ERT), who may increase their risks for breast cancer with even just one drink.)

Fortunately, most women do drink in moderation, that is, they drink less than two drinks a day (a single drink being a 5-ounce glass of wine, a 12-ounce beer, or a 1-ounce shot of distilled spirits). Fewer than 3 percent of adult women have two or more drinks daily. On the other hand, however, heavy drinking, particularly weekend binge-drinking, is more common, especially among teens and carries with it disturbing risks.

Perhaps the best-understood benefit of alcohol is its effect on the cardiovascular system. More than 17 studies performed over the last decade show that alcohol increases the level of high-density lipoproteins (HDLs—the "good" cholesterol), thus helping to prevent the buildup of fatty plaques that cause heart disease. Alcohol also protects the cardiovascular system by reducing the tendency of blood platelets to clump and clot. The Harvard Nurses' Health Study found that women who imbibed three to nine drinks every week were about half as likely to develop heart disease as nondrinkers.

One way that light alcohol consumption protects the heart is by elevating estrogen levels, which provides special benefit to postmenopausal women. As a 1992 article in *Clinical and Experimental Research* stated, "Moderate alcohol use is an important factor for postmenopausal estrogen status and may offer a partial explanation for the reported protective effect of moderate alcohol consumption with respect to postmenopausal cardiovascular risk." Unfortunately, this same boost of estrogen, when compounded with ERT, may pose unacceptable risks for breast cancer: Levels of circulating estrogen in women taking ERT nearly double after drinking just half a glass of wine.

In addition, alcohol consumption also carries other serious risks. Alcohol abuse and the disease of alcoholism ravage the lives of millions of Americans, leading to car accidents, falls, fires, lost jobs, failed relationships, depression, brain damage, birth defects, cirrhosis of the liver, heart disease, and osteoporosis, among many other tragic consequences. Since at least 1910, physicians have reported the link between chronic alcoholism and cancer, including cancers of the esophagus, mouth, pharynx, and liver.

In more than fifty studies, extending over three decades, and involving more than 11,000 women, researchers have explored the relationship between alcohol and breast cancer. The results make it clear that alcohol consumption raises a woman's risk for both pre- and postmenopausal breast cancer. A 1994 report in *Cancer Causes and Control,* based on a pool of prior studies, found that one drink daily posed an 11 percent increase in risk for women of all ages. That means a 50-year-old woman who otherwise has a one in fifty chance of developing breast cancer now has a one in forty-five chance.

Two recent, large-scale studies confirm these findings. The 1995 Nurses' Health study found that consuming one to two drinks daily increases a woman's risk by 37 percent, while another 1995 study showed that one drink a day increases risk by 40 percent, two drinks by 70 percent, and three drinks by more than 200 percent. For the average 50-year-old woman, one drink a day raises her risk from only one in fifty to one in thirty, and three drinks a day quadruples her risk to as high as one in twelve and one-half.

Two groups of women are at even higher risk: Those who drink heavily during adolescence and early adulthood, and post-menopausal women who take ERT. A 1988 study in *Cancer Research,* for instance, showed that women who did most of their drinking before 30 had nearly twice the risk of those who started drinking later in life. A 1989 *International Journal of Epidemiology* study concluded that women who started drinking before the age of 25 experienced an 80 percent increase in risk compared to those who started later in life. In general, studies showing the strongest associations have come from Western European countries that have a higher per capita alcohol intake beginning at an early age.

Unfortunately, heavy drinking appears almost epidemic among young women today in the United States. According to a 1995 *New York Times* article, 80 percent of sorority women are now binge drinkers, consuming five or more drinks at one sitting. A recent review in the journal *Cancer Epidemiology, Biomarkers and Prevention*, concludes:

> *Several studies have explored the effect of early drinking. . . . All have found a significant impact of consumption at a younger age. . . . These findings need to be corroborated, but the consistent implication that drinking at a young age adversely affects the risk of breast cancer warrants serious attention by those interested in prevention. If onset of drinking could be delayed, risk of breast cancer could potentially be markedly reduced.*

Although women who start drinking at an early age have the highest risk of breast cancer, heavy drinking at any age, especially in women who smoke or take ERT, is risky. Both of these activities are themselves risk factors for breast cancer, and may combine with alcohol to cause cancer. As discussed, women on ERT who drink also face special risks: A 1996 study in the *Journal of the American Medical Association* found that levels of estrogen circulating in the blood of women taking ERT surges to more than 300 percent after three glasses of wine.

You may be asking: How does alcohol, which has a such a healthy cardiovascular effect and represents a pleasant cultural and personal tradition, change a healthy breast cell into a cancer cell?

INCREASES OVERALL ESTROGEN LEVELS

Because male alcoholics frequently suffer from gynecomastia (enlarged breasts), experts have long suspected that drinking increases the level of estrogen in the body. In addition, studies show that alcohol causes the liver to metabolize more estrogen from the "good" to the "bad" type. This risk is even greater in women who take ERT, in whom alcohol dramatically raises estrogen levels.

INHIBITS MELATONIN RELEASE

Animal studies and studies of alcoholics show that alcohol inhibits release of the hormone melatonin. Secreted at night by the pineal gland, an endocrine organ at the base of the brain, melatonin protects against breast cancer by decreasing estrogen levels and reducing estrogen receptors located on breast cells. A recent report in *Science News* revealed that the normal amount of melatonin secreted at night is enough to inhibit growth of breast cancer cells. That means that any reduction of the hormone caused by drinking would increase a woman's risk of developing breast cancer.

CONTAINS CARCINOGENIC CONTAMINANTS

Alcoholic beverages contain a fair share of carcinogenic contaminants and ingredients that may well increase breast cancer risk. Here are the most common:

- **Urethane:** Urethane is a contaminant found in high levels in bourbon, whiskey, cream sherry, port wine, Chinese wine, Japanese rice wine (sake), European fruit brandies, and liqueurs; highest levels are found in commercial ales. Urethane has long been known to induce breast cancer in rodents. In one study, cited in *Tainted Booze* by the Center for Science in the Public Interest, urethane caused breast tumors in 100 percent of dosed animals. Urethane also exacerbates the carcinogenic effects of X rays. It is also likely that the carcinogenicity of alcoholic beverages may be due to their combined effects with urethane.

  Urethane is formed by the reaction between certain chemicals (diethylpyrocarbonate and ammonia) in alcohol, particularly alcohol fermented with urea additives. As shown by the Canadian liquor industry, manufacturers can reduce urethane levels sharply by eliminating the use of these additives. In fact, the Canadian liquor industry now systematically tests products for excessive urethane levels and, if found, immediately recalls the products.

The United States liquor industry, on the other hand, trivializes the public health significance of urethane and refuses to reduce exposure levels. In this, it has tacit Food and Drug Administration (FDA) approval.

- **Zearalenone:** Zearalenone, a carcinogenic and estrogenic fungal toxin, is found in homemade beers and beers made from wheat and other grains contaminated with the fungus. Unfortunately, no information exists about current zearalenone levels in United States and European beers.

- **Pesticides:** A wide range of carcinogenic pesticides contaminate American and European wines, including dichlorvos (DDVP), a metabolite of another pesticide called trichlorfon. As highlighted in a review by the International Agency for Research on Cancer, DDVP induces breast cancer in rodents.

DEPRESSES THE IMMUNE SYSTEM

Prolonged binge-drinking has devastating effects on the immune system, which can lead to the development and spread of early breast and other cancers. In rodents given high levels of alcohol, the alcohol inactivates key immune defense cells called natural killer (NK) cells, which search out and destroy circulating virus and tumor cells. According to a 1996 article cited by United Press International, "A single incident of binge drinking may be all it takes to trigger tumor cells to spread throughout the body. Ordinary social drinking will not create the effect. . . . I'd say that if someone had circulating tumor cells, it would be extremely dangerous to drink." The authors concluded that their findings help explain why heavy drinkers have double or higher rates of breast (as well as liver and digestive system) cancer.

AFFECTS ENZYMES

Alcohol stimulates production of enzymes (cytochromes P450) that can raise levels of "bad" estrogen as well as promoting other carcinogens.

HAIR DYES: AN AVOIDABLE RISK

Almost since the beginning of time, and in every culture, women (and men!) have practiced sometimes strange, sometimes dangerous beauty regimens. Asian women bound their feet, causing permanent bone deformities; European and American women wore corsets so tight they could barely breathe (the cause of the "vapors" so common during the Victorian era); and modern women continue to strain their backs, legs, and ankles by wearing high heels. Breast implants, discussed in chapter 6, are the modern equivalent, enhancing as they do a woman's appearance (according to current cultural bias) at the expense of her health. Other modern cosmetic risks are the chemicals used in some hair dyes.

In ancient Egypt, women dyed their hair with henna, a natural substance derived from plants. Ancient Romans dipped their combs in vinegar and walnut stains. In Elizabethan England, women dyed their hair with potash alum and a rhubarb concoction. By the French Revolution, merchants sold some 24 million pounds of starch every year to women to use as a hair color binder. Starting in the nineteenth century, chemists made permanent dyes from coal tar, a distant relative of today's dyes synthesized from petroleum-derived chemicals. Currently, more than 50 million American women—nearly 40 percent of the United States female population aged 18 to 60—dye their hair monthly or bimonthly, and often for decades. Annual United States sales now reach over $1 billion, almost 50 percent of the world market.

A few years ago, women using hair dyes breathed a sigh of relief when the American Cancer Society (ACS) and the FDA announced the results of a study claiming almost "no connection between hair dyes and fatal cancers." That statement, and the study itself, are both misleading in the extreme.

HOW DYES WORK

Three types of dyes are currently in use: permanent, semipermanent, and temporary. About 75 percent of women use permanent dyes, 20 percent semipermanent, and 5 percent temporary color. Temporary hair dyes and rinses contain lead and other heavy metals and dyes that coat but do not penetrate hair. They not only contain fewer toxic chemicals than permanent dyes, they also are not absorbed by the body, which makes them far less likely to pose serious health risks.

Permanent and semipermanent hair dyes, on the other hand, are known as "precursors" or "couplers." During application of permanent coloring products, a key chemical reaction, called oxidation, occurs between "precursors" and another key ingredient, hydrogen peroxide. This reaction leads to the formation of highly reactive compounds (benzoquinonemimines) that penetrate hair fibers. The "precursor" dyes react with the reactive compounds to form the desired color shades. The hydrogen peroxide also decolorizes melanin, the substance that naturally colors the hair, allowing the new color to take hold. Semipermanent colorants work in a similar way, but without the hydrogen peroxide process.

Both animal and human studies show that the body rapidly absorbs chemicals in permanent and semipermanent dyes through the skin during the more than thirty minutes the dyes remain on the scalp. Additionally, the detergents and solvents used to wash and rinse the hair further increase skin absorption.

EVIDENCE OF RISKS

Permanent and semipermanent colors contain a wide range of carcinogenic ingredients and contaminants including diaminotoluene, diaminoanisole, and other phenylenediamine dyes; artificial colors; dioxane, a contaminant in detergents and solvents; nitrosamines formed by the interaction of ethanolamine detergents with nitrite preservatives or contaminants; and formaldehyde-releasing preservatives. Temporary dyes and rinses contain carcinogenic metals and petrochemicals, particularly formaldehyde-releasing preservatives and nitrosamine precursors.

In short, permanent and semipermanent hair dyes are a witches' brew of carcinogens. The potential risks of breast and other cancers posed by these toxic products are well documented—as are also the efforts by the cosmetic industry to ignore and obfuscate the facts while continuing to manufacture and market the dyes (Table 10.1).

A SORRY HISTORY

In 1971, the hair dye industry "voluntarily" removed one of the most widely used phenylenediamine dyes, diaminotoluene (TDA). It did so to avert proposed regulatory action by the government, following findings that the dye induced liver cancer in rodents (see chapter 6 for information on TDA and breast implants). In 1978, the closely related dye diaminoanisole was shown to induce breast and other cancers in rodents, and was removed from hair dyes. By 1979, TDA was also shown to induce breast cancer. In a sly sleight-of-hand, the manufacturers replaced TDA with a closely related chemical (4-ethoxy-m-phenylene sulfate [4-EMPD]). A *Consumer Reports* article cautioned, however, that "There's not one iota of difference between their potential for causing cancer." The FDA subsequently admitted (in response to a recent request under provisions of the Freedom of Information Act) that it has still not obtained information on the carcinogenicity of 4-EMPD.

Although diaminotoluene and diaminoanisole have been removed from hair dyes, no action has been taken with regard to other phenylene dyes in current use. In 1986, para-phenylenediamine—the basic dye used in virtually all permanent and semipermanent hair coloring products today—was found to cause breast cancer in rodents following oxidation with hydrogen peroxide, as occurs during permanent dye treatments. However, no further animal carcinogenity tests have been conducted on para-phenylenediamine, let alone on other suspect ingredients in hair dyes that may also pose cancer and other risks.

TABLE 10.1: CARCINOGENS IN HAIR DYES	
Ingredient	Hazard
Dyes	
C1 disperses Blue 1	Carcinogenic
D&C Red 33	Carcinogenic
Diaminoanisole	Carcinogenic
Diaminotoluene	Carcinogenic
HC Blue No. 1	Carcinogenic
Para-phenylenediamine	Carcinogenic when oxidized
Detergents/Solvents	
Diethanoloamine/ Triethanolamine	Combine with nitrite to form carcinogenic nitrosamines
Ceteareths and Laureths	Contaminated with the carcinogen 1,4-dioxane
Dyes	
Polyethylene glycol	Contaminated with 1,4-dioxane; degrades into the carcinogen formaldehyde
Preservatives	
DMDM-hydantoin, Imidazolidinyl urea, Quarternium 15	All release formaldehyde

Poorly Tested Ingredients in Hair Dyes

Para-phenylenediamine

2-amino-4-nitrophenol

HC Red No.3

2-amino-5-nitrophenol

HC Yellow No. 4

4-amino-2-nitrophenol

Meta-phenylenediamine

HC Blue No. 2

2-nitro-para-phenylendiamine

Moreover, despite the fact that tens of millions of women use dyes, relatively few adequate studies in humans have investigated their cancer risks. Those few that have been undertaken are flawed to varying degrees because other risk factors, such as family history of breast cancer, reproductive issues, or obesity were not recognized and controlled for.

In spite of such limitations, a series of five epidemiological studies in the late 1970s (see page 230) found links between use of permanent or semipermanent dyes and breast cancer. On the basis of these studies, it appears that the age at which women start to use dyes and the period of time they use dyes significantly affect their risk: Women who start at the age of 40 have less than one-third the risk of breast cancer than those who start at age 30. Women who start at the age of 20 have over twice the risk.

Another conclusion is that the darker the shades of permanent and semipermanent dyes, the higher are the risks of breast cancer. Moreover, although diaminotoluene and diaminoanisole were removed from dyes in the 1970s, it is very likely that their past use is responsible for many cases of breast cancer today.

More recently, a report jointly funded by the ACS and the FDA

Hair Dyes and Breast Cancer: The Studies

- A 1976 study in the *New York State Journal of Medicine* reported that 87 of 100 breast cancer patients had been long-term hair dye users.

- A 1977 United Kingdom study in the *British Medical Journal* found an increased risk among hair dye users over the age of 50 whose first pregnancy had occurred after the age of 30.

- A 1979 United States a study in the *Journal of the National Cancer Institute* found a significant relationship between frequency and duration of hair dye use and breast cancer. The relation was even stronger for women with a "low natural risk for breast cancer." Women at greatest risk tended to be 50 to 79 years old, suggesting that the cancer takes decades to develop.

- Another 1979 study in the *The Lancet* found excess breast cancers among American women who had used hair dyes for at least 21 years. Again, one of the key factors in this increased risk was long-term use.

- A well-controlled 1980 study reported in the *Journal of the National Cancer Institute* found that women who dyed their hair to change its color, in contrast to masking grayness, were at threefold risk. These risks were even greater for women with a past history of benign breast disease, and for women aged 40 to 49.

dismissed the connection between permanent hair dyes and cancers. However, the study failed to consider women who used the dyes more than 10 years previously, or who ever used semipermanent dyes. While insisting that hair dyes pose no breast cancer risk, the authors recommended "removal of carcinogens from hair dyes and appropriate labeling of hair coloring products."

While downplaying the potential risk of breast cancer, the ACS/FDA report admitted a fourfold increase in relatively uncommon cancers, including non-Hodgkin's lymphoma (the cancer that killed dark-haired Jacqueline Onassis) and multiple myeloma. Other recent studies show that hairdressers who apply these chemicals have higher than normal rates of bladder cancer (chapter 12). The association between hair dyes and cancer is based on unarguable experimental studies, backed up by highly suggestive human evidence. Nevertheless, this risk is still largely unrecognized. Fortunately, safer alternatives are available.

INACTIVITY AND BREAST CANCER

The United States is rapidly becoming a nation of fat, underexercised adults and children (chapter 9). If you're like most people, you blame yourself for being lazy. However, our mechanized, technology-obsessed society strongly encourages inactivity every step of the way: Your boss measures your productivity by how long you stay in front of your computer. Recreation more often involves watching videos or playing computer games than playing tennis or ice-skating. Your longest walk might be from the elevator on the ground floor to your car in the parking lot. A National Institutes of Health panel recently emphasized, "Physical inactivity afflicts most Americans. Exertion has been systematically engineered out of most occupations. In 1991, 54 percent of adults reported little or no regular leisure physical activity."

Until recently, most physicians even supported this tendency toward sloth in their patients, insisting that frequent exercise might "wear out their bodies." Because manual labor has long been associated with low socioeconomic status, status-seeking Americans used to shun physical activity of any kind. Even today, despite the proliferation of gyms and health spas and exercise and beauty magazines, most of us still fail to exercise on a regular basis. And young women seem even more vulnerable to inactivity than the rest of the population. As of 1990, fewer than 40 percent of girls in their junior and senior high school years enrolled in physical education courses. Fewer than 20 percent participated in vigorous physical activity three or more times a week.

Our tendency toward inactivity continues despite the well-publicized protective effects of exercise on heart disease and osteoporosis. The additional benefits of exercise in preventing breast cancer, while still largely unrecognized, are quite impressive. For instance, a 1989 study of 7,400 women found that the risk of breast cancer was 70 percent greater in inactive than active postmenopausal women. United States and Canadian studies in 1990 concluded that low physical activity markedly increased breast cancer mortality. Further international studies show that women with high-activity jobs have lower rates of breast cancer than those in more sedentary occupations.

How Inactivity Increases Risk

EFFECTS ON REPRODUCTIVE PATTERNS

- Early menarche
- Late menopause

EFFECTS ON ESTROGEN

- Increases total estrogen levels
- Decreases safe estrogen levels
- Decreases estrogen-binding protein levels

DIETARY ASSOCIATIONS

- Often accompanies increased meat and dairy consumption
- Often associated with increased calorie intake
- Often coupled with increased body fat and obesity

Inactivity increases risk of breast cancer in various ways. When women don't exercise vigorously, their bodies produce more estrogen, thus opening the "estrogen window." Inactive young girls tend to have an early menarche and a late menopause. Inactivity also triggers the body to produce more "bad" than "good" estrogen. Additionally, inactivity tends to be associated with high-caloric, high-fat/high animal and dairy product diets, which further increase risk. Fortunately the antidote to inactivity is simple: Add exercise to your life and you effectively close the estrogen window.

THE PROTECTIVE BENEFITS OF EXERCISE

A January 1986 headline in *The New York Times* read "Lower Cancer Risk Found in Athletic Women." In the report cited, researchers studied the association between risk of breast cancer and physical activity in some 5,000 graduates between 1925 and 1981. They concluded that women who began athletic training in youth and maintained a vigorous lifestyle suffered significantly decreased rates of breast cancer—both pre- and postmenopausally—than their sedentary counterparts. Less active women had about twice the rate of breast cancer as well as increased rates of cancers of the uterus, ovary, cervix, and vagina, which together represent 40 percent of all women's cancers. Subsequent reports, including one published in 1987 by the *American Journal of Clinical Nutrition,* confirm these conclusions.

A more recent study, published in the *Journal of the National Cancer Institute,* followed some 1,000 women under age 40. Those who exercised about four hours per week on a consistent basis reduced their risk of breast cancer by about 60 percent—even if they didn't start exercising until after reaching adolescence. Just by exercising, an average 35-year-old woman can decrease her chances of developing breast cancer by more than one-third, from 1 in 622 to 1 in 895. Even greater benefits were found in those who had children and were physically active as teenagers and young adults. Even just two to three hours of exercise per week offers a protective edge. Furthermore, some protection against cancer was evident despite the presence of other risk factors, such as obesity, early menarche, or childlessness. Authors of the study concluded: "Our data strongly suggest that continued participation in a physical exercise regimen can markedly reduce the risk of breast cancer in premenopausal women, and emphasize the importance of beginning an exercise regimen early in life and maintaining it through adulthood."

A study by Dr. Inger Thune of the Institute of Community Medicine in Norway and published in the *New England Journal of Medicine* in 1997 further confirms the protective effects of exercise. The study recruited 26,000 healthy women between the ages of 20 and 54 and questioned them about other risk factors for breast cancer, including diet, weight, and age at menarche, menopause, and childbirth. The women were followed for an average of fourteen years and questioned again about exercise and diet halfway through the study. Vigorous exercise, enough to cause women to break a sweat, for at least four hours weekly, reduced risks of breast cancer in the entire group by 37 percent, and by 50 percent among women who had not reached menopause. Another study on the effects of starting an exercise program after menopause is now underway.

Further evidence on the positive effects of exercise in averting breast cancer exists in the form of animal studies. In a 1991 experiment, scientists injected female rats with a potent breast carcinogen and then divided them into four groups. They placed one group on a low-fat diet, the second on a medium-fat diet, and the third and fourth on high-fat diets. They forced the fourth group to exercise moderately, the equivalent of running one to three miles daily. Even though they consumed more fat and gained more weight than the inactive rats on low-fat diets, the fourth group developed fewer breast cancers. This suggests that exercise may be even more protective than a low-fat diet.

A 1995 rodent study published in the *Journal of the National Cancer Institute* confirmed that moderate to intense exercise is "highly protective against tumor induction." Similar to the 1991 study, female rats were injected with a breast carcinogen and then assigned to four groups with varying degrees of daily exercise for six months. The activity levels ranged from none, a level lower than generally required to improve cardiovascular fitness, an amount sufficient to improve fitness, to a "super-intense . . . sprint" level of exercise at 100 percent of their oxygen capacity. The sedentary

How Activity Decreases Risks

EFFECTS ON REPRODUCTIVE PATTERNS

- Late menarche
- Fewer periods
- Early menopause

EFFECTS ON ESTROGEN

- Decreases total estrogen
- Increases "good" estrogen
- Increases estrogen-binding proteins

DIETARY ASSOCIATIONS

- Increases levels of vegetarianism
- Decreases caloric intake and increased calorie expenditure
- Decreases body fat and obesity

MEDICAL ASSOCIATIONS

- Decreases need for ERT

rodents developed up to five times more breast cancers than their vigorously exercising counterparts.

All this is very good news for women who want to take control of their health: Almost anyone at any age can begin a moderate exercise program that will help reduce breast cancer risk as well as boost overall health. But exactly what is the connection between exercise and breast cancer prevention?

How Exercise Protects

Just as inactivity opens the "estrogen window," prompting a woman's body to produce more estrogen for longer periods of time, exercise closes that window. Physical activity, particularly starting at an early age, is associated with late menarche, fewer periods, and early menopause, all of which reduce breast cancer risk.

Effects on Reproductive Patterns

At the same time that exercise reduces body fat, it suppresses menstruation and ovulation. Delayed menarche is common in lean girls with a low percentage of body weight and body fat. Most experts agree that a girl must have at least 17 percent of total body weight due to fat before menarche can occur. Moreover, a body fat percentage of at least 22 percent is necessary to maintain the menstrual cycle. Studies conducted over several decades confirm that women who exercise enough to reduce body fat to lower than 22 percent experience fewer periods, thereby lowering their levels of estrogen (chapter 2).

Exercise also appears to enhance the protective effects of breast-feeding in women who reached late menarche because they exercised vigorously as children. These women tend to stop menstruating for longer following pregnancy. Women who reached early menarche, on the other hand, menstruated more quickly after pregnancy, even when they breast-fed.

Effects on Estrogens

Physically active women of all ages have decreased levels of body fat and estrogen. Apart from delaying menarche and decreasing frequency of ovulation, a balanced exercise program shifts the balance from the "bad" to the "good" form of estrogen. Exercise also protects a woman's breast tissue by limiting the conversion of testosterone to estrogen and stimulating the production of estrogen-binding pro-teins, which divert estrogen away from sensitive breast cells.

Effects on Diet

Not surprisingly, vigorously active women tend to consume diets low in beef and dairy products. A 1985 report in the *British Journal of Cancer* stated:

> *Young women who began their training before menarche ate in a different pattern than women who began after menarche. . . . The athletes who began very early in life ate less fat and less calories. Something about the exercise lifestyle brings about this beneficial change in the diet, and these athletes who begin at the earliest age simply do not seem to like much saturated fat in their diets.*

It seems that few people, of any age, would want to indulge in a fatty meal after vigorous exercise. In fact, many athletes choose largely vegetarian diets and eat meat only as a side dish, if at all. Such diets are associated with both lower overall levels of estrogen and a balance in favor of "good" estrogen.

THE MIND/BODY CONNECTION

Psychoneuroimmunology—a big word for a new science—is based on a simple but crucial concept. Our mind and emotions—the way we think and how we feel—profoundly influence our physical health. The belief that feeling of stress, anxiety, depression, and hopelessness contribute to cancer and other illnesses dates back to 200 A.D., when the Greek physician, Galen, commented that cancer seems to afflict melancholic women more frequently than those that are happy.

Somewhere along the line, modern Western medicine made a strict and highly artificial division between mind and body. Only recently have scientists begun to investigate the basic connection between them. What they've discovered is that our immune system is profoundly affected by our emotions. Some studies indicate that hopelessness and passivity trigger changes that leave the body more vulnerable to cancer, while others show that aggression or depression do the same.

Indeed, the immune system plays a key role in the relationship between cancer and emotions. The connection between the two is what we commonly call *stress*, a physical and emotional reaction to internal and external events. Stress affects the entire body, particularly the adrenal glands that secrete hormones (corticosteroids) that impair the body's immunity to cancer and other disease. Corticosteroids, which are secreted in response to physical or mental stress, damage white blood cells vital to defending against cancer, as well as lymph glands and the thymus where these cells are programmed. Once the immune system falters, the body becomes more vulnerable to cancer, including breast cancer.

STRESS AND BREAST CANCER

Scientists have studied the mind/body connection in breast cancer in animals and humans. Three studies of animals show the association in interesting and startling ways:

- A 1975 study in *Psychosomatic Medicine* revealed that when the forcible removal of newborn baby mice disrupted the rodents' social order, the incidence of maternal breast cancer increased sharply.

- A 1983 study in the same journal showed that stress directly increased the risk of breast cancer. They did so by subjecting two groups of mice to electric shocks, then allowing one group to escape and trapping the other. Those unable to escape developed high rates of cancer.

- A 1981 study in *Science* showed that 90 percent of mice housed in high-stress cages (those with high levels of noise, vibration, and light intensity) developed full-blown cancer after injections with breast cancer virus, while only 10 percent of mice housed in low-stress cages became ill with cancer.

Some human studies also show a profound connection between stress, emotions, and breast cancer. Most studies show that passive, emotionally suppressed breast cancer patients had a worse prognosis than those with a positive, take-charge attitude. A 1995 *British Medical Journal* article claimed that risks of breast cancer increased by as much as fourfold following severely stressful events in the preceding five years. However, other studies have failed to detect any relation between stress and breast cancer risk or survival in breast cancer patients. Of all the known and suspected risk factors we review in this book, stress appears to be the least important, at least on the basis of available evidence. Nevertheless, you can help improve your overall health and sense of well-being—if not breast cancer in particular—by reducing the stress in your life.

PERSONAL PROTECTION

WHAT YOU CAN DO

- Stop smoking—and stop smoking in front of others.
- Assess with care the risks and benefits of drinking alcohol.
  - Avoid binge-drinking and heavy drinking.
  - Avoid known or suspected carcinogenic contaminants in alcohol.
- Avoid dark permanent and semipermanent hair dyes.
  - Follow safe-use guidelines if you use hair dyes.
  - Use safer alternatives for coloring hair and cosmetics.
- Purchase safe and healthy cosmetics and personal care products.
- Make moderate exercise a regular part of your life.
  - Encourage your daughter to exercise early in life.
- Learn to recognize and manage stress.
- Take control and fight for your health and well-being.

STOP SMOKING

No need to weigh risks and benefits here: Smoking is the single most harmful personal habit. By smoking, you expose your lungs, and those of everyone around you, to some 4,000 toxic and carcinogenic substances. Unfortunately, nicotine is one of the single most addicting substances still legal in the United States. Quitting, then, is easier said than done. However, your local branches of the ACS, the American Lung Association, the YWCA, and other organizations offer "stop smoking" programs that may help you take this most important, life-saving step.

CAREFULLY ASSESS THE RISKS AND BENEFITS OF ALCOHOL

Clearly, drinking alcohol poses risks for breast and other cancers. At the same time, alcohol also provides health benefits, particularly to the heart. While breast cancer is the leading cause of cancer deaths in women, heart disease causes up to ten times as many fatalities in women over the age of 50 than does breast cancer.

If you are at high risk of heart disease due to a family history, hypertension, or high blood levels of cholesterol (particularly low-density lipoproteins [LDLs]), you may consider that the positive effects of moderate drinking—two drinks or less per day—are worth its potential risks.

However, if you are at higher risk for breast cancer, due to family history, prolonged use of oral contraceptives, current use of ERT, early menarche and late menopause, or long-term smoking, you should consider avoiding any alcohol (see chapter 4). Exacerbating your present risks of breast cancer by drinking may not be worth the protective effects of alcohol on your cardiovascular system.

You can further fine-tune your balancing of risks and benefits by taking your age and other individual factors into consideration. Say you are a 30-year-old woman who drinks moderately. A *New England Journal of Medicine* article outlines your risks this way:

[Your risk] of having coronary heart disease and breast . . . cancer in the next 20 years are about 1 percent and 2 percent respectively. . . . Omitting one drink per day would make these risks about 1.5 percent and 1.3 percent, respectively—for a total that is virtually identical. On this basis only, health considerations would slightly favor not drinking. It appears that the risk of cancer is more important in the equation for young women.

The truth is, alcohol does offer protective benefits to your cardiovascular system. However, you could derive equal or higher benefits from safer alternatives, including exercising, eating a low-fat diet, taking antioxidant supplements, and taking aspirin.

Avoid Binge and Heavy Drinking

Whatever health benefits alcohol consumption offers, they remain viable only if drinking is moderate—meaning two drinks or less per day. Unfortunately, binge-drinking has become increasingly common among American youth and should be avoided at any age, and for obvious reasons that extend far beyond the increased risk of breast cancer.

Avoid Known or Suspected Carcinogenic Contaminants in Alcohol

Stay away from commercial ales, sake, bourbon, and European fruit brandies. If you choose to drink, opt for beverages—preferably organic—with the lowest levels of urethane, including wine, champagne, tequila, vodka, and beer. Organic wines are legally defined as coming from grapes not treated with pesticides. However, there is no such definition for beer and hard liquor.

AVOID DARK PERMANENT OR SEMIPERMANENT HAIR DYES

We recommend that you completely avoid black or dark brown permanent or semipermanent hair coloring products since they contain well-known carcinogens. Other shades and products labeled "all natural" may be okay to use.

Determining whether your favorite product is safe is not very difficult. In the United States, women need simply to read the label listing the ingredients. If "phenylenediamine" is listed among the ingredients in any form, the product probably poses a risk of breast and other cancers. Also check to see if the product contains any other carcinogens (listed on page 228). Avoid any product with the following type of disclaimer on the package:

> CAUTION: *This product contains ingredients that may cause skin irritation in certain individuals and a preliminary test according to accompanying directions should first be made.*

Follow Safe-Use Guidelines

If you do decide to use permanent or semipermanent dark dyes, try to wait until you are at least age 50 before doing so, and then choose as light a shade as possible. When applying the dyes, you or your hairdresser should follow these safety steps:

- Always wear gloves.
- Do not leave the hair dye on the scalp longer than absolutely necessary.
- Avoid rubbing the dye into your scalp.
- Wash any dye off facial skin immediately.
- Flood the scalp thoroughly with water immediately after use.
- If possible, frost or highlight the hair using tipping, streaking, painting, or aluminum foil weaves to avoid close contact between dye and scalp.

Use Safer Alternatives

Chadwick's, a beauty salon in Seattle, Washington, is an example of the trend in beauty toward more natural and safer cosmetics, including hair dyes. When owner Cherie Smith found that the chemicals used in her salon were so toxic they were making her and her employees ill, she opened a beauty salon emphasizing safer products.

Among these safer materials is henna, a substance found in plants native to Egypt and used for thousands of years as a semipermanent dye. Some brands of henna cover gray completely, restoring natural, pregray color to the hair. You can buy henna products at most drug or health food stores.

In recent years, manufacturers have been starting to create safe nonhenna products as well. One highly recommended line is Igora Botanic, available at many salons. Their plant-based, semipermanent hair colors contain natural raw materials such as indigo, chamomile, walnut, logwood, cochineal, and guar gum. Another option is a permanent hair coloring product from VitaWave of California. The ingredients are safer than those found in commercial permanent and semipermanent hair coloring products. Finally, Paul Penders of Petaluma, California, has come out with a safer line of hair coloring products. You'll find these at your local natural products supermarket or health food store.

PURCHASE SAFE AND HEALTHY COSMETICS AND PERSONAL CARE PRODUCTS

The only cosmetics free from estrogenic synthetic chemicals such as methylmethacrylate are found in natural product supermarkets or health food stores. These include such brands as Aubrey Organics, Dr. Hauschka, Ecco Bella, and Paul Pendars.

MAKE EXERCISE PART OF YOUR DAILY ROUTINE

Women of all ages benefit from exercise. The consensus of experts today is that 30 minutes of moderate activity every day is the least amount of exercise everyone at every age requires to stay healthy. To achieve this modest goal, you could take a walk or bicycle ride, even work around the yard. For those who currently exercise very little or not at all, easy exercise might be the best way to start. According to the chairman of the 1995 National Institutes of Health consensus panel, Russell V. Leupker, "More than half of adult Americans do not get enough physical activity, and these are the very people who can gain the most by just getting started."

The good news is that even if you're inactive right now, you can help improve your general health and reduce your risks of breast cancer by simply taking a ten-minute walk or climbing the stairs instead of taking the elevator.

If you currently exercise vigorously on a regular basis, another warning might be appropriate. It is possible to be too thin and to have too little body fat. Too much exercise, combined with a diet extremely low in calories and nutrients, increases the risk of osteoporosis. If your doctor determines that your body fat percentage is below 22 percent, you might want to consider gaining some weight, either by reducing your exercise level or increasing your calorie and fat intake.

Encourage Your Daughter to Exercise Early in Life

Most women (and men, for that matter), however, could add some activity to their lives. As they do so, they'll not only be helping achieve their own health goals, but they'll also be setting a good example for their daughters and sons. It is extremely important that we encourage young girls, who currently are underexercised, to get out there and move! Society still sends negative messages to young girls about athletics, discouraging from them competing in sports at school or in their free time.

If you have a young daughter, work with your local Parent Teachers Association (PTA) to ensure that schools encourage participation in strenuous sports like cross-country training, track and field, competitive swimming, gymnastics, ballet, soccer, martial arts, and full-court basketball. The best age for girls to start becoming involved in competitive sports is at about age 9, as long as they find themselves in a supportive, fun atmosphere devoid of undermining pressure that could lead to self-destructive behaviors like anorexia or bulimia.

If a child learns to love being active at a young age, exercise could well become a healthy part of her daily routine throughout her life. Furthermore, she will be more likely to stay connected, emotionally and spiritually, to the physical part of her life. In this day and age of stress and anxiety, that connection becomes ever more important.

LEARN TO RECOGNIZE AND MANAGE STRESS

There is no simple equation when it comes to the mind/body connection to cancer. There is no evidence that staying calm could reduce your risks of developing breast cancer if you are a naturally active and emotional person. However, learning how you react to stress and then figuring out better ways to manage stress will help protect your immune system. Many people find that having a trained professional guide them through the process of identifying and reducing stress can be very helpful. Among the methods available are relaxation therapy, hypnosis, biofeedback, and individual and group counseling.

TAKE CONTROL AND FIGHT FOR YOUR HEALTH AND WELL-BEING

Simply by picking up and reading this book, you've shown that you're willing and able to take control and fight for your health. The more information you absorb, the more answers you demand, the harder you try to change your life to reduce your risks, the healthier you are bound to be.

11

Where You Live

Living near hazardous waste sites, chemical plants, power lines, or nuclear plants poses risks for breast cancer, as does using the cleaning solvents in your kitchen, the pesticides in your garden, your electric blankets, and computers. Identifying these risks, and eliminating or avoiding them as much as possible, will help lower your and your family's risk of breast cancer and other cancers.

"For the first time in the history of the world, every human being is now subjected to contact with dangerous chemicals, from the moment of conception until death. . . . We are living in a sea of carcinogens." So wrote environmentalist Rachel Carson in her 1962 landmark book, *Silent Spring*, in which she warned the world about the risks—not just to humans but to the entire ecosystem—of pesticides and other environmental hazards. Some thirty-five years later, those hazards still exist and still permeate our neighborhoods and homes. In this chapter, we outline those risks and how they may affect your risks for breast cancer.

HAZARDS IN YOUR NEIGHBORHOOD

For thirty years, Rhonda Sylvester lived beside a paint factory in a neighborhood on the west side of Detroit. "I can smell those fumes today. I remember that smell like I still lived there," Rhonda told a reporter from the *Utne Reader* shortly before her death from breast cancer at the age of 37.

Was the development of Rhonda's disease related to her years exposed to toxic fumes, or just a coincidence?

Studies show that where you live—the area of the country and your neighborhood—affects your susceptibility to cancer and other disorders such as asthma and miscarriages. Studies also link increased breast cancer risk directly to living near chemical plants, hazardous waste sites, and nuclear facilities.

You can see the way environmental factors affect people on an international level. Each country in the world has its own different incidence risk pattern of breast cancer. The highest rates of pre-menopausal breast cancer are found in Australia and New Zealand, for instance, while the highest postmenopausal rates occur in the United States. Does that mean the genes of Australian and American women predispose them to breast cancer? Or are national dietary and socioeconomic differences involved? Or could it be that these countries have higher levels of carcinogenic environmental pollutants?

An important 1995 study on immigration and breast cancer rates in the *Journal of the National Cancer* Institute makes it clear that these rates are highly affected by environmental factors. Immigrants to Australia and Canada from other nations were found to develop profound changes in breast cancer mortality rates. Slowly but surely, the immigrants—no matter what age they moved from their country of origin—assumed risks similar to those experienced by native-born women. Indeed, most people tend to emigrate as adults, not as adolescents when risk factors for breast cancer are thought to be most important. In other words, someone who moves from a low-risk nation like Japan to a high-risk nation like Australia or the United States will eventually have higher breast cancer risk than she would have if she had stayed in Japan. And the reverse is equally true, an American woman who moves to Japan decreases her risk of breast cancer—no matter what her age.

These findings have two implications: First, and most positively, these studies show that any woman can reduce her risk at any age.

Breast cancer is rarely predestined at birth, except for pure and dominant genetic factors, but is rather a preventable disease with avoidable risk factors. By following the tips for Personal Protection outlined in this book, for instance, you can significantly lower your risk of breast cancer at age 25, 50, or 70.

Second, these findings make it clear that the environment—the air we breathe, water we drink, and the earth in which our food grows (and hence our diet)—influences our risk for cancer. This influence is probably best validated by looking at breast cancer rates across the United States, where fewer cultural and lifestyle differences exist than might occur between different nations.

UNITED STATES: THE BREAST CANCER PICTURE

NORTHEAST VERSUS SOUTH

In 1977, an important article in the *Journal of the National Cancer Institute* reported different patterns of postmenopausal breast cancer mortality within the United States. Women in the West and Northeast, particularly those living in large urban regions, were found to have higher postmenopausal mortality rates than women in the South. Plainly speaking, the farther north you live, the greater is your risk of breast cancer. In fact, after adjusting for other variables, death rates in the Northeast exceeded those in the South by more than 20 percent. However, no differences were noted for premenopausal cancer, thus incriminating reproductive rather than environmental risk factors.

A 1995 National Cancer Institute (NCI) study concluded that the excess of postmenopausal cancers in the Northeast is due primarily to reproductive risk factors, such as age at menarche and at first birth, and family history (chapter 2). Yet even after adjusting for these influences, postmenopausal rates remained 13 percent higher in the West and Northeast, and eight percent higher in the Midwest than in the South. The study admitted that these remaining excesses might be due to "environmental factors," including exposure to organochlorines and electromagnetic fields (EMFs).

Despite this qualification, an accompanying NCI editorial misleadingly insisted that this study provided definitive proof that reproductive influences account for regional differences in breast cancer death rates and that excess breast cancer deaths in the Northeast are largely due to delayed childbearing patterns: "The findings of the NCI should help allay fears that unknown environmental hazards are responsible for the clustering of elevated breast cancer mortality in the Northeast."

This claim was based on "ecological" studies in which overall comparisons for disease and death rates are made from one geographic area to another. At best, such results can be used only to generate ideas that need further investigation, investigation that requires studies that control for a wide range of other breast cancer risks, such as the Pill and ERT use—factors that this study failed to consider. In this case, significant excesses of breast cancers remained in the West, Midwest, and Northeast even after reproductive influences were compared. In essence, then, this study clearly reveals the need for further examination of environmental influences on breast cancer rates. Although the NCI continues to deny any environmental influences in the regional differences in breast cancer death rates, industrial and hazardous waste pollutants play a significant role in breast cancer risk, as discussed in chapter 9.

The problem with understanding the role that environmental carcinogens play in breast cancer risk by looking at risk differences between regions within the United States is that so many other factors besides environmental ones may be involved. More women of a higher socioeconomic status live in the Northeast than the South, and these women increase their risk by tending to have their babies at an older age than their less wealthy counterparts. More African-American women live in the Northeast, and, because many have poorer access to health care, their breast cancers are diagnosed relatively late and with a resulting higher mortality. Southern women also have higher vitamin D levels, due to their longer exposure to sunlight, which a 1994 *Journal of Nutritional Biochemistry* study suggests is protective against breast cancer. Another factor is diet: Regional surveys indicate that women in the North eat more meat and fat and fewer vegetables than women in the South. Yet even after adjusting for these influences, postmenopausal breast cancer rates remained 13 percent higher in the West and Northeast, and 8 percent higher in the Midwest than in the South.

HAZARDOUS WASTE DISPOSAL

For more than a decade, the people of Long Island, New York have known that something is wrong in their environment: Women there are developing breast cancer at an alarming rate—statistics show that breast cancer mortality in this area has long been higher than in 99 percent of all counties nationwide, and women living in one part of Long Island had twice the incidence of breast cancer from 1978 to 1987 than other New Yorkers—but no one could tell them why.

Geri Rarish was one of those women. Diagnosed with breast cancer on August 1, 1986, Rarish spoke at a New York House of Representatives meeting seven years later, in October 1993. This meeting was convened as a result of grassroots pressure by local women demanding that public officials investigate the potential connection between breast cancer and heavy pesticide use, exposure to radiation from a ring of several nuclear power and weapons plants surrounding the area, and the proliferation of poorly regulated chemical factories and plants in Long Island. In fact, Long Island is home to more than 22 Superfund hazardous waste clean-up sites.

Edolphus Towns, the subcommittee member who listened to Rarish that day, asked a series of probing questions that focused on the issue of environmental influences on cancer:

> *Why is it that researchers find deposits of DDT in the breast tissue of breast cancer patients? How is it that breast cancer rates are higher in areas surrounding nuclear power plants? It is about time that we have*

> *answers. . . . I, along with the American people and the*
> *audience assembled today, want to know how we can*
> *avoid our exposures to industrial carcinogens.*

In response to mounting pressure from activist groups, Congress enacted Public Law 103-43 in 1993. This law mandates a study of the potential causes of breast cancer rates on Long Island, including studies of biological markers for environmental and other risk factors. In April 1995, the NCI announced the launch of a $7 million, four-year study to investigate the impact of environmental hazards on a woman's risk of breast cancer. The focus of the study, being performed by the Columbia University School of Public Health, is Suffolk and Nassau counties in Long Island, New York. For the thousands of women on Long Island already stricken by breast cancer, this advance comes too late, as it does for the millions of women who might have been saved if the cancer establishment had taken seriously the risks posed by environmental hazards decades ago. It should be noted, however, that Fran Visco, president of the National Breast Cancer Coalition, opposes these studies on regional clusters of breast cancer, maintaining that all such decisions should be left to the NCI and not Congress (chapter 13).

Indeed, since the late 1950s, the chemical industry has dumped more than a billion tons of toxic wastes—wastes containing known carcinogens—largely in unprotected ponds, pits, and lagoons in some fifty thousand sites nationwide. Often these sites are illegal and/or abandoned, and range in size from small operations with only a few 55-gallon barrels to large industry operated disposal sites. Some three-quarters of these sites contaminate about 50 percent of the nation's drinking water with pesticides and solvents.

Hazardous wastes disposed of by incineration are as dangerous, if not more so. By 1989, a nationwide network of more than 1,100 commercial and on-site incinerators, cement kilns, and industrial boilers burned nearly eight billion pounds of waste, with resulting large-scale air pollution. These pollutants include incompletely combusted wastes; new chemicals formed during combustion, particularly dioxins; and heavy metals, particularly cadmium, lead, and mercury. Some pollutants, such as dioxin, lead, and cadmium, have profound hormonal effects or are breast carcinogens.

Scientists first identified a relationship between hazardous waste sites and breast cancer in the Northeast. A 1985 study in *Preventive Medicine* found that breast cancer rates were higher in New Jersey— a state in which twenty-one counties contain hazardous waste disposal sites—than elsewhere in the United States. The authors concluded that the excess may be "related to ingestion of carcinogens or carcinogen promoters arising from industrial chemicals or [chemical toxic waste disposal sites]." The study also showed that all counties with hazardous waste sites had higher breast cancer rates, as well as more birth defects. Although published more than a decade ago, these results have not been investigated any further in New Jersey.

A subsequent survey of 340 counties in forty-nine states by the Environmental Protection Agency (EPA) in 1989 confirmed these findings. Published in the *Archives of Environmental Health*, this extensive analysis demonstrated excess breast cancer rates among women living in counties with toxic waste sites. In fact, counties with the highest breast cancer rates housed from four to thirteen times more hazardous waste facilities than elsewhere in the United States. Explanations of these excesses included: "[W]orking for companies that created the waste . . . [as well as] contamination of local food supplies, emissions into the ambient environment, and contaminated water."

In 1994, newspaper reports on the high breast cancer incidence in the San Francisco Bay area related it to "higher exposure to unidentified environmental factors." Judy Brady, a breast cancer activist, reported in the *Women's Cancer Resource* that the Chevron Ortho Chemical Co. (recently purchased by Monsanto) discharges some 57,000 pounds of the breast carcinogen methylene chloride annually into the air that local residents breathe. Brady, herself a breast cancer survivor, suspects environmental influences played significant role in the development of her disease.

A 1997 study in the *Journal of the National Cancer Institute*, however, points to the difficulty in identifying risk factors when it comes to a complex disease like breast cancer. While confirming that the incidence of breast cancer in the San Francisco Bay Area is about 14 percent higher for white women and 10 percent higher for black women than in eight other geographical areas, it could not confirm that environmental factors contributed to this increase. In fact, after adjusting for established and probable risk factors (age at first pregnancy, breast-feeding, age at menarche, age at menopause, and alcohol consumption), the authors of the study concluded that the excess San Francisco rates "can be completely accounted for by regional differences in known risk factors." They further emphasized that well-established reproductive risk factors may be involved in explaining national or other regional differences in breast cancer incidence.

At the same time, however, the study failed to examine the potential role that specific environmental risks factors, such as pesticides or other pollutants, may play in the high rates of breast cancer found in the San Francisco Bay Area population, a fact that dismays breast cancer activists.

Drs. Devra Lee Davis and H. Leon Bradlow offer further insight into the role of environmental pollution on women's health in a 1995 issue of *Scientific American:* "People who live in areas where the air or water is highly polluted by industry or by the dumping of or burning of wastes might take in estrogenic chemicals simply by breathing the air or drinking contaminated water." Indeed, the environmental connection extends far beyond neighborhoods that contain hazardous wastes. Many other areas have high levels of toxic chemicals, too.

OTHER SOURCES OF CHEMICAL POLLUTANTS

The air above the remarkably beautiful Massachusetts Military Reservation on scenic upper Cape Cod is filled not only with seagulls and puffy white clouds on a typical summer day, but also with the military wastes from artillery firing and open-air burning of unused propellants. A 1991 study of women who live in the area by the Boston University School of Public Health offers further evidence of the relationship between pollutants and breast cancer. Women living on upper Cape Cod had significantly higher rates of breast cancer than other Massachusetts women—and women who lived near gun and mortar positions for more than 20 years doubled their expected risk of breast cancer. To put a human face on that startling statistic, a 70-year-old woman living near the reservation has a one in seven chance of developing breast cancer instead of the expected one in fourteen chance at that age.

In fact, the rate of breast cancer throughout all regions of Cape Cod is higher than the rest of the state, so much higher that Cape Cod women created the Massachusetts Breast Cancer Coalition to find out the reasons. Their concerns sparked the Newton, Massachusetts Silent Spring Institute to conduct a $4 million large-scale study of breast cancer on Cape Cod. Julia Brody, executive director of the Institute and the study's director, remarked:

> Breast cancer on the Cape is 21 percent higher than the rest of Massachusetts, and it has been elevated for every year that the Massachusetts Cancer Registry has data, from 1982 to 1992.
>
> People had questions about whether [the increased rate] was due to more frequent mammography screening, but we now have data that shows this is not the explanation. The percentage of tumors diagnosed early on the Cape is nearly identical to the rest of the state. People also raised questions about whether there were socio-demographic explanations. But standardized incidence rates show it is not due to age.
>
> Finally, we asked researchers from the Collaborative Breast Cancer Study, involving three New England states and Wisconsin, to go back to their data and explore differences between women on the Cape and from the rest of Massachusetts. They statistically took

into account a long list of established risk factors for breast cancer, including family, medical, and reproductive history. These alone did not account for the increased rates. That is why we believe environmental influences may hold the key.

Indeed, the very reasons that the Cape is beautiful—the sandy beaches and glorious sea that surrounds it—may hold the key to its high breast cancer rates. Brody remarks:

Nearly all the drinking water on the Cape comes from shallow groundwater. Because of the sandy soil, there is a chance for contaminants to move into the drinking water, including pesticides and detergents. Further, to protect marine life, all wastewater is discharged on land into septic systems where there is potential for these contaminants to leach through the soil. The use of pesticides is also prevalent due to cranberry bogs, and a history of spraying for tree pests. Cape Cod adopted DDT as one of its favorite pesticides.

As you can see, tracking down environmental exposures is a multilayered, complicated process. Another all-too-common source is chemical plants that emit emit toxic and carcinogenic pollutants substances. In April 1994, a preliminary study by the New York State Department of Health reported that postmenopausal women living close to large chemical plants on Long Island had increased risks of breast cancer "about equal to that of having a family history of breast cancer." Ignoring the earlier New Jersey and EPA hazardous waste surveys showing such a connection, the *New York Times* claimed that this study represented the "first credible study outside a laboratory to suggest a possible link between breast cancer and industrial pollution."

As late in the game as this study comes, however, it does reveal some persuasive and compelling information about the dangers posed from having chemical plants in your neighborhood. For one thing, postmenopausal women living less than a mile from a chemical plant had excess breast cancer rates; the farther away they lived from the plant, the lower the rates of breast cancer. And for another, the more chemical plants in the area, the higher the rates of breast cancer. Although it was impossible to relate risks to specific plants or pollutants due to the concentrated clustering of many industries in a small area, the results of the study provide solid evidence that chemical pollution does indeed pose serious risks for breast cancer.

NUCLEAR POWER PLANTS

A series of well-publicized reports by radiation experts Drs. Ernest Sternglass and Jay Gould claim that exposure to radioactive emissions from civilian and military nuclear reactors are major, unrecognized causes of breast cancer. One such study again focused on Long Island and its environs, which in addition to being home to myriad chemical industries is also ringed by four nuclear plants: the Brookhaven plant, operating since the 1950s as a Department of Energy (DOE) weapons facility; the Indian Point plant, operating since 1961; the Haddam Neck facility, operating since 1967; and the Millstone plant in Waterford, at the northern tip of Long Island, operating since 1970.

In the decades that followed start-up of these plants, breast cancer mortality increased by 72 percent in Suffolk County and by 24 percent in Westchester County. They rose in direct connection to peak plant emissions: rates in Nassau and Suffolk counties increased sharply from 1974 to 1976 after the Haddam Neck reactor went on-line and then again from 1983 to 1985 after the Millstone plant started up in 1975.

The highest breast cancer rates in Long Island were noted among Suffolk County residents within 15 miles of the Brookhaven DOE reactor. These rates rose by 40 percent from 1950 to 1989, the largest increase for any major suburban county in the United States. Emissions from the two units at the Millstone plant forced the

Nuclear Regulatory Commission to shut them down in 1996, raising the possibility that women living near the plant are at even higher risk. Shortly following the shutdown of the first two units, regulators found Millstone Unit 3's design deficiencies also placed neighboring women at increased risk for exposure to nuclear fission products.

Women living downwind from reactors elsewhere in the United States appear to have similar increases in breast cancer mortality rates. In counties downwind from the reactor in Hanford, Washington state, for instance, breast cancer rates tripled between the early 1950s and late 1960s. Nearby, but upwind from the reactor, rates actually declined. In Anderson County, Tennessee, downwind from the DOE Oak Ridge reactor, breast cancer rates increased by 28 percent during the decades that followed the start-up, while in nearby Roane County, located upwind from the plant, rates declined. In the South Carolina and Georgia counties of Burke, Aiken, and Savannah River, downwind from the DOE Savannah River facility, breast cancer rates increased by 15 percent. Nationwide, studies in 100 counties with nuclear reactors emitting iodine and strontium fission products show similar increases in breast cancer deaths—increases in sharp contrast to lower rates in counties without nuclear plants or in counties with lower emission levels.

While provocative and suggestive, these studies are flawed by statistical and other problems that caution against drawing definitive conclusions about breast cancer risk. Researchers may have been biased in their selection of the counties to study; some failed to provide back-up meteorological data for classification of "downwind" and "upwind" counties; and virtually all failed to consider the role of other breast cancer risks. Furthermore, the authors made no attempt to investigate the county rates of childhood leukemia, probably the most sensitive indicator of radioactive exposure.

Despite these shortcomings—or perhaps because of them—the need for more studies appears reasonable. The NCI, however, rejects outright any possibility that emissions from nuclear plants put women at risk, and denies the need for further evaluation of the claims by Drs Sternglass and Gould.

ELECTROMAGNETIC FIELD RADIATION

Electromagnetic fields (EMFs)—the emissions from electricity—come from both the environment and manufactured sources. The sun and, to a lesser extent, the Earth's magnetic field, are prominent sources of EMFs. But we also are exposed to emissions from radio and television communication, household appliances (from microwave ovens to personal computers), and power lines. In fact, scientists estimate that more than 20 million Americans are exposed to EMFs from high-power voltage lines at levels high enough to raise safety concerns.

Studies in 1991 by the California Department of Health show that EMFs interfere with natural electrical fields of the body and can damage the immune system. EMFs also suppress production of the hormone melatonin, with a resulting increase in estrogen levels and breast cancer risk. Substantial evidence also strongly suggests the carcinogenicity of EMFs. At least nine studies, dating from 1979 and published in prestigious journals such the *American Journal of Epidemiology, Bioelectromagnetics,* and the *American Journal of Industrial Medicine,* show that women exposed to EMFs before conception or during pregnancy deliver more children who later develop childhood cancers, including leukemia, brain, and nervous system cancers. Other evidence links adult cancer with residential and occupational exposure to high-voltage transmission lines. In fact, at least eighteen occupational studies link EMF exposures to leukemia, five to brain cancer, and thirteen to other cancers, including breast cancer.

Evidence on the breast carcinogenicity of EMFs originally stemmed from studies on occupationally exposed men, but many more recent studies suggest a relationship to female breast cancers as well. A study in 1987 in the *Annals of the New York Academy of*

Sciences shows increased rates of premenopausal breast cancer in women living near electrical transmission lines in Colorado. A subsequent 1991 study from the Boston University School of Public Health also reported a modestly increased risk of breast cancer among women in upper Cape Cod living within 500 feet of electric power substations. The relation between EMF exposure and breast cancer clearly merits extensive investigation.

Ignoring the growing evidence, the ACS dismisses risks posed by EMFs. A 1996 ACS paper concluded without reservation:

> *To date, no form of electromagnetic energy at frequency levels below those of ionizing radiation (X-rays) and ultraviolet radiation has been shown to cause cancer. . . . Numerous epidemiological studies . . . have addressed the topic. None has yet provided fully persuasive results.*

HAZARDS IN THE HOME

Most of us tend to think of home as a safe haven from the dangers of the outside world. However, there is evidence that the cleansers we use to scrub our kitchens and bathrooms, the pesticides we use on our lawns, the fumes we inhale while cooking or heating the home, and the EMFs emitted from myriad household appliances may well be putting our health at risk.

Carcinogenic Chemicals

Indoor air pollution poses one of the greatest environmental health risks: According to a five-year survey of 600 homes in six cities by the EPA's expert Lance Wallace, peak concentrations of twenty toxic or carcinogenic chemicals were up to 500 times higher indoors than outdoors. Four classes of indoor pollutants have been implicated as causes of breast cancer: household products; pesticides; fumes from cooking and heating appliances; and contaminated work clothing (Table 11.1).

TABLE 11.1: INDOOR AIR POLLUTANTS THAT CAUSE BREAST CANCER IN RODENTS	
Carcinogen	Source
Methylene chloride	Spray paints, aerosol strippers, drinking and washing water
Atrazine, DDVP	Pesticides for home and lawn, drinking and washing water
1, 8-dinitropyrene,	Kerosene heaters, gas burners
2-nitrofluorene, benzpyrene, and benzene	Auto exhaust from an attached garage; shower
Asbestos, polyvinyl chloride (PVC), toxaphene, kepone, PCB, DES, cadmium, zearonal, atrazine, benzopyrene, DDT	Contaminated work clothing, battery manufacture, welding, electrical trade, painting, dry cleaning, agriculture, pest control

Household Products

Many chemicals used in household products are highly volatile, which means they easily evaporate and can thus be inhaled. Others, sprayed from aerosol cans or hand pumps, release a shower of microscopic, easily inhaled particles. Specifically, aerosol spray paints and paint strippers may contain the propellant methylene chloride, which is carcinogenic to the breast and other organs in rodents.

Pesticides and Industrial Chemicals

You might not think that caring for your half-acre of lawn would increase your risks for breast cancer, but that all depends on what you use for pesticides. It's important to keep in mind that most people apply lawn pesticides at a remarkable—and potentially toxic— rate of 5 to 11 pounds per acre, while farmland is treated with under 2 pounds per acre. This means that suburban lawns and gardens received heavier pesticide applications than most other land areas in the United States.

The air inside your home is likely to be even more contaminated by pesticides than the air outside. The EPA's 1990 Non-Occupational Pesticide Exposure Study identified at least five pesticides at levels up to ten times greater indoors than outside. Among those most frequently detected is chlordane—used to eradicate termites—a chemical that induces breast and other cancers in rodents. (Professional pesticide applicators used chlordane widely through the late 1980s, when the EPA banned its use.)

Other indoor pesticides posing breast cancer risk are the very common No-Pest Strips, which contain the insecticide dichlorvos (DDVP). DDVP is the active ingredient in No-Pest Strips. Although the EPA initiated a special review of the dangers of DDVP, it remains widely available in hardware and drugstores throughout the United States and in other countries. The EPA estimates that domestic exposure to DDVP from these strips poses cancer risks ten times greater than for pest-control workers who regularly apply this insecticide.

Believe it or not, even showering, washing dishes, and flushing toilets can also be significant sources of exposure to carcinogenic substances that contaminate your water. Many carcinogenic industrial solvents and contaminants, including breast carcinogens such as benzene and methylene chloride, easily pass through the skin into the body during showers, baths, and dishwashing. More important-ly, such carcinogens become gases at room temperature, and can thus be readily inhaled. According to a 1984 *American Journal of Public Health,* and a 1985 *Environmental Health Perspective* article, the amount of such industrial volatiles inhaled during a 15-minute shower with contaminated water is equivalent to drinking about eight glasses of contaminated water.

Heating and Cooking Fumes

Kerosene heaters and gas burners emit pollutants, including 1,8-dinitropyrene, 2-nitrofluorene, and benzopyrene, which induce breast and other cancers in experimental animals. Natural gas cook-ing and heating appliances can also emit benzene.

Contaminated Work Clothing

Many men and women work in petrochemical and other industries that expose them to chemical carcinogenic substances, which they inadvertently carry home on their work clothes, skin, hair, and in their cars. (chapter 12). Families of these workers can thus be chron-ically exposed to such carcinogenic contaminants. These include carcinogens inducing breast and other cancers in rodents, and some have also been shown to be human carcinogens, such as asbestos, PVC, toxaphene, kepone, diethystilbestrol, lead, cadmium, zearanol, atrazine, benzopyrene, and DDT. A 1985 study of five children of workers handling the carcinogen zeranol developed enlarged breasts. In 1995, a report to Congress from the National Institute for Occupational Safety and Health noted that workers' home contam-ination "may be associated with breast cancer."

High-risk occupations and their "carry-home carcinogens" include: Electric and plastic manufacturing (asbestos), agricultural and pest control (atrazine and other carcinogenic and estrogenic pesticides), and radiation and nuclear plant works (radioactive con-taminants).

ELECTROMAGNETIC FIELDS

Exposure to EMFs occurs not only from living near high-voltage power lines and transmission stations, but also from home appliances, including hair dryers, electric blankets, televisions, and even grounding connections to metallic water pipes (Table 11.2). Risks posed by EMFs depend on the distance from sources and duration of exposure. For instance, transmission lines located only 200 or 300 feet away expose people to fewer EMFs than many common domestic appliances.

In a recent test published in *Green Alternatives*, researchers placed a chair in a room where a compact disc player played music, then turned on other appliances elsewhere in the home, including an oven, toaster, and refrigerator. With all appliances running, anyone seated in the room would receive a high exposure of about 3 milliGauss (mG)—greater than that from a 500-kilovolt transmission line at a distance of 300 feet. Similarly, the EPA reported that the use of electric blankets involves continuing exposure to EMFs at levels of up to 100 mG, higher than exposure resulting from proximity to power lines. And while a washing machine emits 20 mG at 6 inches, this drops to only 1 mG at 2 feet.

There is growing evidence that EMFs in the home may pose risks of breast cancer. For example, a 1991 *American Journal of Epidemiology* article showed a modest increased risk among premenopausal women using electric blankets:

> *There was potential for underestimation of risk. . . .*
> *Thus, the elevated estimate of risk for the most frequent*
> *users of electric blankets and the potential public health*
> *significance of electromagnetic fields exposure associat-*
> *ed with even a modest increase in risk suggest that fur-*
> *ther inquiries be pursued of breast cancer, especially*
> *premenopausal cases.*

The National Institute of Environmental Health Sciences is now funding research on magnetic fields and breast cancer in rats treated with low doses of carcinogens. However, the American Cancer Society report dismissed these risks outright.

TABLE 11.2: ELECTROMAGNETIC FREQUENCY EXPOSURES (MG) AT DISTANCES FROM APPLIANCES*

Distance from Source	6"	1'	2'	4'
Kitchen				
Dishwasher	20	10	4	—
Microwave ovens	200	40	2	—
Bathroom Sources				
Hair Dryers	300	1	—	—
Electric Shavers	100	20	—	—
Living/Family Room Sources				
Ceiling Fans		3	—	—
Window Air Conditioners		3	1	—
Tuners/Tape Players	1	—	—	—
Color TVs		7	2	—
Black-and-White TVs		3	—	—
Laundry/Utility Room Sources				
Electric Clothes Dryers	3	2	—	—
Washing Machines	20	7	1	—
Irons	8	1	—	—
Portable Heaters	100	20	4	—
Vacuum Cleaners	300	60	10	1

(continued)

Distance from Source	6″	1′	2′	4′
Bedroom Sources				
Air Cleaners	180	35	5	1
Digital Clocks		1	—	—
Analog (Conventional Clock-Face) Clocks	15	2	—	—
Baby Monitors	6	1	—	—
Electric Blankers (Conventional)	22			
Electric Blankets (Low-Magnetic-Field)	1			

— = *Exposures are normal background levels. An empty cell indicates no measurement recorded.*

United States Environmental Protection Agency. EMF In Your Environment. Magnetic Field Measurements of Everyday Electrical Devices. Office of Radiation and Indoor Air, Radiation Studies Division, Washington, DC, December 1992.

LIGHT AT NIGHT

Reports in the *American Journal of Epidemiology, the American Journal of Public Health,* and elsewhere suggest that exposure to near-constant bright artificial light at night (LAN) may increase risks of breast cancer by inhibiting the pineal gland's secretion of melatonin, a hormone that in turn inhibits estrogen production. Other suggestive evidence comes from a 1991 study in *Epidemiology,* in which blind women were found to have relatively low rates of breast cancer, presumably due to their higher melatonin levels.

As LAN expert B.B. Harrell wrote in a *New York Times* Letter to the Editor:

> *We think nothing of switching on an unnatural 100-watt bulb to change the baby or go to the bathroom . . . thereby interrupting the estrogen-lowering darkness in a manner unthinkable to most of the third world, and to most of our grandparents. . . . Every time we turn on a light we are inadvertently taking a drug. . . . We think Thomas Edison had a bigger effect on the human body than anyone realized.*

PERSONAL PROTECTION

Without question, your environment influences your risks of breast cancer. You can reduce your risk of breast cancer by making changes to your environment. Women of all ages can take reasonable precautions to reduce avoidable environmental risks in their homes and neighborhoods.

WHAT YOU CAN DO

- Avoid living near pollution sources.
- Make where you live safer.
- Reduce domestic exposure to breast carcinogens and EMFs.
- Avoid light at night.

AVOID LIVING NEAR POLLUTION SOURCES

If at all possible, avoid buying or renting a home near chemical and nuclear plants and waste sites as well as high-intensity EMF sources when choosing a new home. If you already live in such locations, consider moving to safer area.

MAKE WHERE YOU LIVE SAFER

First of all, get to know your neighborhood. Is there a pulp and paper mill upstream from where you or your family fish? Are there dairies located near a nuclear reactor? Is your tap water from an aquifer or surface locale nearby a pollution source? If the answer to any of these questions is yes, you must try to make the necessary changes to reduce your increased risk of breast and other cancers.

Protect Your Home

If you are moving to a new home or apartment, avoid these hazards. If they exist in your home now, eliminate them as soon as possible:

- Asbestos ceilings and pipes
- Dwellings treated with chlordane for termite treatment, unless tested and found to be contaminant-free
- Use of No-Pest Strips containing DDVP
- Basement oil or gas heaters (look for ones located outside the house)
- Contaminated private or public water supply
- High EMF readings inside or outside
- Contaminated clothing

If finding a safer place to live is not possible for financial or other reasons, make every effort to reduce exposure to environmental pollutants. Avoid drinking local water unless it is filtered by activated carbon and reverse osmosis systems. Also avoid eating beef, dairy, fish, produce, and grains if you know the food comes from areas close to pollution sources.

Get involved with local environmental groups to fight toxic dumping or other sources of environmental pollution in your community. A recent federal court ruling in a suit brought against the Chemical Manufacturers Association in the District of Columbia affirmed a law requiring chemical companies and refineries to publicly disclose their emissions. The court sided with the EPA's addition of some 300 chemicals, nearly doubling the existing number, to the government-mandated Toxic Release Inventory, required by the Emergency Planning and Community Right-to-Know Act. In a May 2, 1996 article, the *New York Times* emphasized the importance of such legislation, writing, "The annual disclosures of emissions, by factory and town, have long been considered a major incentive driving the industry to cut pollution, although the law does not require that the pollution be controlled."

REDUCE DOMESTIC EXPOSURE TO BREAST CARCINOGENS

Be aware that the home can be the source of exposure to breast carcinogens. Likely sources include household products, pesticides, heating and cooking fumes, contaminated clothing, and EMFs.

- **Household products:** Eliminate the use of toxic chemicals in the home whenever possible. Properly store and dispose of those that cannot be eliminated; discourage family members from visiting areas when such chemicals are in use. Avoid any use of spray paints and strippers and other aerosols, especially those with methylene chloride propellants. Similarly, avoid art-supply paints containing breast carcinogens such as hexachlorobenzene. Instead, purchase readily available nontoxic brands.

People who work at home as artists or craftspeople need to be especially aware of the potential for contamination. Separate craft and hobby areas from living quarters; try to work as far from a living area as possible. Even better, work in a separate structure unattached to the home if using toxic chemicals.

■ **Pesticides and industrial chemicals:** Never use DDVP home-pest strips. Avoid any lawn pesticides, including atrazine and 2,4-dichlorophenoxy acetic acid (2,4-D), which are estrogenic or carcinogenic. Avoid use of any pesticides in the home and garden other than pyrethrum extracts, fatty acid soaps, boric acid, and other safe and natural alternatives such as beneficial insects, superior horticultural oils, physical barriers, and pheromone traps. Use a filter to reduce exposure to pesticides and industrial chemicals contaminating drinking water. At about $2,000, a better, more costly solution is filtering the entire residence's water with a whole house filter.

■ **Heating and cooking fumes:** Always make sure to turn off kerosene heaters and gas burners when you are not using them. Ventilate your kitchen well by keeping windows open whenever possible. Wear warmer clothing instead of turning the heat on or up.

■ **Contaminated clothing:** You or your spouse may work in industries that expose you to carcinogenic and toxic exposures. Change your clothes before going home from work and, if possible, have your employers wash them at the plant. Store your street clothes in a separate closet from work clothes to prevent cross-contamination. Leave toxic substances, contaminated items, and containers at the workplace, and wash your hands, face, and other exposed skin with care.

REDUCE DOMESTIC EXPOSURE AND ELECTROMAGNETIC FIELDS

We are not going to get rid of our refrigerators, stoves, or televisions and other electrical appliances. However, you can reduce exposures without inconvenience.

Replace electrical with nonelectrical appliances when feasible. For example, you could replace an electric can-opener with a hand-held one without suffering too great a hardship. Use a hand, rather than electric, whisk for cooking, try two blankets or a down-filled comforter instead of an electric blanket, and let your hair dry naturally instead of using a blow-dryer.

Maintain distance from electrical appliances whenever possible, as EMFs' intensity drops off rapidly the further the distance. In particular, avoid sitting too close to the television set and use a leaded EMF shield to reduce emissions from home computer display terminals. And remember, EMFs pass through walls, so be aware of what electric appliances are running in every part of the house, and make sure to turn off EMF-emitting appliances when you're finished with them.

AVOID ARTIFICIAL LIGHT AT NIGHT

To stimulate maximum production of melatonin, it's important that you sleep in true darkness: When you are ready for bed, turn off all inside lighting and televisions, and mute outside lamps with adequate blinds.

12

Hazards in the Workplace

Some occupations expose women to toxic chemicals that increase their risk of breast cancer. Among the most dangerous are those in the petrochemical, nuclear, and electrical industries. Protect yourself from exposure by either avoiding high-risk industries or insisting on safe work practices.

A leading expert on occupational cancer at a 1993 international conference on Women's Health and Cancer stated, "Almost nothing is known about the potential risk of breast cancer among women associated with occupational exposures and changes in job status across the life spectrum." Decades after women first started working in high-risk occupations in the manufacturing and chemical industries, neither the cancer establishment nor the public has recognized the risks of breast cancer involved.

Since World War II, women have been moving into the workforce in increasing numbers numbers. According to the National Institute for Occupational Safety and Healthy (NIOSH), more than four million women now work in industries that expose them to chemicals well recognized as causes of occupational cancer in men. Yet research on women's occupational cancer—particularly occupational causes of breast cancer—remains minimal.

At the 1993 Conference on Women's Health, Sheila Hoar-Zahm, Ph.D., reported on a review of some 1,200 publications on occupational cancer and concluded that only 14 percent specifically studied women. She further stated that such studies "tended to use weaker methodologies . . . and were less able to provide convincing data on the occupational cancer risks of women [than men] and minorities."

A 1997 review of some 115 studies on occupational cancer—conducted over the last twenty-five years and published in the *American Journal of Industrial Medicine*—reveals the paucity of information. Its authors conclude that "Few high-quality occupational studies directed specifically toward women have been carried out to allow the unambiguous identification of occupational risk factors for breast cancer." In fact, the overwhelming majority of these studies provide no information on any risk factors other than poorly documented occupational exposures.

But even what little we know about occupational causes of breast cancer is disturbing. More than fifty occupational carcinogens induce breast cancer in experimental animals, and are thus likely to do the same in women exposed to them in the workplace (Table 12.1).

WORKERS AT RISK

The vast majority of workplace exposures to industrial chemicals known to cause breast cancer in rodents involves just four high-volume carcinogens: benzene, methylene chloride(dichloromethane), ethylene oxide, and phenylenediamine dyes. In total, nearly one million women working in the petrochemical, manufacturing, or cosmetology industries are exposed to these four carcinogens (Table 12.2).

Small-scale epidemiological studies (see Table 12.1) also show increased breast cancer rates in certain jobs. However, because these studies generally fail to evaluate personal risk factors, they do not necessarily prove a direct connection. Nevertheless, such findings are a strong basis for concern, especially because many of the chemicals involved have been shown to cause breast cancer in experimental animals.

TABLE 12.1: OCCUPATIONAL EXPOSURES TO KNOWN OR SUSPECTED BREAST CARCINOGENS

Carcinogen	Occupation
Dyes	
Cl. Acid Red 114	Engineering technicians; textile machine operators
4-aminobiphenyl	Contaminant in manufacture of 2-aminobiphenyl
Cl. Basic Red 9 Monohydrochloride	Biological and life scientists; medical scientists; clinical laboratory technologists
2,4-diaminoanisole	Cosmetologists; dyeing furs, leather, and textiles
2,4 diaminotoluene	Cosmetologists, manufacturing and formulating toluene diisocyanate elastomers, and dyes
3,3'-dimethoxy-benzidine	Manufacturing and formulating dyes
3,3'-dimethoxy-benzidine dihydrochloride	Manufacturing and formulating dyes
Hydrazobenzene	Dye manufacturing; pharmaceuticals
Para-phenylenediamine	Cosmetologists and hair dressers

(continued)

Carcinogen	Occupation
Polymers	
Acrylamide	Paper and pulp; construction; foundry; oil drilling; textiles; cosmetics; food processing; plastics; mining; agricultural industries
Acrylonitrile	Manufacture of synthetic fibers; also used in fumigants
1,3-butadiene	Chemical, rubber, and plastics manufacturing
Vinyl chloride	Manufacture of flame retardants and polyvinyl chloride (PVC)
Ethylene oxide	Manufacture of industrial products including glycol ethers, polyester fibers, hospital sterilant; ethanolamines, detergents, heavy-duty home laundry detergents and soaps and their ingredients, and textile chemicals
Toluene-2,6-diisocyanate	Welding; assembling; industrial painting; electrical equipment manufacturing
Polyurethane foam	Industrial insulation, breast implants
Pesticides (manufacture, formulation, and application)	
Aldrin (no longer manufactured in the United States)	
Atrazine	

Carcinogen	Occupation
Pesticides	
1,2-dibromo-3-chloropropane	
Chlordane	
Cyanazine	
DDT (breast tumor accelerator)	
Dichlorvos	
Dieldrin	
Sulfallate	
Polycyclic Hydrocarbons (transportation and fuel handling industries)	
Benz(a)pyrene	
Dibenz(ah)-anthracene	
3-methylchol-anthrene (3-MCA)	

(continued)

Carcinogen	Occupation
6-nitrochrysene (6-NC)	
1-nitropyrene	
Pharmaceuticals (manufacture, formulation, and handling)	
Adriamycin (doxorubicin)	Handling by health professions
Cisplatin	Chemotherapeutic production and handling by health professions
Estrogens (estradiol-17; estrone; ethinylestradiol; mestranol)	Drug manufacturing for pharmaceuticals, feed additives, and cosmetics
Metronidazole	Manufacture, formulation, packaging, administration
Nitrofurazone, powder	Managers and administrators; veterinarians; health technologists and technicians; janitors and cleaners; animal caretakers (except farm)
Procarbazine hydrochloride	Drug manufacture; administration of chemotherapeutic drugs
Progestins (norethisterone, progesterone)	Drug manufacturing for pharmaceuticals, feed additives, and cosmetics
Reserpine	Drug manufacturing

Carcinogens	Occupation
Pharmaceuticals	
Toluamide, N-isopropyl-alpha-(2-methylhydrazine)-, para-monohydrochloride	Physicians; pharmacists
Industrial Chemicals and Solvents	
Benzene	Petrochemical; electrical equipment industries; printing; assemblers; hand painting, coating, and decorating
1,1-dichloroethane	Chemical technicians
1,2-dichloroethane	Chemical technicians; health services; garment workers (textile sewing and pressing machine operators); industrial painting; naval; assemblers
Methylene chloride	Machinists; electrical equipment manufacturing; petrochemical; molding and casting machine operators; metal plating; printing; textiles; photography; assembling; hand packers
1,2-dichloro-propane	Assemblers; chemists; industrial painters

(continued)

Carcinogen	Occupation
Other Classification	
Benzidine, 3,3'-dimethyl-dihydrochloride	Science technicians
Acetophenon, 2-chloro	Biological technicians; mixing and blending machine operators; hand packers and packagers
Benzidine, 3,3'-dimethoxy-dihydrochloride	Clinical laboratory technologists and technicians
Propanol, 2,3-epoxy-,1-	Punching and stamping press machine operators; assemblers
2,4-toluene-diisocyanate	Welders; textiles
1,2,3-trichloro-propane	Chemical technicians
Anthranilic acid, 4-chloro-N-furfuryl-5-sulfamoyl	Health professions
Ochratoxin A	Handling and storing grains, nuts, corn, cereals, and animal feeds

National Institute for Occupational Safety and Health (NIOSH). National Occupational Exposure (1981-83) Survey. Unpublished Provisional Data as of July 1, 1990. Cincinnati, OH: U.S. Department of Health and Human Services, Division of Surveillance, Hazard Evaluations and Field Studies Surveillance Branch, Hazard Section.

Carcinogen	Occupation	Approximate Number Exposed
TABLE 12.2: NUMBERS OF WOMEN WORKERS EXPOSED TO COMMON BREAST CARCINOGENS		
Benzene	Solvents; petrochemical synthesis; electrical equipment industries; printing; hand painting, coating, and decorating	143,000
Ethylene oxide	Manufacture of products including detergents, glycol ethers, polyester fibers, and textile chemicals; past major use as hospital sterilant	121,000
Methylene chloride	Solvents; petrochemical manufacturing; electrical equipment; molding and casting machine operators; metal plating; printing; textile; and photography	353,000
Phenylene-diamine dyes	Manufacture and formulation dyes; cosmetologists	200,000

PETROCHEMICAL WORKERS

A 1991 study in the *American Journal of Industrial Medicine* show that women working in petrochemical industries have high rates of breast cancer—up to four times those of other women.

Employment in these industries involves exposure to various carcinogens and carcinogenic contaminants (benzene, benzopyrene, benzanthracene, 1-nitropyrene, and methylene chloride) that induce breast cancer in rodents. Even though these studies failed to control for personal risk factors, the absence of such excess rates in twenty other industries—which did not expose women to these particular carcinogens—further emphasizes their significance.

A 1977 study revealed the risks another workplace carcinogen, the plastic polyvinyl chloride—which is manufactured from and contaminated with its carcinogenic precusor vinyl chloride—poses of breast cancer in women who work with it. Studies of animals that show that the lowest amount of vinyl chloride tested induces breast cancer confirm this result: Since vinyl chloride concentrates in fatty tissues, including the breast, breast cancer among women exposed to vinyl chloride is "biologically plausible."

Other women at high risk are textile workers exposed to petroleum-based dyes and solvents, chemical and gas handlers, and workers in industries that use carbon tetrachloride, formaldehyde, styrene, and methylene chloride. Of particular interest is methylene chloride, a chemical used by some 350,000 women in the manufacturing and textile industries, and in photography, printing, molding and casting, and other industries. In a 1988 *American Journal of Industrial Medicine* report, scientists incriminated methylene chloride and related hydrocarbon solvents as causes of breast cancer among women manufacturing lamps for Canadian General Electric from before 1960 until 1975. This finding was supported by a 1991 study showing a strong association between exposure to methylene chloride and excess breast cancer mortality among aircraft maintenance employees.

Similar increases in breast cancer rates have been found in women working in electrical equipment and printing industries, aircraft maintenance employees exposed to chlorinated organic solvents and Freons, and health care workers exposed to ethylene oxide gas used as a sterilant. A study on health care workers is noteworthy because it found that the exposed group of women "as a whole appeared to be largely free of known risk factors for breast cancer."

A recent review further incriminates carcinogenic organic solvents as occupational risks factors for breast cancer and also helps explain the mechanisms involved. Organic solvents are known to accumulate and concentrate in breast fat, then migrate into breast lobules and ducts. The solvents are then activated by enzymes in the breast called P-450 to produce highly reactive and carcinogenic products. However, the breast, unlike the liver and kidney, lacks detoxifying enzymes that would render the carcinogens harmless. Therefore, the carcinogenic products persist unchanged in breast tissue.

Despite the fact that we know a great deal about the carcinogenic and estrogenic effects of many pesticides in experimental animals, some causing breast cancer, only a few studies have been carried out on women involved in their manufacture, formulation, and application. For example, atrazine, a widely used herbicide found in rural drinking water and one of the commonest water pollutants in the United States and Western Europe, induces breast cancer in rodents. While women occupationally exposed to atrazine have high rates of ovarian cancer, scientists have not yet investigated the chemical's relationship to breast cancer.

Within a group of about 400 German women exposed to the potent carcinogen dioxin, a contaminant in trichlorophenol (TCP) and 2,4,5-trichlorophenoxyacetic acid herbacides, four women developed breast cancer. Because the study involved such a small number of people, it is hard to reach conclusions about the breast cancer risks of dioxin. Furthermore, while dioxin is carcinogenic in numerous animal species, it induces cancers at sites other than the breast.

COSMETOLOGISTS

More than 200,000 women work in the cosmetology industry today and are thus exposed (or have been exposed) to carcinogenic hair dyes on a daily basis (chapter 10). While the studies on hair dye risk are generally small and poorly controlled, taken together they clearly suggest increased breast cancer risk (see box below). While a few studies show no such association, the overall weight of evidence clearly warrants immediate reduction of exposure to dyes in the beauty industry to the maximum extent feasible. Thus, large-scale, well-controlled studies on hairdressers are critically needed, especially since we know that common hair dyes—diaminoanisole and diaminotoluene in the past, and para-phenylenediamine today—induce breast cancer in rodents and are thus likely to do the same in humans.

Breast Cancer Risk among Hairdressers

- Several studies from Great Britain in the late 1950s show significantly higher risks among unmarried hairdressers.

- In 1972, the International Agency for Research on Cancer found an increase of breast cancer among cosmetologists based on a review of Social Security disability lists between 1969 and 1972.

- A 1990 Japanese study also found an increase in breast cancer among hairdressers.

- A 1992 Finnish study reported excesses of breast and ovarian cancers among hairdressers.

- A 1993 Washington state study presented at the 1993 International Conference on Women's Health found excess breast cancers among cosmetologists.

Pharmaceutical Workers

Pharmaceutical workers also suffer from excess rates of breast cancer. While scientists are unsure what causes this increased risk, evidence suggests that exposure to estrogens and progestins in their manufacture, formulating, and handling by pharmacists is implicated. An interesting report in 1977 on acute hormonal effects in workers at a plant manufacturing oral contraceptives in Puerto Rico adds substance to this supposition. More importantly, these hormones have also been clearly shown to induce breast cancer in experimental animals and in women, as evidenced by numerous studies on oral contraceptives and ERT (chapters 3 and 6).

Pharmacists also handle antihypertensive and antibiotic drugs known to increase breast cancer risk, including reserpine, Aldactone, hydrazaline, Flagyl, and Furacin. Cancer drugs, handled both by pharmacists and health care professionals, have also been incriminated (chapter 8).

METAL WORKERS

The *Journal of Occupational and Environmental Medicine* recently published studies linking exposure to individual metals such as lead and cadmium and to "overlapping" combinations of metals, including chromium, arsenic, beryllium, nickel, and solder, to higher risks for breast cancer. Since such exposures are likely to be "overlapping," only a few metals may be responsible. A 1991 *British Journal of Industrial Medicine* report, for instance, showed that aircraft workers exposed to solder alone were at higher risk for breast cancer. Increased risks of breast cancer have also been reported among women exposed to metalworking fluids for pressing and cutting metals, due to the methylene chloride and other related solvents found in such fluids, and also their contamination with benzene and benzpyrene.

ASBESTOS WORKERS

Asbestos, long associated with lung cancer, may also be a risk factor for breast cancer. A 1985 review in the *British Journal of Industrial Medicine* showed high rates of breast cancer among 700 workers manufacturing asbestos products prior to 1967. High concentrations of asbestos have also been found in lungs of women with breast cancer. More recent studies further confirm an excess rate of breast cancer among asbestos workers.

ARTISTS

Practicing the fine art of painting involves prolonged exposure to a wide range of carcinogens, including benzene, which induces breast cancer in experimental animals, and methylene chloride, linked to breast cancer in both animal and human studies. Oil paints from Grumbacher Corporation, one of the nation's major manufacturers, contain PCBs, which are both carcinogenic and estrogenic and which selectively concentrate in breast cancer tissue.

A preliminary NCI study of some 1,600 artists reported significant excesses of breast, rectum, and lung cancer. Risks of breast cancer were as high for married as single women, suggesting that reproductive influences were not responsible.

RADIATION WORKERS

In chapter 5 on mammography, we described the breast cancer risks of radiation in some depth, so it should come as no surprise that radiation workers have excess rates of breast cancer.

Ionizing Radiation

We know from decades of research that the breast, particularly the premenopausal breast, is highly sensitive to the carcinogenic effects of X rays. The first clear-cut evidence came from the British "luminizer worker study." According to studies later published in *The Lancet*, the *Journal of Occupational Medicine*, and elsewhere, women painting luminous radium on instrument dials before the 1930s accumulated about 0.5 rads exposure per week. While some exposure was internal (following ingestion by mouth from painting and tipping brushes), most was external and at relatively high doses. High rates of breast cancer developed in these women, particularly those exposed in their twenties.

Despite these well-known findings, little information exists on risks to women working in modern radiation industries. A 1988 Chinese study in the *Journal of the National Cancer Institute* reported significant excesses of breast cancer among some 27,000 diagnostic X ray workers employed between 1950 and 1980. This risk may well increase as these workers are followed for longer periods. A 1993 study found a "small excess" of breast cancer among workers at the Hanford nuclear weapons plant; the risk was three times higher among nuclear than other plant workers. Among women working on one particular nuclear-related task, the risk was sixfold. This means that a 60-year-old woman increased her chances for developing breast cancer from one in twenty-four women to as much as one in four. While scientists claimed that these results were not related to exposure levels, they did admit "a good deal of measurement error." Finally, a well-controlled 1992 *British Journal of Medicine* study found "significantly raised risks" of both breast and bone cancer among Finnish airline cabin attendants, risks attributed to relatively low levels of cosmic radiation.

Despite these findings, the NCI failed to publish results of its investigation of mammography and radiation technicians until 1994. While researchers identified no excess risk, this study was seriously flawed by the absence of any information on exposure other than duration of employment.

All these findings are strongly supported by both animal studies and human evidence of excess breast cancer among atom bomb survivors and women exposed to diagnostic and therapeutic radiation. As discussed in chapter 5, radiation also increases the carcinogenicity of estrogens.

Electromagnetic Fields

Electricity creates biologically active, long radiation waves called electromagnetic fields (EMFs). These EMFs are literally everywhere, indoors and outdoors, but mostly at such low levels they pose no health risk. Women in occupations involving EMF exposure, however, appear to have increased risks of breast cancer. These occupations include police officers using radar guns, and telephone switching and power line workers.

However, the evidence on EMFs remains contradictory. Two studies, based on small numbers of women in a various occupations, found no excess risk. In contrast, two other studies, specifically designed to investigate the relation between breast cancer and EMF exposure levels, did find excess mortality among those with higher levels of exposure. The first study, on telephone mechanics-repairers and engineers-technicians and published in the *British Journal of Industrial Medicine* in 1993, concluded that "possible exposure to technological advancement in the modern telephone industry may account for excess risks observed, particularly among younger women."

The *Journal of the National Cancer Institute* reported in 1994 that women employed in electrical occupations associated with strong EMF exposure were nearly 40 percent more likely to die of breast cancer than women in occupations without such exposure. Specifically, electrical engineers suffered an increased risk of 73 percent, while telephone installers, repairers, and line workers had even higher rates. On the basis of such evidence, a 1996 ACS review admitted that a statistically significant relationship exists between occupational exposure to EMFs and breast cancer risk.

Other studies further incriminate EMFs, revealing excess breast cancers among women working as railway and tram drivers, electricians, and telephone installers. Additionally, one nonoccupational study suggested an excess of breast cancer among women exposed to EMFs from electric blankets (chapter 11).

Experimental studies also support the EMF-breast cancer association. Electromagnetic fields suppress production of the hormone melatonin, secreted by the pineal gland, which helps the body to regulate estrogen levels and maintain normal balances and is protective against breast cancer. The office and manufacturing workplaces are common sources of EMF exposures. The distance from an EMF source is crucial: The closer you are to an EMF-emitting appliance, the greater your exposure (Table 12.3) For example, while a copy machine emits as much as 90 milliGauss (mG, the standard measurement for EMFs) at a distance of 6 inches, this drops to only 1 mG at a distance of 4 feet.

TABLE 12.3: ELECTROMAGNETIC FIELDS EXPOSURES (MG) AT DISTANCES FROM WORKPLACE SOURCES*

Distance from Source	6"	1'	2'	4'
Plant				
Battery chargers	30	3	—	—
Drills	150	30	4	—
Power saws	200	40	5	—
Electric screwdrivers (while charging)	—	—	—	—
Office				
Air cleaners	180	35	5	1
Copy machines	90	20	7	1
Fax machines	6	—	—	—
Fluorescent lights	40	6	2	—
Electrical pencil sharpeners	200	70	20	2
Video display terminals (PCs with color monitors)	14	5	2	—

— = *Exposures are no greater than normal background levels.*

United States Environmental Protection Agency. EMF In Your Environment. Magnetic Field Measurements of Everyday Electrical Devices. Office of Radiation and Indoor Air, Radiation Studies Division, Washington, D.C., December 1992.

TEACHERS AND OTHER PROFESSIONALS

Strangely enough, many professional women, especially teachers, appear to be at increased breast cancer risk. A recent study in the *American Journal of Public Health* focused on excess breast cancer rates among teachers in the United States and Canada. Personal factors alone do not appear to account for this excess, as female physicians, who have similar reproductive patterns as teachers, have lower breast cancer mortality. Based on these considerations, the authors of the study concluded that "The increased breast cancer mortality that we observed in teachers and other professionals may represent the deaths that remain even after adequate screening and medical care."

One possible cause could be the routine, often intensive, application of carcinogenic pesticides in schools. However, other professionals, including clergywomen, mathematicians, computer scientists, and dietitians, have similar increases in risks of breast cancers. In most cases, the related risk factors are probably personal rather than job-related. Most professional women delay childbirth and have more prolonged use of oral contraceptives than their blue-collar peers. Indeed, women with five or more years of college education are more likely to become professionals, to have their first births from the ages of 30 to 44, and to either limit or avoid breast-feeding, a pattern associated with excess cancer risk.

Another connection among these professions is their largely sedentary nature. Two studies suggest that excess risks could be due to the inactive nature of their jobs and associated tendency to obesity. A 1987 study in the *American Journal of Clinical Nutrition* specifically related an increased risk of breast cancer to sedentary work. A more recent 1993 Chinese investigation in *Cancer* showed that women in occupations involving low physical activity had higher risks of breast cancer than women in high-activity jobs (chapter 10).

PERSONAL PROTECTION

Occupation is, in principle at least, an avoidable cause of breast cancer: In an ideal world, we would all be able to choose the safest possible jobs. In reality, however, most of us are not able to change jobs very easily, even for safety reasons. If your work puts you at high risk, it is up to you and your co-workers to demand a safe environment.

WHAT YOU CAN DO

■ **Avoid exposure to carcinogens.**

■ **Insist on a safe workplace.**

AVOID EXPOSURE TO CARCINOGENS

Do not take a job that exposes you to any known occupational carcinogens. If you currently face risk in the workplace, consider switching to another, safer occupation if at all possible. If you work in schools that use pesticides, lobby the school board to remove them as soon as possible (an information brochure entitled *Pesticides In Our Homes and Our Schools* can help you do just that). And if you work in a sedentary environment, make sure you exercise vigorously every day before or after work.

INSIST ON A SAFE WORKPLACE

If avoiding carcinogenic exposures at work is not feasible or practical, insist that your employer put strict safety measures in place. While these recommendations particularly apply to blue-collar workers, others may also find them protective:

■ **Label hazardous chemicals clearly:** Know which chemicals you work with and if they are carcinogenic. Request a Material Safety Data Sheet (MSDS), which your employer must make available to you, that provides basic information on workplace chemicals and their toxic effects. While often incomplete and biased, the MSDS does provide some helpful information. Also use reference materials from the International Agency for Research on Cancer, NIOSH, or the EPA. Demand clear labeling, complete with the chemical name (not code words, complex names, or brand names) and comprehensive information on all hazards. You can also anonymously call the regional office of NIOSH and request that the agency perform Health Hazard Evaluation at your plant.

- **Closed systems:** Confining the handling of carcinogens to a specific, closed area will minimize exposure of other workers.

- **Adequate area ventilation:** The entire plant must be well ventilated to reduce exposure to carcinogens as well as the spread of toxic substances from one work area to another.

- **Local exhaust ventilation:** The immediate area in which workers directly handle carcinogens should also be thoroughly vented through an efficient local exhaust hood.

- **Use of protective clothing and equipment:** All workers handling carcinogens or other toxins should wear impermeable work clothing, respirators, gloves, and goggles. Protective equipment should be NIOSH-approved for the particular carcinogens with which you work. Such safety equipment, however, does not replace safe work practices, including ventilation and labeling of hazards. Workers dealing with X rays must also take special precautions to reduce exposure whenever possible. EMF-exposed workers should reduce exposure by shielding or positioning themselves away from high-emitting EMF sources. Office workers, for instance, should sit far away from electrical equipment, or use a lead glass shield that reduces EMF exposures from computer display monitors.

- **Air quality control:** Air concentrations of carcinogens may vary widely from area to area within the plant and even within specific work areas. Your employer must measure the air quality directly in your work space on a regular basis, using detection limits sensitive enough to detect relatively low levels of contaminants in the parts per billion (ppb) range. If your employer refuses or neglects to take such measurements, contact your state Occupational Safety and Health Administration (OSHA) and your union's Medical Surveillance. Radiation workers should use an X-ray badge to monitor their environment. EMF workers may use a Gauss meter.

- **Work surface control:** Because carcinogenic material may contaminate work surfaces, frequent monitoring is essential, using the same guidelines described above.

- **Medical surveillance:** Your employer should monitor the effects of toxic chemicals on your health by providing regular medical examinations, complete with urinalysis, blood analysis, hair analysis, and breath analysis. If any examination reveals the presence of such chemicals in your body fluids or evidence of genetic damage to blood cells, you must demand immediate action from your employer. If none is forthcoming, take action yourself by discussing the problem with your supervisors, leaving employment until exposure is reduced, contacting NIOSH or OSHA officials, and taking legal action. If you run into resistance from your employer, try to involve local or national union and women's groups. As a last resort, quit your job and find a safer one. No job is worth losing your health over.

- **Clean, uncontaminated clothing:** Wash all work clothing outside the home and apart from all other clothing in order to avoid carrying toxins into the home and contaminating other clothing (chapter 11). If possible, run the washer through two extra cycles between washings. Better yet, demand that your employer wash your clothing and provide fresh, clean, uncontaminated clothing on a daily basis.

- **Self-employed workers:** If you are self-employed, as are many artists and craftspeople, take responsibility for your own safety. Know the hazards of the materials with which you work. Read labels carefully, request MSDSs on all products from the manufacturer, and know what precautions, safety gear, and clean-up procedures will help you avoid contamination. Use the safest materials and procedures possible. Stay current on new developments in your art or craft; safer, less toxic alternatives are being devised for many activities. Ventilate your workspace and keep it as clean as possible. Separate work and living areas and avoid eating, drinking, or smoking in your work space.

PART IV

Finding Out the Truth About Breast Cancer

13

The Politics of Breast Cancer: Setting a New Agenda

> *The Breast Cancer Prevention Program* presents the facts about all known and suspected causes of breast cancer. It emphasizes, as much as possible, the risks under your direct personal control—the risks you can avoid. You can begin today to reduce your risks for developing this devastating disease by making changes in the way you eat, exercise, and manage your health care.

After reading this book and seeing that the statistics and studies cited come from decades of available scientific literature and government reports, you are probably asking yourself some important questions. Why, for instance, are you just now hearing about all these avoidable risks? Why have United States government agencies like the NCI and FDA or powerful private charities like the ACS not publicized studies showing that mammograms can trigger the development of breast cancer? Or that ERT indeed increases risk for breast cancer? Why have the NCI or ACS not undertaken an educational campaign that focuses on dietary, environmental, and occupational contaminants known to cause breast cancer?

In this chapter, we answer those questions by looking at the politics of breast cancer: The behind-the-scenes agendas of the major breast cancer organizations that actively prevent you from receiving life-saving information about risk factors for breast cancer. Then we will show you how to take the initiative, lobby for change, and help develop national educational and action programs that have a true commitment to preventing breast cancer.

UNDERSTANDING THE CANCER ESTABLISHMENT

Two organizations, the NCI (the semiautonomous branch of the federal National Institutes of Health) and the ACS (the world's largest tax-exempt charity), control virtually all aspects of prevention, research, diagnosis, and treatment of breast and other cancers. Together with their extensive national network of well-funded clinics at major hospitals, universities, and cancer centers, these organizations comprise what we have termed the "cancer establishment."

How is it that the cancer establishment, with its overwhelming medical, educational, media, and financial resources, has failed to act on substantial scientific information about reducing risks of breast cancer? Perhaps the most fundamental reason is that both organizations retain a narrow and shortsighted fixation on diagnosis, treatment, and genetic research rather than on preventing avoidable causes of breast cancer. Another problem is that both organizations have developed strong links, both financial and scientific, to transnational pharmaceutical companies that manufacture, market, and promote anticancer drugs. Cancer treatment is big business, with multibillion-dollar annual cancer drug sales. Cancer prevention is very much less profitable, at least to big business.

Finally, the ACS, a so-called "charity," often places a higher priority on fund-raising than on good science, and often values money above the public's right to know the facts. This situation leaves American women with a cancer establishment that ignores their needs—even harms them—while claiming to protect them.

THE NATIONAL CANCER INSTITUTE

Since 1971, when President Richard Nixon inaugurated the "War On Cancer" and the National Cancer Program, taxpayers' dollars have lavishly funded the NCI. Today, its annual budget is more than $2 billion, of which it allocates less than 5 percent—less than $50 million—to primary prevention programs for all cancers.

The NCI's remarkable indifference to prevention led the federal General Accounting Office to warn that "there has been no progress in preventing the disease." In fact, even as NCI funding sharply increased over recent decades, the incidence of breast and other cancer has escalated to epidemic proportions. Nor has our ability to treat and cure most cancers materially improved.

In 1992, a group of sixty-five scientists (under the chairmanship of author Epstein), including Eula Bingham, Ph.D., former Assistant Secretary of Labor, OSHA; David Rall, M.D., Ph.D., former assistant Surgeon General; and Anthony Robbins, M.D., past director of the NIOSH, demanded that the government hold the NCI accountable for its lavish funding. The scientists urged that the NCI shift at least 50 percent of its $2 billion budget to programs directly aimed at the prevention of avoidable cancer:

> *We express grave concerns over the failure of the "war against cancer." . . . This failure is evidenced by the escalating incidence of cancer to epidemic proportions over recent decades. Paralleling and further compounding this failure is the absence of any significant improvement in the treatment and cure of the majority of all cancers. Notable exceptions are the successes with some relatively rare cancers, particularly those in children.*
>
> *A recent report by the American Hospital Association predicts that cancer will become the leading cause of death by the year 2,000 and the "dominant specialty" of American medicine. The costs in terms of suffering and*

*death and the inflationary impact of cancer, now esti-
mated at $110 billion annually (nearly 2 percent of the
GNP), is massive. These costs are major factors in the
current health care crisis, with per-case Medicare pay-
ments exceeding those of any other disease.*

*We express further concerns that the generously
funded cancer establishment, the NCI, the ACS, and
some twenty comprehensive cancer centers, have misled
and confused the public and Congress by repeated
claims that we are winning the war against cancer. In
fact, the cancer establishment has continually minimized the evidence for increasing cancer rates which it
has largely attributed to smoking and dietary fat, while
discounting or ignoring the causal role of avoidable
exposures to industrial carcinogens in the air, food,
water, and the workplace.*

*Furthermore, the cancer establishment and major
pharmaceutical companies have repeatedly made
extravagant and unfounded claims for dramatic
advances in the treatment and "cure" of cancer. Such
claims are generally based on an initial reduction in
tumor size ("tumor response") rather than on prolon-
gation of survival, let alone on the quality of life which
is often devastated by highly toxic treatments.*

Faced with mounting criticisms, the NCI finally admitted that it
had lost the war against cancer in its 1994 *Cancer at the Crossroads*
report. However, the NCI blamed not its own misdirected priorities,
but lack of funding from the White House and Congress. The NCI's
President's Cancer Panel Special Commission on Breast Cancer
urged that the NCI needed still more financial support for basic science research, but maintained that breast cancer was "*simply not a
preventable disease.*" The message from the NCI despaired:

*At this time, there are no proven methods of preventing
breast cancer. Advances in basic science have raised the*

realistic hope that more specific methods can be developed to treat . . . breast cancer. . . . Women in the United States should be provided with accurate, up-to-date and culturally sensitive information about the risks of breast cancer and how it is best detected. . . . Research funding of no less than $500 million [more] per year [is needed] for this program until these goals are achieved.

Excessive and disproportionate priority on basic science at the expense of prevention—if not indifference to prevention—is clearly evidenced by the candid views of the nation's leading basic molecular scientists and recipients of the cancer establishment's multimillion-dollar funding. In 1988, author Natalie Angier, in her book *Natural Obsession: The Search for the Oncogene*, quoted molecular biologist and Nobel Laureate David Baltimore as saying, "I have no idea when we'll know enough to develop anything that's clinically applicable, and I don't know who's going to do it. . . . It's not a high priority in my thinking." In the same book, molecular biologist M. Barbacid said, "If you're giving me money, I'll talk about cures. Since you're not, I won't. Talking about cures is absolutely offensive to me. In our work, we never think about such things even for a second."

Nobel Laureate Harold Varmus, now director of the National Institutes of Health (NIH), who determines the policies of the NCI and strongly influences those of the Department of Health and Human Services, was equally revealing about the NCI's priorities. He told Angier:

> *You can't do experiments to see what causes cancer. It's not an accessible problem, and it's not the sort of thing scientists can afford to do. You've got to live, and you've got to eat, you've got to keep your postdocs happy. Everything you do can't be risky.*

These and other leading cancer establishment scientists need only look at the highly successful campaign to reverse rates of heart disease to recognize the deep, if not irresponsible, flaws in their thinking. The

American Heart Association, together with the National Institute for Heart and Lung Diseases, constantly alert Americans about the need to exercise, stop smoking, and change their eating habits. They successfully lobbied to put pressure on the FDA to ensure that the amount of fat, cholesterol, and other nutrients on all food product labels are prominently indentified. However, no such labels identify breast or other carcinogens in food, nor do Americans receive warnings about the connections between a sedentary life-style, high-animal-fat and high-calorie diets, environmental pollutants, premenopausal mammograms and their risks for breast and other cancers.

Another problem with the NCI is that it continues to ignore the important role of environmental and occupational hazards as risk factors for breast and other cancers. Contrary to the explicit requirements of the 1971 National Cancer Act that no less than five members of the NCI's Advisory Board "shall be individuals knowledgeable in environmental carcinogenesis," its eighteen-member board remains virtually devoid of scientists and others concerned with and knowledgeable about environmental and occupational causes of cancer. Similarly lacking in such expertise is the current, and past, three-member executive President's Cancer Panel that controls NCI policies and priorities.

Of critical significance has been and remains the NCI's consistent refusal to provide any guidance to Congress and to regulatory agencies on scientific principles of cancer prevention and on the paramount need both to reduce avoidable and unknowing exposures to environmental and occupational carcinogens, and to inform the public of such avoidable exposures.

Noted epidemiologist and ex-senior NCI scientist Dr. John Bailar, now chairman of the Department of Health Sciences at the University of Chicago Medical School, echoed these criticisms of NCI's indifference to cancer prevention. At recent hearings by Senator Arlen Spector's (R-PA) subcommittee on Labor, Health, and Human Services, Dr. Bailar testified, "I'm convinced that a major emphasis in cancer research should be shifted from cancer treatment to cancer prevention. . . . The argument that the 'cure is just around the corner' is old now."

REVEALING THE CONFLICT OF INTEREST

A poorly recognized but basic conflict of interest further com-pounds the NCI's problems. For decades, powerful groups of inter-locking financial interests, with the highly profitable cancer drug industry at its hub, have dominated the war on cancer. By linking their priorities with those of major pharmaceutical companies (whose interest is focused on making a profit on cancer treatment and not on prevention), the NCI has directed its own priorities away from prevention.

The NCI's prototype Comprehensive Cancer Center, New York's Memorial Sloan-Kettering Hospital, represents just one example of how entrenched is this conflict of interest. Jointly funded by the NCI and ACS, the Sloan-Kettering annual budget exceeds $350 million—the equivalent of the combined total budgets of the nation's ten largest environmental organizations. Bristol-Myers Squibb, the world's largest manufacturer of cancer drugs and past manufacturer of carcinogenic breast implants, along with other major pharmaceutical companies, controls key positions on Memorial Sloan-Kettering's board. Other board members have close affiliations with oil, petrochemicals, and other industries, and the media. Further examples of this basic conflict of interest show up in employment and funding practices.

An Employment Revolving Door

A revolving door of employment between the cancer establishment and drug industry raises disturbing questions about conflict of interest among senior executives. Dr. Stephen Carter, now head of drug research and development at Bristol-Myers Squibb, for instance, previously served as director of NCI's Division of Cancer Treatment. He was followed in August 1994 by Dr. Richard Adamson, former Director of the Division of Cancer Etiology, who later left NCI to head the Washington office of the National Soft Drinks Association, an organization that vigorously promotes the use of artificial sweeteners, including the carcinogenic substance saccharin. After six years as NCI Director, Samuel Broder, M.D., resigned in April 1995 to become Vice President and Chief Scientific

Officer of IVAX Co. of Miami, a major manufacturer of cancer drugs. Broder was recruited to this new job by Dr. Phillip Frost, CEO of IVAX and key member of an NCI Advisory Board.

This pattern is not new. The late Dr. Frank Rauscher, who was appointed NCI Director by President Nixon to spearhead his "War On Cancer," resigned in 1976 to become Senior Vice President for Research of the ACS and moved from there in 1988 to become Executive Director of the Thermal Insulation Manufacturers Association, which promotes the use of carcinogenic fiberglass and fights against regulation of this material. The late oil magnate Armand Hammer, chairman of Occidental Petroleum, a major manufacturer of carcinogenic industrial chemicals and pesticides, chaired the President's Executive Cancer Panel of NCI in the 1980s. The previous chairman, for over a decade, was Benno C. Schmidt, an investment banker, senior drug company executive, and member of the Board of Overseers of the Memorial Sloan-Kettering Comprehensive Cancer Center. Not surprisingly, both Schmidt and Hammer showed little interest in cancer prevention research and programs.

Drug Development and Marketing

Using taxpayers' money, the NCI paid for the research and development of Taxol, an anticancer drug now manufactured by Bristol-Myers Squibb. Following the completion of clinical trials—an extremely expensive process in itself—the public paid further for developing the drug's manufacturing process. Once completed, NCI officials gave Bristol-Myers Squibb the exclusive right to sell Taxol at an inflationary price. As investigative journalist Joel Bleifuss wrote in a 1995 *In These Times* article, "Bristol-Myers Squibb sells Taxol to the public for $4.87 per milligram, which is more than 20 times what it costs to produce."

Taxol is not the only drug involved in such murky funding practices. Bristol-Myers Squibb now sells nearly one-third of the approximately thirty-five cancer drugs currently available, often with inflated profits, and often developed with taxpayer funds. In

1995, NIH director Harold Varmus decided that "reasonable pricing" clauses, which protect against pharmaceutical industry profiteering from drugs developed with taxpayer dollars, were driving away private industry. So he struck these from agreements between industry and the NCI. Now no controls on prices for cancer drugs made at taxpayers' expense exist. James P. Love of Ralph Nader's Center for Study of Responsive Law has extensively investigated conflicts of interest between the NIH, the NCI, and the cancer drug industry. In testimony before the Subcommittee on Regulation of Business Opportunity, and Technology of the Committee on Small Business of the United States House of Representatives, Love protested:

> *It is just one more example of NIH's efforts to accommodate the pharmaceutical industry's interest in a wide range of matters. . . . NIH sees itself as a partner with industry, and it has become highly sympathetic of the industry views on issues such as drug pricing and reporting requirements. Why is it that the U.S. government does not collect data on drug prices, does not routinely collect data on drug development costs, even for drugs developed with government funding, and does not express the slightest interest in these matters? There are . . . less benign reasons. NIH officials often seek employment in the private sector after their government service, or anticipate lucrative consulting arrangements with the private sector if they obtain a university appointment. What's good for the industry may eventually be good for them too. Indeed, as Dr. Robert Wittes has shown in the case of Taxol, one can work on a research project for NIH, then leave the government to help a drug company commercialize the discovery, and then return to the same government agency and begin a new research project.*

THE AMERICAN CANCER SOCIETY

Marching in lockstep with the NCI in its "war" on cancer is its "ministry of information," the ACS. With powerful media control and public relations resources, the ACS is the tail that wags the dog of the policies and priorities of the NCI. In addition, the approach of the ACS to cancer prevention reflects a virtually exclusive "blame the victim" philosophy. It emphasizes faulty lifestyle rather than unknowing and avoidable exposure to workplace or environmental carcinogens. Giant corporations, which profit handsomely while they pollute the air, water, and food with breast and other carcinogens, are greatly comforted by the silence of the ACS.

Indeed, despite promises to the public to do everything to "wipe out cancer in your lifetime," the ACS fails to make its voice heard in Congress and the regulatory arena. Instead, the ACS repeatedly rejects or ignores opportunities and requests from congressional committees, regulatory agencies, unions, and environmental organizations to provide scientific testimony critical to efforts to legislate and regulate a wide range of occupational and environmental carcinogens. This history of ACS unresponsivenes is a long and damning one, as shown by just a few examples:

- In 1977, the ACS called for a congressional moratorium on the FDA's proposed ban on saccharin and even advocated its use by nursing mothers and babies in "moderation" despite clear-cut evidence of its carcinogenicity in rodents. This reflects the consistent rejection by the ACS of the importance of animal evidence as predictive of human cancer risk.

- In 1978, Tony Mazzocchi, senior representative of the Oil, Chemical and Atomic Workers International Union, stated at a Washington, D.C., roundtable between public interest groups and high-ranking ACS officials: "Occupational safety standards have received no support from the ACS."

- In 1978, Congressman Paul Rogers censured the ACS for doing "too little, too late" in failing to support the Clean Air Act.

- In 1982, the ACS adopted a highly restrictive cancer policy that insisted on unequivocal human evidence of carcinogenicity before taking any position on public health hazards. Accordingly, the ACS trivializes or rejects evidence of carcinogenicity in experimental animals, and has actively campaigned against laws (the 1958 Delaney Law, for instance) that ban deliberate addition to food of any amount of any additive shown to cause cancer in either animals or humans.

- In 1983, the ACS refused to join a coalition of the March of Dimes, American Heart Association, and the American Lung Association to support the Clean Air Act.

- In 1993, just before PBS, *Frontline* aired the special, "In Our Children's Food," the ACS came out in support of the pesticide industry. In a damage-control memorandum sent to some forty-eight regional divisions, the ACS trivialized pesticides as a cause of childhood cancer, and reassured the public that carcinogenic pesticide residues in food are safe, even for babies. When the media and concerned citizens called local ACS chapters, they received reassurances from an ACS memorandum by its Vice President for Public Relations:

    The primary health hazards of pesticides are from direct contact with the chemicals at potentially high doses, for example, farm workers who apply the chemicals and work in the fields after the pesticides have been applied, and people living near aerially sprayed fields. . . . The American Cancer Society believes that the benefits of a balanced diet rich in

> *fruits and vegetables far outweigh the largely theo-*
> *retical risks posed by occasional, very low pesticide*
> *residue levels in foods.*

Charles Benbrook, former director of the National Academy of Sciences Board of Agriculture, worked on the pesticide report by the Academy of Sciences that the PBS special would preview. He charged that the role of the ACS as a source of information for the media representing the pesticide and product industry was "unconscionable." Investigative reporter Sheila Kaplan, in a 1993 *Legal Times* article, went further: "What they did was clearly and unequivocally over the line and constitutes a major conflict of interest."

TRACK RECORD OF THE AMERICAN CANCER SOCIETY ON BREAST CANCER PREVENTION

The track record of the ACS on breast cancer prevention, shared in general by the NCI, is equally dismal. It continually ignores or trivializes research on avoidable causes of breast cancer, in essence preventing American women from access to potentially life-saving information:

- In 1971, when studies unequivocally proved that diethylstilbestrol (DES) caused vaginal cancers in teenaged daughters of women administered the drug during pregnancy, the ACS refused an invitation to testify at congressional hearings to require the FDA to ban its use as an animal feed additive. It gave no reason for its refusal.

- In 1977 and 1978, the ACS opposed regulations proposed for hair coloring products that contained dyes known to cause breast cancer. In so doing, the ACS ignored virtually every tenet of responsible public health, as these chemicals were clear-cut liver and breast carcinogens.

- In 1992, the ACS issued a joint statement with the Chlorine Institute in support of the continued global use of organochlorine pesticides—despite clear evidence that some were known to cause breast cancer. In this statement, Society Vice President Clark Heath, M.D., dismissed evidence of this risk as "preliminary and mostly based on weak and indirect association." Heath then went on to explain away the blame for increasing breast cancer rates as due to better detection: "Speculation that such exposures account for observed geographic differences in breast cancer incidence or for recent rises in breast cancer occurence should be received with caution; more likely, much of the recent rise in incidence in the United States . . . reflects increased utilization of mammography over the past decade."

In its 1997 *Cancer Facts and Figures*, the ACS continues to insist that there are no known avoidable causes of breast cancer, and that there is little—except perhaps stopping smoking and reducing fat intake—that any individual woman can do to reduce her risk. Nonetheless, women and men alike continue to contribute to this short-sighted agency, making it one of the richest nonprofits in the world.

THE WORLD'S WEALTHIEST NONPROFIT AGENCY

The ACS is accumulating great wealth in its role as a "charity." According to James Bennett, professor of economics at George Mason University and recognized authority on charitable organizations, the ACS held a fund balance of over $400 million with about $69 million of holdings in land, buildings, and equipment in 1988. Of that money, the ACS spent only $90 million—26 percent of its budget—on medical research and programs. The rest covered "operating expenses," including about 60 percent for generous salaries, pensions, executive benefits, and overhead. By 1989, the cash reserves of the ACS were worth more than $700 million. In 1991, Americans, believing they were contributing to fighting cancer, gave nearly $350 million to the ACS, 6 percent more than the previous year. Most of this money comes from public donations of $100 or less. However, over the last two decades, an increasing proportion of the ACS budget comes from large corporations, including the pharmaceutical, cancer drug, telecommunications, and entertainment industries.

In 1992, *The Chronicle of Philanthropy* reported that the ACS was "more interested in accumulating wealth than in saving lives." Fundraising appeals routinely stated that the ACS needed more funds to support their cancer programs, all the while holding more than $750 million in cash and real estate assets.

Another 1992 article, this one in the *Wall Street Journal*, by Thomas DiLorenzo, professor of economics at Loyola College and veteran investigator of nonprofit organizations, revealed that the Texas affiliate of the ACS owned more than $11 million worth of assets in land and real estate, as well as more than fifty-six vehicles, including eleven Ford Crown Victorias for senior executives and forty-five other cars assigned to staff members. Arizona's ACS chapter spent less than 10 percent of its funds on direct community cancer services. In California, the figure was 11 percent, and under 9 percent in Missouri:

> *Thus for every $1 spent on direct service, approximately $6.40 is spent on compensation and overhead. In all ten states, salaries and fringe benefits are by far the largest single budget items, a surprising fact in light of the characterization of the appeals, which stress an urgent and critical need for donations to provide cancer services.*

Salaries and overhead for most ACS affiliates exceeded 50 percent, although most direct community services are handled by unpaid volunteers. DiLorenzo summed up his findings by emphasizing the hoarding of funds by the ACS:

> *If current needs are not being met because of insufficient funds, as fund-raising appeals suggest, why is so*

much cash being hoarded? Most contributors believe their donations are being used to fight cancer, not to accumulate financial reserves. . . . More progress in the war against cancer would be made if they would divest some of their real estate holdings and use the proceeds—as well as a portion of their case reserves—to provide more cancer services.

Today the cash reserves of the ACS approach one billion dollars. Yet its aggressive fund-raising campaign continues to lament the lack of available money for cancer research, while ignoring efforts to prevent cancer by phasing out avoidable exposures to environmental and occupational carcinogens. Meanwhile, the ACS is silent about its intricate relationships with the wealthy cancer drug, chemical, and other industries.

CONFLICTS OF INTEREST

Of the members of the ACS board, about half are clinicians, oncologists, surgeons, radiologists, and basic molecular scientists—and most are closely tied in with the NCI. Many board members and their institutional colleagues apply for and obtain funding from both the ACS and the NCI. Substantial NCI funds go to ACS directors who sit on key NCI committees. Although the ACS asks board members to leave the room when the rest of the board discusses their funding proposals, this is just a token formality. In this private club, easy access to funding is one of the "perks," and the board routinely rubber-stamps approvals. A significant amount of ACS research funding goes to this extended membership. Such conflicts of interest are evident in many ACS priorities, including their policy on mammography and their National Breast Cancer Awareness campaign.

Mammography

The ACS has close connections to the mammography industry. Five radiologists have served as ACS presidents, and in its every move, the ACS reflects the interests of the major manufacturers of mammogram machines and film, including Siemens, DuPont, General Electric, Eastman Kodak, and Piker. In fact, if every woman were to follow ACS and NCI mammography guidelines, the annual revenue to health care facilities would be a staggering $5 billion, including at least $2.5 billion for premenopausal women (chapter 5).

Promotions of the ACS continue to lure women of all ages into mammography centers, leading them to believe that mammography is their best hope against breast cancer. A leading Massachusetts newspaper featured a photograph of two women in their twenties in an ACS advertisement that promised early detection results in a cure "nearly 100 percent of the time." An ACS communications director, questioned by journalist Kate Dempsey, responded in an article published by the Massachusetts Women's Community's journal *Cancer*:

> *The ad isn't based on a study. When you make an advertisement, you just say what you can to get women in the door. You exaggerate a point. . . . Mammography today is a lucrative [and] highly competitive business.*

In addition, the mammography industry conducts research for the ACS and its grantees, serves on advisory boards, and donates considerable funds. DuPont also is a substantial backer of the ACS Breast Health Awareness Program; sponsors television shows and other media productions touting mammography; produces advertising, promotional, and information literature for hospitals, clinics, medical organizations, and doctors; produces educational films; and, of course, lobbies Congress for legislation promoting availability of mammography services. In virtually all of its important actions, the ACS has been strongly linked with the mammography industry, ignoring the development of viable alternatives to mammography.

The ACS exposes premenopausal women to radiation hazards from mammography with little or no evidence of benefits (chapter 5). The ACS also fails to tell them that their breasts will change so much over time that the "baseline" images have little or no future releveance. This is truly an American Cancer Society crusade. But against whom, or rather for whom?

National Breast Cancer Awareness Month

The highly publicized "National Breast Cancer Awareness Month" campaign further illustrates these institutionalized conflicts of interest. ACS and NCI representatives help sponsor promotional events, hold interviews, and stress the need for mammography every October. The flagship of this month-long series of events is National Mammography Day on October 17 in 1997.

Conspicuously absent from the public relations campaign of the National Breast Cancer Awareness Month is any information on environmental and other avoidable causes of breast cancer. This is no accident. Zeneca Pharmaceuticals—a spin-off of Imperial Chemical Industries, one of the world's largest manufacturers of chlorinated and other industrial chemicals, including those incriminated as causes of breast cancer—has been the sole multimillion-dollar funder of National Breast Cancer Awareness Month since its inception in 1984. Zeneca is also the sole manufacturer of tamoxifen, the world's top-selling anticancer and breast cancer "prevention" drug, with $400 million in annual sales (chapter 7) Furthermore, Zeneca recently assumed direct management of eleven cancer centers in United States hospitals. Zeneca owns a 50 percent stake in these centers, known collectively as Salick Health Care.

The link between NCI and Zeneca is especially strong when it comes to tamoxifen. The NCI continues aggressively to promote the tamoxifen trial, which is the cornerstone of its minimal prevention program. On March 7, 1997, the NCI Press Office released a four-page "For Response to Inquiries on Breast Cancer." The brief section on prevention reads:

> *Researchers are looking for a way to prevent breast cancer in women at high risk. . . . A large study [is underway] to see if the drug tamoxifen will reduce cancer risk in women age 60 or older and in women 35 to 59 who have a pattern of risk factors for breast cancer. This*

study is also a model for future studies of cancer prevention. Studies of diet and nutrition could also lead to preventive strategies.

Since Zeneca influences every leaflet, poster, publication, and commercial produced by National Breast Cancer Awareness Month, it is no wonder these publications make no mention of carcinogenic industrial chemicals and their relation to breast cancer. Imperial Chemical Industries, Zeneca's parent company, profits by manufacturing breast-cancer-causing chemicals. Zeneca profits from treatment of breast cancer, and hopes to profit still more from the prospects of large-scale national use of tamoxifen for breast cancer prevention. National Breast Cancer Awareness Month is a masterful public relations coup for Zeneca, providing the company with valuable, if ill-placed, good will from millions of American women.

MAINSTREAM WOMEN'S GROUPS

The National Alliance of Breast Cancer Organizations (NABCO) is an extensive network of breast cancer organizations providing information, assistance, and referral services. Established in January 1986, the network now numbers over 350 organizations and thousands of individual members. NABCO retains close links with the cancer establishment, the cancer drug industry, and other industry trade groups such as the Cosmetic, Toiletry and Fragrance Association and the breast implant industry.

In January 1991, NABCO played a major role in forming the National Breast Cancer Coalition, a national advocacy movement loosely modeled on AIDS activist groups. Shortly after its formation, Fran Visco, president of the coalition, testified before Congress that "women have declared war on breast cancer, and they'd better find a way to fund that war."

By June, the NCI and members of Congress joined the coalition to announce a challenge: To find the cause and reduce the incidence of breast cancer by 50 percent by the year 2000. In October 1993, 200 members of the coalition met with the President and Mrs. Clinton and Secretary of Health and Human Services Donna Shalala to deliver more than 2.6 million signatures in support of the coalition goal. The President accepted the signatures and, as a first step in the design of a National Action Plan on Breast Cancer, asked Secretary Shalala to host a summit that December.

Nearly five years later, the coalition's tremendous impact on breast cancer research is evident: Total federal spending on research, about $90 million a year in 1991, now approaches over $550 million, with more than $350 million coming from the NCI and the remainder from the Department of Defense. As an article in *Science* pointed out: "The Coalition's most spectacular success was to persuade Congress in 1992 to add $200 million to the Department of Defense's budget to fund a new breast cancer research program."
In addition, several coalition leaders now sit on the President's Cancer Panel and the National Cancer Advisory Board. Unfortunately, although its fund-raising techniques have proved splendid, the coalition remains as focused, like its partner the NCI, on diagnosis and treatment rather than prevention.

THE NATIONAL BREAST CANCER COALITION'S MISDIRECTED PRIORITIES

Like the cancer establishment, the coalition's research agenda and recommendations largely focus on genetic research and mammography, with minimal emphasis on prevention. The coalition's *Research Agenda* recently concluded: "We are unable to prevent breast cancer as little is known of its cause(s)."

When it does discuss prevention, the coalition calls for an indepth look at chemoprevention, development of a breast cancer vaccine, psychological and social support services, and investigation into the relationship between stress and breast cancer. The coalition makes no mention of phasing out breast-cancer-causing contaminants from air, water, food, and the workplace; avoiding premenopausal mammography; or understanding the dangers of hormonal contraceptives, ERT, and permanent dark hair dyes. By doing so, the coalition fails to tell women how to prevent breast cancer. The coalition's growing dependence on funding from such corporations as Revlon, Rhone-Poulenc, and Bristol-Myers Squibb makes it most unlikely that its emphasis will change in the future.

In a disturbing illustration of the coalition's policies and mindset, its president and member of President Clinton's Cancer Panel Special Commission on Breast Cancer, Fran Visco, strongly opposes congressional efforts to investigate environmental causes of breast cancer in scattered nationwide locations where high rates or clusters have been reported. She told a *New York Times* reporter in June 1997, "That's Congress deciding which science should be supported and which particular ideas warrant attention." Visco's views is that all such decisions should be left entirely to the NCI.

Although the coalition represents a welcome trend toward organized women's involvement in public health, its current goals remain too narrowly defined within the context of cancer establishment policies. The coalition needs broader and more radical strategies if it is to reverse the modern epidemic of breast cancer.

ACTIVIST GROUPS

Members of NABCO and the National Breast Cancer coalition include a loose network of regional and national activist women's groups with sharply differing priorities. These include National Women's Health Network, in Washington, D.C.; Women's Community Cancer Project in Boston; Women's Environment Development Organization; Breast Cancer Action in San Francisco; Massachusetts Breast Cancer coalition; and the Long Island Adelphi Breast Cancer Support Program.

Since 1993, the Women's Environment and Development Organization (WEDO) has worked to build coalitions among grassroots breast cancer activist groups, environmental organizations, and environmental justice groups throughout the nation. Led by former Congresswoman Bella Abzug, WEDO has held public hearings in New York City, Ann Arbor, Albuquerque, and Boston, among other United States cities. In collaboration with Canadian breast cancer activists, WEDO held a World Conference on Breast Cancer in Kingston, Ontario, July 12-17, 1997. More than 650 women from fifty-four countries met to hear presentations by leading scientists on environmental connections to breast cancer. Nancy Evans of San Francisco's Breast Cancer Action testified on behalf of the United States:

> *We are losing the war on cancer because we are fighting the wrong enemies. The cancer establishment has taught us to look for the enemy within—within our genes, or our unwise reproductive choices, or our stressful lifestyles. Although these factors may contribute to breast cancer and other cancers, our real enemies are faceless transnational corporations that spread their poisons around the globe in the name of free trade. . . .*

Together with other groups, notably the Cancer Prevention coalition in Chicago, activist groups like WEDO continue to attempt to redirect emphasis from diagnosis and treatment to prevention.

Spearheaded by the Cancer Prevention coalition, some groups are now calling for a boycott of the ACS to protest its indifference to prevention and its appalling conflicts of interest. Others continue to organize and conduct conferences that publicize information on avoidable risks of breast cancer. How much activists can influence the activities of mainstream groups, however, remains to be seen.

PERSONAL PROTECTION

WHAT YOU CAN DO

- Remain skeptical of the cancer establishment and its priorities.
- Become involved at the grassroots level.
- Lobby to change the cancer establishment and its practices.

LEARN ALL YOU CAN—AND GET INVOLVED

You are the best hope for the future of breast cancer prevention. As you have seen, the cancer establishments most of us look toward for direction—the NCI and the ACS—fail abysmally to provide objective and available information to the American public. Their priorities remain skewed by their interest in continued funding, as well as their ties to industries that make a profit from cancer. The next time you read a pamphlet from the NCI or ACS, keep this bias in mind.

In view of this, other organizations must become more involved in disseminating a wide range of available information on breast cancer prevention. The insurance industry, independent health care professional societies, and women's and public health activist organizations can all play a part in this effort. Without doubt, a huge step in the right direction would be to start educating our children about making sound lifestyle decisions that will help reduce their chances of developing breast or other cancers. You can become involved by lobbying any of the following groups or—even better—joining or starting an activist group yourself:

- **Schools and universities:** Breast cancer prevention should begin at a young age, and you can help make your local Parent Teachers Association aware of this. As soon as a young girl starts school, her teachers should encourage her to play sports and stay active. Her health education should include information about the relationship between unsafe food, weight, and exercise and breast cancer risk. Middle and high schools must provide information about the dangers of hormonal contraception, as well about safer and more effective methods of birth control. Parents and teachers alike should discuss alcohol use with adolescents, particularly the dangers of increasingly common weekend binge-drinking. Girls should learn how to perform breast self-examination from a trained nurse.

  These same fundamental methods of prevention should also be stressed in college, university, and adult education. Breast self-examination should be taught in community classes and its use emphasized as an alternative to mammography.

- **The insurance industry:** Another important source of information is the insurance industry, which often responds more quickly to public health needs than the government. By sponsoring a breast cancer prevention agenda, insurance companies would save the substantial money they now spend on treatment. Mutual of Omaha now funds a preventive approach to heart disease based on the work of nutrition specialist Dr. Dean Ornish. It is time to do the same for breast cancer prevention. Write a letter (or two or three!) to the president of your insurance company to offer that suggestion.

- **Activist public health groups:** The American Public Health Association, especially with its new activist president, Dr. Quentin Young, as well as the large, loose national network of public interest, environmental, labor, social justice, and women's groups, all should provide information to women through rallies, symposia, literature, and advertising. Help set the new agenda by joining (or starting) a group in your own neighborhood.

- **The religious community:** Churches, synagogues, and other religious groups should take an important lead in disseminating educational information, featuring speakers, offering courses, and providing educational materials. If you belong to a church or synagogue, discuss the matter with fellow members or religious leader. After all, cancer prevention is as much a concern of social justice and community standards as of science.

LOBBY TO CHANGE THE MEDICAL ESTABLISHMENT AND ITS PRACTICES

- **Reform medical consent forms:** Women must demand informed consent on a wide range of medical procedures and drugs, including premenopausal mammography, hormonal contraceptives, and ERT. In *The Journey Beyond Breast Cancer*, author V.M. Soffa, reveals that: "It seems women are still a long way from participating in truly informed consent. Although there are informed-consent laws in most states . . . some researchers report that 80 percent of patients are not told their options."

Informed consent requires that evidence of both benefits and risks be explicitly detailed to patients before they are administered or prescribed a medical drug or procedure. This is a legal, besides ethical, responsibility of all clinicians and the hospitals or institutions where they work. Neither the tamoxifen trial nor premenopausal mammography tests provide women with anything that currently meets even the minimal criteria of informed consent.

- **Pressure the consumer product industry to label all carcinogens:** Until the government makes consumer product labelling of carcinogens a reality, you should boycott foods and other consumer products known or suspected to contain carcinogenic ingredients and contaminants, and buy safer products. Get others in your neighborhood involved and pressure your local supermarket managers to make organic and nontoxic brands more available. More and more stores stock organic foods as demand for them grows. By voting with your shopping dollar, individually and collectively, you can reward companies that protect your health while punishing those that act with reckless disregard.

- **Reform the cancer establishment:** The policies and priorities of the NCI and ACS remain virtually unchanged after decades. Both remain committed to diagnosis, treatment, and basic genetic research and indifferent to cancer prevention. The 1992 coalition of scientists (see page 299) urged the NCI to shift at least 50 percent of its $2 billion budget to programs that have the control and prevention cancer as their primary goals. Their statement read, in part:

> *This major shift in direction should be initiated immediately and completed within the next few*

years. . . . A high priority for the cancer prevention program should be a large-scale and ongoing national campaign to inform and educate the media and the public, besides Congress, the Administration, and the industry, that much cancer is avoidable and due to past exposures to chemical and physical carcinogens in air, water, food, and the workplace, as well as to lifestyle factors.

There is no conceivable likelihood that such reforms will be implemented without legislative action. The National Cancer Act should be amended explicitly to re-orient the mission and priorities of the NCI to cancer cause and prevention. Compliance of the NCI should then be assured by detailed and ongoing Congressional oversight and, most critically, by House and Senate Appropriation committees. However, only strong support by the independent scientific and public health communities, together with concerned grassroots citizen groups, will convince Congress and Presidential candidates of the critical and immediate need for such drastic action.

One important step you can take to help reform the NCI is to lobby your representative in Congress—and urge members of your community to do so also. Well-organized pressure by grassroots groups targeted at the Senate and House Appropriations committees could help redirect the NCI's bloated budget, especially in view of unarguable evidence of escalating cancer incidence rates. Such scrutiny and accountability represents the only realistic method of forcing the NCI to redirect its priorities away from treatment and toward programs designed to reduce avoidable environmental and occupational exposures to breast and other carcinogens. You should urge congressional appropriation committees to progressively allocate 10 percent of the NCI's annual budget for exclusive use in primary prevention programs until funding for prevention reaches the same level as for all other programs combined.

The NCI continues to resist all such efforts. As an 1995 article in *Science* points out, the NCI could not even hit the NIH's mandate that 10 percent of its funds must be spent on prevention programs, and has asked Congress to drop the requirement. The government should enforce at least this minimal requirement. The annual budget of the NCI must be contigent upon a major shift in priorities and resources into cancer prevention—a shift independently verified by objective outside sources.

Reforming the ACS is more easily and directly achievable. Boycott the ACS and instead give your charitable contributions to public interest and environmental groups involved in prevention of breast and other cancers. The Women's Community Cancer Project, Breast Cancer Action, and the Cancer Prevention Coalition have already taken early steps in this direction. Such a boycott is well overdue, and will send the only message the ACS cannot ignore.

We hope this book has helped you achieve a sense of personal power and control over your health. We also hope that you take this sense of empowerment and act to change public policy and public attitudes. As Gloria Steinem wrote in her classic book, *Revolution from Within*, "In the '70s and '80s, we learned that the personal is political. In the '90s, the world must learn: the political is personal."

Appendix A: Resources

2: ESTROGEN: THE COMMON LINK

BREAST-FEEDING

These organizations provide important information and support for women who are breast-feeding.

> International Lactation Consultants Association
> 201 Brown Avenue
> Evanston, IL 60202
> (847) 492-1648

> *Provides referrals to board-certified breast-feeding counselors.*

> La Leche League International
> 9696 Minneapolis Avenue
> Franklin Park, IL 60131
> (708) 455-7730 or 1-(800)-LA LECHE

> *Provides information on breast-feeding.*

> Mothercare: The National Association of Postpartum Care Services
> Diana McQuiston
> 4414 Buston Court
> Indianapolis, IN 46254
> (317) 293-7763

> *Provides professional referrals.*

4: ESTROGEN REPLACEMENT THERAPY: PROS AND CONS

> American Menopause Foundation, Incorporated
> Madison Square Station
> P.O. Box 2013
> New York, NY 10010
> (212) 475-3107

> *Excellent source of information on alternatives to estrogen replacement therapy.*

9: EATING FOR HEALTH AND LONGEVITY

Many types of organic foods are now available by mail order and in stores. Contact the following purveyors for information on delivery to your area or for stores where their products can be found.

ORGANIC MEAT

Coleman Natural Meats
5140 Race Court, Unit 4
Denver, CO 80216
(303) 297-9393
(800) 442-8666

Organically raised beef and lamb available at stores nationwide. Call for retail outlet nearest you.

Garden Spot Distributors
438 White Oak Road
Box 729A
New Holland, PA 17557
(717) 354-4936

A wide variety of organic meat and poultry products, including whole chickens and turkeys, chicken and beef hot dogs, ground beef and bologna. No nitrites, coloring, fillings, or binders in any products. All organic grains fed to their animals. Will ship to some areas.

Harris Ranch Beef Company
P.O. Box 220
Selma, CA 93662
(800) 742-1955

Certified hormone-free meat. Call for retail outlet nearest you.

Homestead Farm
N1237 Chestnut Road
Pulaski, WI 54162
(920) 822-1998

Chicken, beef, and lamb free from hormones and antibiotics for the Green Bay and Shawano, Wisconsin, areas.

The Piper's Ranch of Maine
RR #1, Box 2180
Buckfield, ME 04220
(207) 336-2325

Walnut Acres
Penns Creek, PA 17862
(800) 433-3998
(717) 837-0601

Organic beef and poultry. Will ship to some areas.

Wolfe's Neck Farm
10 Burnett Road
Freeport, ME 04032
(207) 865-4469

Certified organic beef (air-shipped).

The Humane Farming Association
1550 California Street
San Francisco, CA 94109
(415) 771-CALF

Information on cruelty-free veal and other naturally raised farm animals.

ORGANIC DAIRY

Brier Run Farm
Route 1, Box 73
Birch River, WV 26610
(304) 649-2975

Organic goat cheese sold by mail nationwide. Also carried by many retail stores; call for specific locations.

Horizon Organic Dairy
P.O. Box 17577
Boulder, CO 80308
(303) 530-2711

Organic milk and yogurt available at health food stores nationwide and some supermarkets.

ORGANIC PRODUCE

Blooming Prairie Warehouse, Incorporated
2340 Heinze Road
Iowa City, IA 52240
(319) 337-6448

Organic produce by mail to Midwestern region.

Ecology Sound Farm
42126 Road 168
Orosi, CA 93647
(209) 528-3816

Organically grown navel and Valencia oranges, plums, Asian pears, Fuyu persimmons, and kiwi fruit available by mail nationwide.

Garden Spot Distributors
438 White Oak Road, Box 729A
New Holland, PA 17557
(717) 354-4936

Organically grown nuts, dried fruits, seeds, and beans. In shops, look for their retail brand name Shiloh Farms.

Jaffe Brothers
P.O. Box 636
Valley Center, CA 92082
(619) 749-1133

Organically grown dried fruits, nuts, and seeds by mail.

Star Organic Produce, Inc.
P.O. Box 561502
Miami, FL 33256-1502
(305) 262-1242

Tropical fruits organically grown in Florida.

Walnut Acres
Penns Creek, PA 17862
(800) 433-3998
(717) 837-0601

A wide variety of fresh produce available by mail. Walnut Acres is the exclusive mail-order distributor of Earth's Best organic baby food.

ORGANIC BABY FOOD

Earth's Best
P.O. Box 887
Middlebury, VT 05753
(800) 442-4221

ORGANIC WINE

Chartrand Imports
P.O. Box 1319
Rockland, ME 04841
(800) 473-7307
(207) 594-7300

Mail-order distributor for French and Californian organic wines.

Four Chimneys Farm Winery
R.D. 1, Hall Road
Himrod-on-Seneca, NY 14842
(607) 243-7502

Vintage wines with no added sulfites, available by mail throughout the country.

Frey Vineyard
14000 Tomki Road
Redwood Valley, CA 95470
(707) 485-5177

Organic wines available nationwide. Call for information on local retail outlets.

The Organic Wine Company
54 Genoa Place
San Francisco, CA 94133
(415) 433-0167

Mail-order distributor for French and Californian organic wines.

ORGANIC COFFEE

Royal Blue Organics
P.O. Box 21123
Eugene, OR 97402
(503) 689-1836
(800) 392-0117

CERTIFIERS OF WATER FILTERS

National Sanitation Foundation
3475 Plymouth Road
P.O. Box 130140
Ann Arbor, MI 48105
(313) 769-8010

Provides third-party certification of water filters. Ask for their list of certified products.

Water Quality Association
4151 Naperville Road
Lisle, IL 60532
(708) 505-0160

Will send you general information about water quality problems and point-of-use technologies that can be used in the home or office.

10: LIFESTYLE RISK FACTORS AND COPING STRATEGIES

The following companies manufacture hair dyes and cosmetics that are free of the carcinogens sometimes found in conventional products. Call each company directly to find the retail outlet nearest you.

SAFE HAIR COLORING PRODUCTS

Light Mountain Henna Gray
Lotus Brands, Inc.
P.O. Box 325
Twin Lakes, WI 53181
(414) 889-8561

Henna products for gray hair.

Paul Penders
1340 Commerce Street
Petaluma, CA 94954
(707) 763-5828
Fax: (707) 763-5839

Herbal rinse-in colors.

Schwarzkopf, Incorporated
5701 Buckingham Parkway
Suite E
Culver City, CA 90230
(800) 234-4672

Herbal hair colorings.

VitaWave
P.O. Box 5206
Ventura, CA 93005
(818) 886-3808

(805) 981-1472

Permanent hair coloring.

SAFE COSMETIC LINES

Aubrey Organics
4419 N. Manhattan Avenue
Tampa, FL 33614
(800) 282-7394

Full line of cosmetics.

Ecco Bella Botanicals, Incorporated
1133 Route 23
Wayne, NJ 07470
(201) 696-7766

Complete line of safe cosmetics.

11: WHERE YOU LIVE

These companies are sources for safer cleaning products free of potential breast carcinogens.

Allergy Relief Shop
2932 Middlebrook Pike
Knoxville, TN 37921
(423) 522-2795

Offers a wide range of products by mail.

Seventh Generation
49 Hercules Drive
Colchester, VT 05446
(802) 655-3116
(800) 456-1177

Products sold in health food stores and by mail.

12: HAZARDS IN THE WORKPLACE

For information on safety in the workplace, contact these organizations.

National Institute for Occupational Safety and Health
1-(800)-35-NIOSH

For information on occupational safety and health problems, ask for the free comprehensive NIOSH Pocket Guide to Chemical Hazards.

Center for Safety in the Arts
5 Beekman Street, Suite 1030
New York, NY 10038

Offers information on the use of safe artists' materials and methods.

Arts, Crafts and Theater Safety
181 Thompson Street, #23
New York, NY 10012

Offers information on the use of safe artists' materials and methods.

National Coalition Against the Misuse of Pesticides
701 East Street, SE
Washington, D.C. 20003
(202) 543-5450

Publishers excellent materials on pesticides in our schools.

Appendix B. Activist Breast Cancer Groups

Bay Area Breast Cancer Network
4010 Moore Park Avenue
San Jose, CA 95117
(408) 261-1425

Boston Women's Health Book Collective
240A Elm Street
Sommerville, MA 02144
(617) 625-0277

Breast Cancer Action
55 New Montgomery Street, Suite 323
San Francisco, CA 94105
(415) 243-9301

Cancer Control Society
2043 North Berendon Street
Los Angeles, CA 90027
(213) 663-7801

Cancer Prevention Coalition
520 North Michigan Avenue, Suite 410
Chicago, IL 60611
(312) 467-0600

Greenpeace
847 West Jackson Boulevard
Chicago, IL 60607
(312) 563-6060

Jacobs Institute of Women's Health
409 12th Street SW
Washington, DC 20024
(202) 863-4990

Long Island Breast Cancer Action Coalition
Nassau County Medical Center
2201 Hempstead Turnpike
East Meadow, NY 11554
(516) 357-9622

Massachusetts Breast Cancer Coalition
Pioneer Valley
P.O. Box 536
Leeds, MA 01053
(413) 585-1222

Men's Crusade Against Breast Cancer
4502 Fidelity Court
Annandale, VA 22003
(703) 978-3336

Mothers for Natural Law
P.O. Box 1177
Fairfield, IA 52556
(515) 472-2809

National Black Women's Health Project
1211 Connecticut Avenue NW, Suite 310
Washington, DC 20036
(202) 835-0117

National Organization for Women
1000 16th Street NW
Suite 700
Washington, DC 20036
(202) 331-0066

National Silicone Implant Foundation
4416 Willow Lane
Dallas, TX 75244
(972) 490-0800

National Women's Health Network
1325 G Street NW
Washington, DC 20005
(202) 347-1140

Save Our Selves
P.O. Box 214479
Sacramento, CA 95821
(916) 334-2273

Triad Silicone Network
P.O. Box 7631
Greensboro, NC 27417
(910) 854-5338

United Silicone Survivors of the World
6940 Silver Ridge Circle
Alexandria, VA 22315
(703) 922-5260

Women's Cancer Resource Center
1815 East 41st Street, Suite C
Minneapolis, MN 55407
(800) 908-8544

Women's Community Cancer Project
46 Pleasant Street
Cambridge, MA 02139
(617) 354-9888

Women's Environment & Development Organization
845 Third Avenue, 15th Floor
New York, NY 10022
(212) 759-7982

Women's Issues Network Foundation
359 West Chicago Avenue, Suite 201
Chicago, IL 60610
(312) 944-4868

Notes

INTRODUCTION

Page x   What we've learned doesn't translate into public health advice: Willet, W. cited in Liebman, B. "Breast cancer." *Nutrition Action Health Letter*, 1996;23(1):1, 4–7.

1: DETERMINING YOUR RISK

Page 6   Women may not be able to alter their personal risk factors: *Cancer Facts and Figures*. American Cancer Society, 1996.

Page 13   A woman carrying one of three alterations: Nelson, N.J. "Cancer risk high, but lower than expected with breast cancer genes." *New England Journal of Medicine*, 1997;89(10):680–681.

Page 13   Researchers linked increased breast cancer risk to CYP1: "Estrogen gene tied to breast cancer." *The New York Times*, March 26, 1997:A17.

Page 13   Breast density is risk factor: Pankow, J.S., *et al.* "Genetic analysis of mammographic breast density in adult women: Evidence of a gene defect." *Journal of the National Cancer Institute*, 1997;89(8): 549–556.

Page 15   Rather than thinking of DNA as a rigid structure: PR Newswire. "Potentially cancer-causing damage common in breast." January 8, 1995.

Page 15   Where you live and breast cancer risk: Kliewer, E.V., and Smith, K.R. "Breast cancer mortality among immigrants in Australia and Canada." *Journal of the National Cancer Institute*, 1995;87(15): 1154–1161.

Page 15   Risk for developing breast cancer changes dramatically with age: Marshall, E. "Epidemiology. Search for a killer: Focus shifts from fat to hormones." *Science*, 1993;259(5095):618–620.

2: ESTROGEN

Page 22   Estrogen-dependent breast cancer increase of 130 percent: Glass, A.G. "Rising incidence of breast cancer: Relationship to state and receptor status." *Journal of the National Cancer Institute*, 1990; 82(8):693–696.

Page 22   DHEA is also involved in the onset of puberty: Marano, H.A. "Puberty may start at 6 as hormones surge." *The New York Times*, July 1, 1997:B1.

Page 26   The body produces two different chemical types of estradiol: Davis, D.L., and Bradlow, H.L. "Can environmental estrogens cause breast cancer?" *Scientific American*, October 1, 1995; Bradlow, H.L., *et al*. "16a–hydroxylation of estradiol: A possible risk marker for breast cancer." In *Endocrinology of the Breast: Basic and Clinical Aspects*, ed. A. Angeli, *et al. Annals of the New York Academy of Sciences*, 1986:464:138; Bradlow, H.L., *et al*. "Re; estrogen metabolism and excretion in oriental and caucasian women." *Journal of the National Cancer Institute*, 86(21):1643–1644; Taioli, E., *et al*. "Ethnic differences in estrogen metabolism in healthy women." *Journal of the National Cancer Institute*, 1996;86:617.

Box

Page 26   Taking the birth control pill increases your risk: Rinzler, C.A. *Estrogen and Breast Cancer: A Warning to Women*. New York: Macmillan, 1993.

Page 26   In 1991: Steinberg, K.K., *et al*. "A metaanalysis of the effect of estrogen replacement therapy on the risk of breast cancer." *Journal of the American Medical Association*, 1991;265:1985–1990.

Page 26   In 1995: Brinton, L.A. "Oral contraceptives and breast cancer risk among young women. *Journal of the National Cancer Institute*, 1995;87(11):827–835.

End Box

Page 27   Pseudoestrogens trigger both normal and abnormal cell divisions: Sotao, A.M., and Sonnenschein, C. "The role of estrogen in the proliferation of human breast tumor cells (MCF-7)." *Journal of Steroid Biochemistry*, 1985;23:87–94.

Page 27   Pseudoestrogens stimulate the production of "bad estrogen": Davis, D.L., and Bradlow, H.L. "Avoidable environmental links to breast cancer." In *Reducing Breast Cancer Risk in Women*, ed. B.A. Stoll. Dordrecht, Netherlands: Kluwer Academic Publishers, 1995:231–235.

Page 27   Certain plants contain chemicals that act like estrogen: Kaldas, R.S., and Hughes, C.L. "Reproductive and general metabolic effects of phytoestrogens in mammals." *Reproductive Toxicology*,

1989;3:81–89; Aldercreutz, H., *et al.* "Determination of urinary lignans and phytoestrogen metabolites, potential antiestrogens and anticarcinogens, in urine of women on various habitual diets." *Journal of Steroid Biochemistry*, 1986;24(5b):791–797.

Page 27   Phytoestrogens increase production of "bad estrogen": Davis, D.L., and Bradlow, H.L. "Can environmental estrogens cause breast cancer?" *Scientific American*, 1995;273(4):167–172.

Page 27   Estrogen ends up being scavenged by proteins: Physicians Committee for Responsible Medicine. "Estrogen dangers *before* and after menopause." Press release, Washington, D.C., June 23, 1995.

Page 29   Exposure to estrogenic pollutants: Dewailly, É, *et al.* "Could the rising levels of estrogen receptor in breast cancer be due to estrogenic pollutants?" *Journal of the National Cancer Institute*, 1997;89(12):888.

Page 29   Estrogen receptors have profound influences: *Ibid.*

Page 29   Your "natural estrogen window": Korenman, S.G. "Estrogen window hypothesis of the aetiology of breast cancer." *The Lancet*, 1980:700–701.

Page 30   Fewer than 30 percent of breast cancer cases related to genetic or reproductive risk factors: Madigan, M.P., *et al.* "Proportion of breast cancer cases in the United States explained by well-established risk factors." *Journal of the National Cancer Institute*, 1995;87(22):1681–1686.

Page 30   Most women who have breast cancer have few traditional risk factors: Reuter, K.L., *et al.* "Risk factors for breast cancer in women undergoing mammography." *American Journal of Roentgenology*, 1992;158:273–278.

Page 32   Average age of menarche has declined: Giddens-Herman, M.E., *et al.* "Secondary sexual characteristics and menses in young girls seen in office practice." *Pediatrics*, 1997;88(4):505–511.

Page 33   Earlier menstruation elevates risk: Kelsey, J.L., *et al.* "Reproductive factors and breast cancer." *Epidemiologic Reviews*, 1993;338: 389–394.

Page 33   Early menarche doubles risk compared to late menarche: Willet, W. "The search for the causes of breast and colon cancer." *Nature*, 1989:338:389–394.

Page 33   High fiber, low animal fat diets, and later menarche: Hughes, R.E. "A new look at dietary fiber." *Human Nutrition: Clinical Nutrition*, 1986;40C:81–86.

Page 34   Breast cancer mortality and high birth rates: Blot, W.J., *et al.* "Geographic patterns of breast cancer in the U.S." *Journal of the National Cancer Institute,* 1977;59(5):1407–1411.

Page 34   20 to 70 percent higher risk in childless women over the age of 45: Kelsey, J.L., *et al.* "Reproductive factors and breast cancer." *Epidemiological Reviews,* 1993;15(1):36–47.

Page 34   Initial estrogen surge at the very beginning of pregnancy: *Ibid.*

Page 35   Progesterone helps to mature breast cells: Petrakis, N.L., *et al.* "Influence of pregnancy and lactation on serum and breast fluid esterogen levels: Implications for breast cancer risk." *International Journal of Cancer,* 1987;40:587–591.

Page 35   A strong connection exists between later ages of childbearing: Frazier, A.L., and Colditz, G.A. "Shifting the time frame of breast cancer prevention to youth." In *Reducing Breast Cancer Risk in Women,* ed. B.A. Stoll. Dordrecht, Netherlands: Kluwer Academic Publishers, 1995.

Page 35   The younger you are when you have your first child: Kelsey, J. *et al.* "Reproductive factors and breast cancer." *Epidemiology Reviews,* 1993;15:36–47; MacMahon, B. "Breast cancer at menopausal ages: An explanation of observed incidence changes." *Cancer,* 1957;10:1037–1044; Hahn, R.A., and Moolgavkar, S.H. "Nulliparity, decade of first birth, and breast cancer in Connecticut cohorts, 1855 to 1945: An ecological study." *American Journal of Public Health,* 1989;79(11):1503–1507; Blot, W.J., *et al.* "Geographic patterns of breast cancer in the U.S." *Journal of the American Cancer Institute,* 1977;59(5):1407–1411.

Page 35   Women who have their first child after age 35: MacMahon, B., *et al.* "Age at first birth and breast cancer risk." *Bulletin of World Health Organization,* 1970;43:209–221.

Page 36   Increased risk with late first pregnancy is short-lived: Bruzzi, P., *et al.* "Short term increase in risk of breast cancer after full-term pregnancy." *British Medical Journal,* 1988;47:757–762.

Page 36   Women who have five full-term pregnancies: LaVecchia, C.L., *et al.* "Reproductive factors and breast cancer: An overview." *Soz Praventivmed,* 1989;34:101–107.

Page 36   "Women with a positive family history": Colditz, G.A., *et al.* "Risk factors for breast cancer according to family history of breast cancer." *Journal of the National Cancer Institute,* 1996;88(6): 365–371.

Page 36   Abortion doubles risk of breast cancer in women under 33: Pike, M.C., *et al.* "Oral contraceptive use and early abortion as risk factors for breast cancer in young women." *British Journal of Cancer*, 1981;43:72–76.

Page 36   An analysis of twenty-three studies of abortion: *The New York Times*, October 12, 1996:8.

Page 37   Pregnancy terminated by a surgical abortion: Brinton, L.A., *et al.* "Reproductive factors in the aetiology of breast cancer." *British Journal of Cancer*, 1983;47:757–762; Daling, J.R., *et al.* "Risk of breast cancer among young women: Relationship to induced abortion." *Journal of the National Cancer Institute*, 1994;86(21): 1584–1592.

Page 37   Rats who had interrupted pregnancies suffered accelerated breast cancer development: Russo, J., *et al.* "Susceptibility of the mammary gland to carcinogenesis. I Differentiation of the mammary gland as determinant of tumor incidence and type of lesion. II Pregnancy interruption as a risk factor in tumor incidence." *American Journal of Pathology*, 1980;100:497–512;721–736.

Page 38   Breast-feeding for seventeen months reduced risk by 30 percent: Brinton, L.A., *et al.* "Breast-feeding and breast cancer risk." *Cancer Causes and Control*, 1995;6:199–208.

Page 38   Breast-feeding and lower levels of DDE in breast milk: Dewailly, É., *et al.* "Protective effect of breast-feeding on breast cancer and body burden of carcinogenic organochlorides." *Journal of the National Cancer Institute*, 1994;86(10):803.

Box

Page 39   In 1977: Petrakis, N.L., et al. "Breast secretory activity in non-lactating women, postpartum involution, and the epidemiology of breast cancer." *National Cancer Institute Monograph*, 1977;47: 161–164.

Page 39   In 1986: Newcomb, P.A. "Pregnancy termination in relation to risk of breast cancer." *Journal of the American Medical Association*, 1986;275;4:283–287.

Page 39   In 1988: Yuan, J.M., *et al.* "Risk factors for breast cancer in Chinese women in Shanghai." *Cancer Research*, 1988;48:1949–1953.

Page 39   In a 1989 issue: Siskind, V., *et al.* "Breast cancer and breast-feeding: Results from an Australian case-control study." *American Journal of Epidemiology*, 1989;130:229–236.

Page 39   In 1992: Yoo, K.Y., *et al.* "Independent protective effect of lactation against breast cancer in young women." *American Journal of Epidemiology*, 1992;135(7):726–733.

Page 39   In 1993: United Kingdom National Case-Control Study Group. "Breast-feeding and risk of breast cancer in young women." *British Medical Journal*, 1993;307:17–20.

Page 39   In 1994: Newcomb, P.A., *et al.* "Lactation and a reduced risk of premenopausal breast cancer." *New England Journal of Medicine*, 1994;330(2):81–87

END BOX

Page 41   Women with a family history of breast cancer: Colditz, , G.A., *et al.* "Risk factors for breast cancer according to family history of breast cancer." *Journal of the National Cancer Institute*, 1996;88(6):365–371.

Page 42   Only 50 percent of American women breast-fed their babies in 1994: Short, R.V. "Breast-feeding." *Scientific American*, 1994;250(4):35–41.

3: THE PILL

Page 45   "No Link Is Found": Gilbert, S. "No link is found between pill and breast cancer." *The New York Times*, September 25, 1996:B6.

Page 45   Relationship between "breast cancer risk and hormone exposure": "Breast cancer and hormonal contraceptives: Collaborative reanalysis of individual data on 53,297 women with breast cancer and 110,239 women without breast cancer from 54 epidemiological studies." *The Lancet*, 1996;347(9017):1713–1727.

Page 48   Medical establishment and press endorsed FDA's approval: Epstein, S.S. *The Politics of Cancer.* San Francisco: Sierra Club, 1978.

Page 48   The American Medical Association official stamp of approval: Lawless, E.W. *Technology and Social Shock.* New Brunswick, NJ: Rutgers University Press, 1977:30.

Page 48   Barbara Seaman investigated the industry: Seaman, B. *The Doctors' Case Against the Pill.* Alameda, CA: Hunter House, 1995 (originally published in 1969).

Page 49   A massive endocrinologic experiment: Asbell B. *The Pill: A Biography of the Drug that Changed the World.* New York: Random House, 1995:305.

Page 49   More than 11 million women are currently using the Pill: "Facts in brief." *Alan Guttmacher Institute Journal*, March 15, 1993.

Page 50   Six rhesus monkeys given standard doses: Hertz, R. "The problem of oral contraceptives on cancer of the breast." *Cancer*, 1969: 1140–1145.

Page 50   Inadequate knowledge concerning the relationship of estrogen to cancer: *Ibid.*

Page 51   "No other drug effect so readily reproducible": "The 'new' esterogens: Are they safer?" *Medical Letter*, 1976;18(11):45–46.

Page 51   More than twenty well-controlled studies demonstrated clear risks: Wolfe, S.M., *et al. Women's Health Alert.* Washington, D.C.: Public Citizen Health Research Group, 1991:133; Paffenbarger, R.S., *et al.* "Cancer risk as related to use of oral contraceptives during fertile years." *Cancer*, 1977;39:1887–1891; Pike, M.C., *et al.* "Oral contraceptive use and early abortion as risk factors for breast cancer in young women." *British Journal of Cancer*, 1981;43:72–76; Harris, N.V., *et al.* "Breast cancer in relation to patterns of contraceptive use." *American Journal of Epidemiology*, 1982;116:643–651; Meirik, O., *et al.* "Oral contraceptive use and breast cancer in young women. A joint national case-control study in Sweden and Norway." *The Lancet*, 1986;ii:650–654; Lipnick, R.J. *et al.* "Oral contraceptives and breast cancer. A prospective cohort study." *Journal of the American Medical Association*, 1986;225(1):58–61; McPherson, K., *et al.* "Early contraceptive use and breast cancer: Results of another case control study." *British Journal of Cancer*, 1987;56:653–660; Kay, C.R., and Hannaford, P.C. "Breast cancer and the Pill—a further report from the Royal College of General Practitioners' oral contraceptive study." *British Journal of Cancer*, 1988;58:675–680; Ravnihar, B., *et al.* "A case-control study of breast cancer in relation to oral contraceptive use in Slovenia." *Neoplasia*, 1988;35(1):109–121; Stadel, B.V. "Oral contraceptives and premenopausal breast cancer in nulliparous women." *Contraception*, 1988;38(3):287–299; Olsson, H., *et al.* "Early oral contraceptive use and breast cancer among premenopausal women: Final report from a study in southern Sweden." *Journal of the National Cancer Institute*, 1989;81:1000–1004; UK National Case-Control Study Group. "Oral contraceptive use and risk of breast cancer in young women." *The Lancet*, 1989;1:974–982; Romieu, I., *et al.* "Prospective study of oral contraceptive use and risk of breast cancer in women." *Journal of the National Cancer Institute*, 1989;81(17):1313–1321; Miller, D.R., *et al.* "Breast cancer before age 45 and oral contraceptive use: New findings." *American Journal of Epidemiology*, 1989;129:269–280; Standford, J.L., *et al.* "Oral contraceptives and breast cancer: Results from an expanded case-control study." *British Journal of Cancer*, 1989;60:375–381; Romieu, I., *et al.* "Oral contraceptives and breast cancer. Review and metaanalysis." *Cancer*, 1990; (66)2253–2263; Thomas, D.B. "The WHO collaborative study of neoplasia and steroid contraceptives: The influence of combined oral contraceptives on risk of neoplasms in developing and developed countries." *Contraception*, 1991;43(6):695–710; White, E., *et al.* "Breast cancer among young U.S. women in relation to oral contraceptive use." *Journal of the National Cancer Institute*, 1994;86(7);505–514; Brinton, L.A. "Oral contraceptives and breast cancer risk among younger women." *Journal of the National Cancer Institute*, 1995;87(11):827–835.

Page 51   Postmenopausal women are also at increased risk: Associated Press. "New link between pill and cancer reported." *The New York Times*, May 6, 1989:8Y; McGonigle, K.F., and Huggins, G.R. "Choosing hormone contraception." In *Reducing Breast Cancer Risk in Women*, ed. B.A. Stoll; Dordrecht, Netherlands: Kluwer Academic Publishers, 1995:155–164; Romieu, I., *et al.* "Oral contraceptives and breast cancer: Review and metaanalysis." *Cancer*, 1990; 66:2253; Paul, C., *et al.*, "Oral contraceptives and risk of breast cancer." *International Journal of Cancer*, 1990;46:366; Kay, C.R., and Hannaford, P.C. "Breast cancer and the pill—a further report from the Royal College of General Practitioners' oral contraceptive study." *British Journal of Cancer*, 1988;58:675.

Box

Page 51   In 1977: Paffenberger, R.S., *et al.* "Cancer risk as related to use of oral contraceptives during fertile years." *Cancer*, 1977;39: 1887–1891.

Page 51   A 1981 study: Pike, M.C., *et al.* "Oral contraceptive use and early abortion as risk factors for breast cancer in young women." *British Journal of Cancer*, 1981;43;72–76.

Page 52   In 1982: Harris, N.V., *et al.* "Breast cancer in relation to patterns of contraceptive use." *American Journal of Epidemiology*, 1982; 116:643–651.

Page 52   In 1986: Meirik, O., *et al.* "Oral contraceptive use and breast cancer in young women. A joint national case-control study in Sweden and Norway." *The Lancet*, 1986;ii:650–654.

Page 52   A 1987 study: McPherson, K., *et al.* "Early contraceptive use and breast cancer: Results of another case control study." *British Journal of Cancer,* 1987;56:653–660.

Page 52   A 1988 study: Ravnihar, B., *et al.* "A case-control study of breast cancer in relation to oral contraceptive use in Slovenia." *Neoplasia,* 1988;35(1):109–121.

Page 52   In 1988: Stadel, B.V. "Oral contraceptives and premenopausal breast cancer in nulliparous women." *Contraception,* 1988;38 (3):287–299.

Page 52   In 1989: Olsson, H., *et al.* "Early oral contraceptive use and breast cancer among premenopausal women: Final report from a study in southern Sweden." *Journal of the National Cancer Institute,* 1989;81:1004.

Page 52   In 1990: Romieu, I., *et al.* "Oral contraceptives and breast cancer. Review and metaanalysis." *Cancer,* 1990:2253–2263.

Page 52   In 1991: Thomas, B.D. "The WHO (World Health Organization) collaborative study of neoplasia and steroid contraceptives: The influence of combined oral contraceptives on risk of neoplasms in developing and developed countries." *Contraception,* 1991;43 (6):695–710.

Page 53   In 1994: White, E., *et al.* "Breast cancer among young U.S. women in relation to oral contraceptive use." *Journal of the National Cancer Institute,* 1994;86(7);505–514.

Page 53   In 1995: Brinton, L.A. "Oral contraceptives and breast cancer risk among young women." *Journal of the National Cancer Institute,* 1995;87(11):827–835.

END BOX

Page 53   Stroke and blood clots risk: Royal College of General Practitioners. *Oral Contraceptives and Health.* New York: Pitman, 1974; Seaman, B., and Seaman, G. *Women and the Crisis in Sex Hormones.* New York: Bantam Books, 1977:85–86, 98–99, 107–112, 151–152.

Page 53   Heart attack risk: Drife, J. "Benefits and risks of oral contraceptives." *Advances in Contraception,* 1990, suppl. 6:15–25.

Page 53   Diabetic-type changes risk: Seaman, B., and Seaman, G. *Women and the Crisis in Sex Hormones.* New York: Bantam Books, 1977:87–88, 117–118, 133, 138.

Page 53   Gallbladder disease risk: *Ibid.*: 125–126.

Page 53   Liver cancer risk: Baum, J.K., *et al.* "Possible association between benign hepatomas and oral contraceptives." *The Lancet,*

1973;2(835):926–929; Stauffer, J.Q., *et al.* "Focal nodular hyperplasia of the liver and intrahepatic hemorrhate in young women on oral contraceptives." *Annals of Internal Medicine,* 1975;83 (3):301–306; Antoniades, K., *et al.* "Liver cell adenoma and oral contraceptives. Double tumor development." *Journal of the American Medical Association,* 1975;234(6):628–629; Americks, J.A., *et al.* "Hepatic cell adenomas, spontaneous liver rupture, and oral contraceptives. *Archives of Surgery,* 1975;110(5)548–557; Sherlock, S. "Hepatic adenomas and oral contraceptives." *Gut,* 1975;16(9):753–756.

Page 53   Depression risk: Seaman, B., and Seaman, G. *Women and the Crisis in Sex Hormones.* New York: Bantam Books, 1977:99, 123–124, 132–133, 135.

Page 53   Increased susceptibility to venereal disease: Rosenberg, M.J., and Gollub, E.L. "Commentary: Methods women can use that may prevent sexually transmitted disease, including HIV." *American Journal of Public Health,* 1992;82:1473–1478.

Page 54   Increased risk of breast cancer through breast-feeding: Ekbom, A., *et al.* "Evidence of prenatal influences on breast cancer risk." *The Lancet,* 1992;340:1015–1018.

Page 54   Lower hormone doses have not solved all problems: Seaman, B. *The Doctors' Case Against the Pill.* Alameda, CA: Hunter House, 1995:212–238.

Page 54   Accumulated effect by age 60 is worse: Wolfe, S.M., *et al. Women's Health Alert.* Washington, DC: Public Citizen Health Research Group, 1991:135.

Page 55   Questions about the Pill's association with cancer: Asbell, B. *The Pill: A Biography of the Drug that Changed the World.* New York: Random House, 1995:310.

Page 55   The third-generation Pill may be just as dangerous or more so: Moore, S.D. "Oral contraceptive draws warning in Germany, U.K." *Wall Street Journal,* October 24, 1995:B8.

Page 56   Women taking progestin-only contraceptives run a 30 percent increased risk: Cancer and Steroid Hormone Study of the Centers for Disease Control and the National Institute of Child Health and Human Development. "Oral contraceptive use and the risk of breast cancer." *New England Journal of Medicine,* 1986; 315:405–411.

Page 56   Progestin increases incidence of breast cancer in dogs: Weisz, J., and Stolley, P.D. Letter to Frank Young, Commissioner, Food and Drug Administration. August 4, 1989.

Page 56   Norplant is "one of the most potent progestational compounds": International Agency for Research on Cancer. *Sex Hormones.* Lyon, France: World Health Organization, IARC Monograph. 1979; 21:485.

Page 56   6,000 complaints about Norplant to FDA: Anonymous. "Norplant update." *Breast Implants,* 1995;3(8):1–3.

Page 57   Users of Norplant sign a "patient acknowledgment form": "Norplant users now must sign warning." *Medical Legal Aspects of Breast Implants,* 1995;3(12):1–12.

Page 57   Depo-Provera also increases risks of breast cancer: Lee, N.C., *et al.* "A case-control study of breast cancer and hormonal contraception in Costa Rica." *Journal of the National Cancer Institute,* 1987;79:1247–1254; Paul, C., *et al.* "Depo medroxyprogesterone (depoprovera) and risk of breast cancer." *British Medical Journal,* 1989;299:759–762; WHO Collaborative Study of Neoplasia and Steroid Contraceptives. "Breast cancer and depo-medroxyprogesterone acetate: A multinational study." *The Lancet,* 1991; 338;8771:833–838.

Page 57   Women using Depo-Provera increased risk within five years: Skegg, D.C., *et al.* "Depo medroxyprogesterone acetate and breast cancer. A pooled analysis of the World Health Organization and New Zealand studies." *Journal of the American Medical Association,* 1995;273(10):799–804.

Page 57   Oral contraceptives containing progesterone-derived progestogens were taken off the market: Young, F.E. "Letter to Paul Stolley, M.D., Ph.D., professor of medicine, Clinical Epidemiology Unit, University of Pennsylvania School of Medicine." October 18, 1989.

Page 58   20 or 30 years needed to see effects of long-term Pill use: Kolata, G. "Cancer experts see a need for caution on use of birth pill." *The New York Times,* January 7, 1989:1.

Page 59   Ortho-Novum package insert reassures doctors and users: *Physicians' Desk Reference.* Montvale, NJ: Medical Economics Data Production Company, 1996:1872–1880.

Page 59   Those who use Norplant "may need to be checked more often": *Ibid.:* 2759–2764.

Page 62   Need for better contraceptive methods: "Suits and regulations stall contraceptive advances." *The New York Times,* December 27, 1995:A1, A9.

4: ESTROGEN REPLACEMENT THERAPY

Page 65   Just as baby boomers hit middle age: Love, S. *The New York Times,* March 20, 1997:A19.

Page 66   All postmenopausal women are castrates: Wilson, R.A. *Feminine Forever.* New York: M. Evans, 1966.

Page 67   "Estrogen Replacement: More Important than Ever": Anonymous. "Estrogen replacement, more important than ever." *Consumer Reports on Health,* November, 1995;7(11):1–2.

Page 68   "The pendulum . . . is now clearly on the side of women taking [estrogen supplements]. . . .": Brody, J.E. "Personal health: A new television series helps to explode the many damaging myths about menopause." *The New York Times,* December 1, 1993:B9.

Page 70   Synthetic progestins tend to be stronger than natural progestins: Jordan, V.C., *et al.* "The estrogenic activity of synthetic progestins used in oral contraceptives." *Cancer,* 1993;71:1501–1505. Stanford, J.J., and Thomas, D.B. "Exogenous Progestins and Breast Cancer." *Epidemiologic Reviews,* 1993;15:98–107.

Page 71   Testosterone increases estrogen and breast cancer risks: Berrino, F., *et al.* "Serum sex hormone levels after menopause and subsequent breast cancer risk." *Journal of the National Cancer Institute,* 1996;88(5):291–296.

Page 72   Three times as many women die of heart disease than breast cancer: Stampfer, M. "Women who use estrogen reduce cardiac risk." *The New York Times,* March 27, 1997:A22.

NOTE: While the drug industry and cancer establishment maintain a clear bias in favor of ERT, ERT opponents have a bias as well. A notable, and puzzling, example comes from the noted and compassionate breast cancer surgeon, Dr. Susan Love, co-founder of the National Breast Cancer Coalition and author of *Dr. Susan Love's Breast Book* and *Dr. Susan Love's Hormone Book.* In a March 20, 1997, *New York Times* editorial attacking ERT, Dr. Love stated, ". . . the data on heart disease are inconclusive. It is important to note that in women younger than age 75, there are actually three times as many deaths from breast cancer as there are from heart disease."

Her statistics are simply false. As pointed out in a March 27, 1997, letter to *The New York Times* from Harvard epidemiologist Dr. Meier Stampfer, 96,000 women between the ages of 35 and 74 died of heart disease while 38,000 died of breast cancer in 1993. Most readers of Dr. Love's editorial believed that she had just made an honest mistake. Unfortunately, this is not the case. When challenged with the facts by a reporter from *The New Yorker*, Dr. Love refused to retract her comment and insisted there are three times as many deaths from breast cancer as from heart disease in women under age 75.

Love, Susan. "Sometimes mother nature knows best." *The New York Times*, March 20, 1997:A19; Stampfer, M. "Women who use estrogen reduce cardiac risk." *The New York Times*, March 27, 1997:A22; Gladwell, Malcolm. "The Estrogen Question." *The New Yorker*, June 9, 1997:54.

Page 73   Osteoporosis causes more than one million fractures annually: *The Surgeon General's Report on Nutrition and Health*. U.S. Department of Health and Human Services. Washington, DC: U.S. Government Printing Office, 1988:312.

Page 74   "For long-term preservation of bone mineral density": Felson, D.T., *et al.* "The effect of postmenopausal estrogen therapy on bone density in elderly women." *New England Journal of Medicine*, 1993; 329(16):1141–1146.

Page 74   Women starting ERT in their 60s: Brody, J.E. "Hormone Therapy Can Increase Bone Mass." *The New York Times*, November 6, 1996:A10.

Page 75   Current use of estrogen provides the most benefits: Schneider, D.L., *et al.* "Timing of postmenopausal estrogen for optimal bone mineral density: The Rancho Bernardo study." *Journal of the American Medical Association*, 1997;227(1):543–547.

Page 75   ERT may cut colon cancer risks in half: Newcomb, P.A., and Storer, B.E. "Postmenopausal hormone use and risk of large bowel cancer." *Journal of the National Cancer Institute*, 1995;87(14): 1067–1071. Potter, J.D. "Hormones and colon cancer." *Journal of the National Cancer Institute*, 1995;87(4)1039–1040.

Page 76   ERT users had only a 7 percent incidence of Alzheimer's: Johnson, R. "Estrogen/Alzheimer's link found." *Medical Tribune*, December 9, 1993:1.

Page 76   Estrogen reduces risk by 50 percent: Brody, J.E. "Estrogen and Alzheimers." *The New York Times*, June 18, 1997:B10.

Page 77   Estrogen also appears to protect brain cells against amyloid: Wickelgren, I. "Estrogen stakes claim to cognition." *Science*, 1997; 276:675–678.

Page 77   ERT eases urinary tract dysfunction: Makinen, J.I., et al. "Trans-
           dermal estrogen for female stress urinary incontinence in post
           menopause." *Maturitas*, 1995;25(3):233–235.

Page 79   "Should cancer be the price we pay for reduced risk of heart disease
           and fractures?": Colditz, G.A. "Estrogens and breast cancer."
           American Association for the Advancement of Science 1994
           Annual Meeting, San Francisco, February 22, 1994.

Page 79   ERT remains one of the most commonly prescribed drugs: Wallis,
           C. "The estrogen dilemma." *Time*, June 26, 1995:46–54.

Page 79   Estrogenization is a major factor in rising rates of female cancers:
           Seaman, B., and Seaman, G. *Women and the Crisis in Sex Hormones*.
           New York: Bantam Books, 1977:14, 41–42, 60, 97, 115–116, 132,
           407–411.

Page 80   Package insert for Premarin pills claims no connection to breast
           cancer: *Physician's Desk Reference*. Monvale, NJ: Medical
           Economics Data Production Company, 1996:2789–2791.

Page 80   The manufacturer of Estrace concurs: *Ibid*.:2792–2794.

Page 80   The National Alliance of Breast Cancer Organizations trivializes
           evidence of ERT's risk: "HRT and breast cancer: More data needed."
           NABCO News, October, 1995:1, 5.

Box

Page 81   In 1991: Grady, D., and Ernester, V. "Invited commentary: Does
           postmenopausal hormone therapy cause breast cancer?" *American
           Journal of Epidemiology*, 1991;134(12):1396–1401

Page 81   In 1991: Steinberg, K.K., *et al*. "A metaanalysis of the effect of estro-
           gen replacement therapy on the risk of breast cancer." *Journal of the
           American Medical Association*, 1991;265:1985–1990.

Page 81   A follow-up to this review: *Ibid*.

Page 81   Another pooled analysis: Steinberg, K.K., *et al*. "Breast cancer risk
           and duration of estrogen use: The role of study design in meta-
           analysis." *Epidemiology*, 1994;5:415–421.

Page 81   In 1995: Colditz, G.A., *et al*. "The use of estrogens and progestins
           and the risk of breast cancer in postmenopausal women." *New
           England Journal of Medicine*, 1995;332(24):1589–1593.

Page 81   A large-scale study: Brody, J.E. "Hormone use helps women." *The
           New York Times*, June 19, 1997:A1.

END BOX

Page 82   Progesterone as part of ERT increased risk more than 400 percent: Bergkvist, L., et al. "The risk of breast cancer after estrogen-progestin replacement." *New England Journal of Medicine*, 1989; 321:293–297.

Page 82   A 1995 study showed a 40 percent increase in risk: Colditz, G.A., et al. "The use of estrogens and progestins and the risk of breast cancer in postmenopausal women." *The New England Journal of Medicine*, 1995; 332(24):1589–1593.

Page 82   ERT sharply increases risk of uterine and ovarian cancer: Centers for Disease Control and Steroid Hormone Study. "Oral contraceptive use and the risk of endometrial cancer." *Journal of the American Medical Association*, 1983;249:1600.

Page 83   Ovarian cancer rates increased by 40 percent after six years: Rodriguez, C., et al. "Estrogen replacement therapy and fatal ovarian cancer." *American Journal of Epidemiology*, 1995;141(9): 828–835.

Page 83   A woman taking ERT is more likely to obtain a false-negative test: McDougall, J.A. *McDougall's Medicine: A Challenging Second Opinion.* Clinton, NJ: New Win Publishing, 1985:81; Laya, M.B., et al. "Effect of estrogen replacement therapy on the specificity and sensitivity of screening mammography." *Journal of the National Cancer Institute*, 1996;88(10):643–649; Black, W.C., and Fletcher, S.W. "Effects of estrogen on screening mammography: Another complexity." *Journal of the National Cancer Institute*, 1996; 88(10):627–628.

Page 85   "It is patronizing to assume": Physicians Committee for Responsible Medicine. Press release. "Estrogen dangers *before* and after menopause." Washington, D.C., June 23, 1995.

Page 86   Women who put off estrogen still receive bone-conserving benefits: Schneider, D. L., et al. "Timing of postemenopausal estrogen for optimal bone mineral density: The Rancho Bernardo study." *Journal of the American Medical Association*, 1997;227(1):543–547.

Page 88   Fresh fruits and vegetables reduce levels of homocystein: Brody, J.E. "Many people are learning to lower their cholesterol by changing their patterns of eating and exercise." *The New York Times*, January 3, 1996:B7.

Page 90   Supplemental magnesium can increase bone density up to 8 percent: Anonymous. "Magnesium found to deter postmenopausal bone loss." *Medical World News*, August 1993:13.

Page 91   High intake of vitamin E lowers risk by 65 percent: Knekt, P., *et al.* "Antioxidant vitamin intake and coronary mortality in a longitudinal population study." *American Journal of Epidemiology*, 1994;139:1180–1189.

Page 91   Vitamin E as treatment for menopause symptoms: Kavinosky, N.R. "Vitamin E and the control of climacteric symptoms. Reports of results in one-hundred-seventy-one women." *Annals of Western Medicine and Surgery*, 1950;4(1):27–32.

Page 91   47 grams of soy protein a day lowers cholesterol up to 20 percent: Anderson, J.W., *et al.* "Metaanalysis of the effects of soy protein intake on serum lipids." *New England Journal of Medicine*, 1995;333(5):276–282.

Page 92   Phytoestrogens in soy increase HDL: *Ibid.*

Page 94   Women who took two or more aspirin weekly: Manson, J.E., *et al.* "A prospective study of aspirin use and primary prevention of cardiovascular disease in women." *Journal of the American Medical Association,* 1991;266(4):521–527.

5: MAMMOGRAPHY

Page 99   "I've always believed in telling people": Brawley, O., cited in Kolata, G. "Same data, 3 different mammogram recommendations." *The New York Times*, March 28, 1997:A16.

Page 100   90 percent of all breast cancers are found during breast self-examination: Ross, W.S. *Crusade: The Official History of the American Cancer Society.* New York: Arbor House, 1987:96.

Page 101   Density tends to mask small early tumors: Byrne, C. "Studying mammographic density implications for understanding breast cancer." *Journal of the National Cancer Institute*, 1997;89(10): 531–533.

Page 101   During the early 1970s, women who underwent mammography: Epstein, S.S. "Mammography radiates doubts." *Los Angeles Times,* January 28, 1992:B7.

Page 101   The average single-exposure dose was about 8 rads in PA: Bailer, J.C. "Screening for early breast cancer: Pros and cons." *Cancer,* 1977;39:2783–2795.

Page 103   A Swedish study showed single-view mammography every two to three years reduces mortality: Dempsey, K., *et al. Screening Mammography: What the Cancer Establishment Never Told You.* The Women's Community Cancer Project, Cambridge, MA, May 5, 1992:9.

Page 103   A Netherlands study reported a 50 percent reduction in mortality: Fletcher, S.W., *et al.* "Report of the international workshop on screening for breast cancer." *Journal of the National Cancer Institute,* 1993;85(20):1644–1656.

Page 103   "Exam for exam, women in the U.S.": Dempsey, K., *et al. Screening Mammography: What the Cancer Establishment Never Told You.* The Women's Community Cancer Project, Cambridge, MA, May 5, 1992:9.

Page 104   Congress passed the 1992 National Mammography Standards Quality Assurance Act: Davis, D.L., and Love, S.M. "Mammographic screening." *Journal of the American Medical Association,* 1994;271(2):152–153.

Page 105   "Screening is always second best": Roberts, M.M. "Breast screening: Time for a rethink?" *British Medical Journal,* 1989;299:1153–1155.

Page 106   From 1987 to 1992, the percentage of Americans having mammograms rose: *Morbidity and Mortality Weekly Report.* "Trends in cancer screening—United States, 1987 and 1992." 1996;45: 57–61.

Page 106   Over the same five-year period: Davis, D.L., and Love, S.M. "Mammographic screening." *Journal of the American Medical Association,* 1994;271(2):152–153.

Page 106   75 percent of women aged 40 to 49 followed ACS guidelines: Smigel, K. "Perception of risk heightens stress of breast cancer screening." *Journal of the National Cancer Institute,* 1993; 85(7):525–526.

Page 106   Fewer postmenopausal women submit to mammograms today: Davis, D.L., and Love, S.M. "Mammographic screening." *Journal of the American Medical Association,* 1994;271(2):152–156.

Page 106   The link between radiation and breast cancer is a strong one: Bertell, R. "Breast cancer and mammography." *Mothering,* Summer 1992:49–52.

Page 106   Rates are highest among survivors who were ten years old: Wanebo, C.K., *et al.* "Breast cancer after exposure to the atomic bombings of Hiroshima and Nagasaki." *New England Journal of Medicine,* 1968;279:667–671.

Page 106   Two-decade lag time between exposure and cancer: Jablon, S., *et al.* "Studies of the mortality of A-bomb survivors: Radiation dose and mortality, 1950–1970." *Radiation Research,* 1972;50:649–698. National Academy of Sciences–National Research Council

Advisory Committee on Biological Effects of Ionizing Radiation. *Report on the Effects on Populations of Exposure to Low Levels of Ionizing Radiation.* Washington, D.C., 1972.

BOX

Page 107   In 1965: Mac Kenzie, I., "Breast cancer following multiple fluorosopies." *British Journal of Cancer,* 1965;19:1–8.

Page 107   In 1971: Janower, M. and Miettinen, O. "Neoplasms after childhood irradiation of the thymus gland." *Journal of the American Medical Association,* 1971;215:753–756; Gofman, J.W. *Preventing Breast Cancer: The Story of a Major, Proven, Preventable Cause of This Disease.* San Francisco: Committee for Nuclear Responsibility, 1995.

Page 107   Reports published in the Canadian Medical Association Journal: Grundy, G.W., and Uzman, B.G. "Breast cancer with repeated fluoroscopy." *Journal of the National Cancer Institute,* 1973;51: 1339–1340; Cook; D.C., *et al.* "Breast cancer following multiple chest fluoroscopy: the Ontario experience." *Canadian Medical Association Journal,* 1974;111:406–409; Iknayan, H.F. "Carcinoma associated with irradiation of the immature breast." *Radiation,* 1975;114:431–433; Deutsch, M., *et al.* "Carcinoma of the male breast following thymic irradiation." *Radiology,* 1975;116:413–414; Shore, R.E., *et al.* "Breast neoplasms in women treated with x-rays for acute postpartum mastitis." *Journal of the National Cancer Institute,* 1977;59(3):813–822.

Page 107   In 1989: Hoffman, *et al. Journal of the National Cancer Institute,* 1989;81(17):1307–1312.

Page 107   Another 1989 study: Modan, B., *et al.* "Increased risk of breast cancer after low-dose radiation." *The Lancet,* 1989;629–631.

Page 107   In 1996: Bhatta, S., *et al.* "Breast cancer and other second neoplasms after childhood Hodgkin's disease." *New England Journal of Medicine,* 1996;334(12):745–751.

Page 107   Past medical radiation is the single most important cause of the breast cancer epidemic: Gofman, J.W. *Preventing Breast Cancer: The Story of a Major, Proven, Preventable Cause of This Disease.* San Francisco: Committee for Nuclear Responsibility, 1995.

Page 107   An editorial attacked this conclusion as "incredible": Skolnick, A.A. "Claims that medical x-rays caused most U.S. breast cancers found incredible." *Journal of the American Medical Association,* 1995; 274(5):367–368.

END BOX

Page 108 — Patients undergoing procedures such as cardiac catheterization were developing radiation-induced skin burns: Food and Drug Administration. "Avoidance of serious x-ray-induced skin injuries to patients during fluoroscopically-guided procedures." FDA Public Health Advisory, September 30, 1994.

Page 108 — People who carry the gene are highly sensitive to radiation: Swift, M. "Ionizing radition, breast cancer, and ataxia-telongiectasia." *Journal of the National Cancer Institute,* 1994;86(21): 1571–1572.

Page 108 — Women carrying the ataxia-telongiectasia (A-T) gene may account for 20 percent of breast cancer cases: *Ibid.*; Bridges, B.A., and Arlett, C.F. "Risk of breast cancer in ataxia-telangiectasia." *New England Journal of Medicine,* 1992;326(20):1357.

Page 109 — "There is no evidence that screening" reduces mortality: Neugut, A.I., and Jacobson, J.S. "The limitations of breast cancer screening for first-degree relatives of breast cancer patients." *American Journal of Public Health,* June, 1995;85(6):832–834.

Page 109 — Women who have higher levels of estrogen are more susceptible: Shore, R.E., *et al.* "Synergism between radiation and other risk factors for breast cancer." *Preventive Medicine,* 1980;9:815–822.

Page 109 — Radiation enhances the carcinogenic effects of estrogen: Shellabarger, C.J., *et al.* "Experimental carcinogenesis in the breast" pp. 169–180; Shore, R.E. "Carcinogenic effects of radiation on the human breast" pp. 279–291. In *Radiation Carcinogenesis,* ed. A.C. Upton, *et al.* New York: Elsevier, 1986.

Page 109 — Somewhere between none and ten women of 10,000 in their forties would prolong their lives: Kolata, G. "Mammogram talks prove indefinite." *The New York Times,* March 24, 1997:A1.

BOX

Page 111 — A Swedish study involving 42,000 women: Elwood, J.M., *et al.* "The effectiveness of breast cancer screening by mammography in younger women." *Online Journal of Current Clinical Trials,* 1993;(2)32.

Page 111 — Another Swedish study of 60,000 women: *Ibid.*

Page 111 — A pooled analysis: *Ibid.*

END BOX

Page 112   "Both the [ACS] and the NCI will gain . . . publicity": Berlin, N. Quoted in Greenberg, D. "X-ray mammography: A background to decision." *Medicine and Public Affairs*, 1976(1973);295:739–740.

Page 112   A story in London's *Sunday Times*: "Breast Scans Boost Risk." *London Times*, June 2, 1991:1.

Page 112   "The 44 deaths from breast cancer": Watmouth, D.J., and Quan, K.M. "X-ray mammography and breast compression." *The Lancet*, 1992;340:122.

Page 113   Premenopausal women who enrolled in the HIP trial received no benefit: Randal, J. "Mammoscam." *New Republic*, October 12, 1992: 13–14.

Page 113   No basis for the promotion of mammographic screening: Elwood, J.M., *et al.* "The effectiveness of breast cancer screening by mammography in younger women." *Online Journal of Current Clinical Trials*, February 25, 1993;(2);32.

Page 114   Its published report concluded no evidence of benefit from screening under 49: Fletcher, S.W., *et al.* "Report of the international workshop on screening for breast cancer." *Journal of the National Cancer Institute*, 1993;85(20):1644–1656.

Page 114   Only two of the seven studies involved *annual* screening: Kolata, G. "Same data, 3 different mammogram recommendations." *The New York Times*, March 28, 1997:A16.

Page 115   NCI and ACS relied on studies based on chronological age: Paykel, J., Wolberg, H. "Concerns about recommended routine screening mammograms for women aged 40–49 years." *Journal of the National Cancer Institute*, 1997;89(12):786–788.

Page 115   At best, mammography only marginally reduced mortality: Eddy, D.M. "Screening for breast cancer." *Annals of Internal Medicine*, 1989;11(1):389–399.

Page 115   Panel of health experts warned physicians against mammograms: Leary, W.E. "Health experts urge reduced use of some medical tests." *The New York Times*, December 13, 1995:A12.

Page 115   Four subsequent trials showed no significant benefit in any age group: Wright, C.J., and Mueller, C.B. "Screening mammography and public health policy: The need for perspectives." *The Lancet*, 1995;346(8966):29–32.

Page 116   Some women have received as much radiation from mammogra-
                phy as from an atom bomb blast: Weed, S. *Breast Cancer? Breast
                Health! The Wise Woman Way.* New York: Ash Tree Publishing,
                1996.

Page 116   "X-ray and nuclear exposures are cumulative in effect": Bertell, R.
                "Breast cancer and mammography." *Mothering*, Summer 1992:
                49–57.

Page 117   False-negative results are common: Miller, A.B. "More on breast
                cancer screening." *Cancer Forum*, 1988;1(3):1–4; Dodd, G.D.
                "Present status of thermography, ultrasound, and mammography
                in breast cancer detection." *Cancer*, 1977;39:2796–2805; Dodd,
                G.D. "Mammography: State of the art." *Cancer*, 1984;53:652–657;
                Bird, R., *et al.* "Analysis of cancers missed at screening mammog-
                raphy." *Radiology*, 1992;613–617; Vogel, V.G. "Screening younger
                women at risk for breast cancer." *Journal of the National Cancer
                Institute Monograph No. 16*, 1994:55–60.

Page 117   "A new study has raised serious questions about radiologists' relia-
                bility": Brody, J.E. "Mammogram interpretations are questioned in
                a report." *The New York Times*, December 2, 1994;A1.

Page 117   About 20 percent of women on ERT develop higher breast densi-
                ties: Laya, M.B., *et al.* "Effect of estrogen replacement therapy on
                the specificity and sensitivity of screening mammography." *Journal
                of the National Cancer Institute*, 1996;88(10):643–649; Black, W.C.,
                and Fletcher, S.W. "Effects of estrogen on screening mammogra-
                phy: another complexity." *Journal of the National Cancer Institute*,
                1996;88(10):627–628; Jenks, S. "Dense breast tissues may hold
                increased cancer risk for some." *Journal of the National Cancer
                Institute*, 1994;86(8):578–580.

Page 118   Implants make the identification of early cancers difficult:
                Silverstein, M.J., *et al.* "Breast cancer in women after augmentation
                mammoplasty." *Archives of Surgery*, 1988;123:681–685; Handel, N.,
                et al. "Factors affecting mammographic visualization of breast after
                augmentation mammoplasty." *Journal of the American Medical
                Association*, 1992;268(14):1913–1917.

Page 118   From 17 to 77 percent of premenopausal cancers surfaced quickly:
                Spratt, J.S., and Spratt, S.W. "Legal perspectives on mammography
                and self-referral." *Cancer*, 1992;69(2):599–600.

Page 118   This type of cancer can double in size in one month: Gofman, J.W.
                Preventing Breast Cancer. San Francisco: Committee for Nuclear
                Responsibility, 1995.

Page 118   Radiologists mistakenly identify lesions as cancer: Skrabanek, P. "Shadows over screening mammography." *Clinical Radiology*, 1989;40:4–5.

Page 119   Only one of ten biopsies recommended because of mammography will be cancerous: Davis, D.L., and Love, S.M. "Mammographic screening." *Journal of the American Medical Association*, 1994; 271(2):152–153.

Page 119   Some 23,000 American women were diagnosed with this cancer: Kolata, G. "Ability to find a tiny tumor poses dilemma." *The New York Times*, March 27, 1996:A1, B8.

Page 119   Doctors should handle cancerous breasts with care: Quigley, D.T. "Some neglected points in the pathology of breast cancer, and treatment of breast cancer." *Radiology*, 1928:383–386.

Page 119   Mammography may rupture blood vessels and spread cancer cells: Watmough, D.J., and Quan, K.M. "X-ray mammography and breast compression." *The Lancet*, 1992;340:122.

Page 119   Metastases can increase up to 80 percent when a tumor is manipulated mechanically: *Ibid.*; Smatchlo, K., *et al.* "Ultrasonic treatment of tumors: Absence of metastases following treatment of a hamster fibrosarcoma." *Ultrasound in Medicine and Biology*, 1979;5:45–49.

Page 119   The screened group had nearly 30 percent more deaths: Anderson, I., *et al.* "Mammographic screening and mortality from breast cancer: The Malmo mammographic screening trial." *British Medical Journal*, 1988;297:943–948.

Page 120   No standards for force used during mammographic procedures: Watmough, D.J., and Quan, K.M. "X-ray mammography and breast compression." *The Lancet*, 1992;340:122.

Page 120   90 percent of women discover their tumors themselves: Ross, W.S. *Crusade: The Official History of the American Cancer Society.* New York: Arbor House, 1987:96; Frank, J.W., and Mai, V. "Breast self-examination in young women: More harm than good." *The Lancet*, 1985;654–656.

Page 120   Breast self-examination leads to earlier detection and improved survival: *Ibid.*

Page 120   Women who perform self-examinations find smaller tumors, earlier: Smigel, K. "Perception of risk heightens stress of breast cancer screening." *Journal of the National Cancer Institute*, 1993;85 (7):525–526.

Page 121   Self-examinations resulted in a 30 percent decrease in breast cancer mortality: Gastrin, G., *et al.* "Preliminary results of primary screening for breast cancer with incidence and mortality from breast cancer in the Mama program." *Sozial- und Praventivmedizin,* 1993:38(5)280–287.

Page 121   80 percent of abnormalities found on self-examination are benign: Frank, J.W., and Mai, V. "Breast self-examination in young women: More harm than good." *The Lancet,* 1985:654–656.

Page 121   Training increases reported breast self-examination frequency: Hall, D.C., *et al.* "Improved detection of human breast lesions following experimental training." *Cancer,* 1980;46(2): 408–414.

Page 121   Sensor Pad increases tactile ability: Associated Press. "F.D.A. approves use of pad in breast exam." *The New York Times,* December 25, 1995:9Y; Langreth, R. "Maker of device to detect breast lumps wants to sell it without a prescription." *Wall Street Journal,* December 27, 1995:17; Bowers, B. "How a device to aid in breast self-exams is kept off the market. Other nations approved it, but U.S. demands proof simple pad isn't risky. Nine-year battle with FDA." *Wall Street Journal,* April 12, 1994:A1.

Page 122   Regular clinical examinations represent the most effective screening method: Wolfe, S.M. *Women's Health Alert.* New York: Addison-Wesley, 1991:12.

Page 122   Transillumination is a sensitive indicator of breast disease: Lafreneiere, R., *et al.* "Infared light scanning of the breast." *American Surgeon,* 1986;52(3):123–128; Greene, F.L., *et al.* "Mammography, sonomammography, and diaphanography (lightscanning): A prospective, comparative study with histologic correlation." *American Surgeon,* 1985;51(1):58–60.

Page 122   Transillumination is more effective for women with scarring from previous biopsies: Elwood, J.M., *et al.* "The effectiveness of breast cancer screening by mammography in younger women." *Online Journal of Current Clinical Trials,* 1993;32.

Page 123   [Thermography] may reduce need for routine mammograms: Lapayowker, M.S., and Revesz, G. "Thermography and ultrasound in detection and diagnosis of breast cancer." *Cancer,* 1980;46: 933–938.

Page 123   Scantek indicates an abnormality and the need for further screening: Cohen, E. "Keeping abreast of technology." *Lear's,* June 1992:36; Lange, D. "New breast test." *Allure,* September 1992:68.

Page 123   Ultra-sonography may well replace mammography in the future: Lapayowker, M.S., and Revesz, G. "Thermography and ultrasound in detection and diagnosis of breast cancer." *Cancer*, 1980;46:933–938.

Page 123   30 percent of cancers have variable ultrasound characteristics: Cole-Beuglet, C., *et al.* "Ultrasound analysis of 104 primary breast carcinomas classified according to histopathologic type." *Radiology*, 1983;147:191–196.

Page 123   Ultrasound offers another option besides biopsy: Phillips, P. "Ultrasound can cut breast biopsy need." *Medical Tribune*, December 9, 1993:4.

Page 123   FDA approval of high-definition digital ultrasound: Associated Press, "Ultrasound breast cancer test approved." *The New York Times*, April 14, 1996:14.

Page 124   Tests to evaluate overall estrogen and ratio of good and bad estrogen: Carroll, L. "Breast cancer may soon be spotted in blood and urine." *Medical Tribune*, September 22, 1994:18.

Page 124   Estrogen tests may identify high-risk women: Taoli, E., *et al.* "Ethnic differences in estrogen metabolism in healthy women." *Journal of the National Cancer Institute*, 1996;88:617.

Page 125   Springer test may be useful: Springer Test source: Heather M. Bligh Cancer Research Laboratories; Chicago Medical School, Chicago, IL 60064. (708) 578–3435.

Page 125   AMAS test can detect cancer up to nineteen months earlier: Abrams, M.B., *et al.* "Early detection and monitoring of cancer in daily practice with the anti-malignin antibody test." *Cancer Detection and Prevention*, 1994;18(1):65–78; Pfeiffer, N. "UK to try blood test to screen for early cancers." *Oncology Times*, 1992;14(1):4.

Page 125   AMAS test had a 96 percent sensitivity: *Ibid.*

Page 126   Gene damage screening can identify precancerous changes in DNA: Press release newswire. "Pacific Northwest Research Foundation: DNA damage linked to risk of breast cancer spread." March 18, 1996.

Page 126   Gene-damage screening may prevent women with cancer *in situ* from submitting to mastectomies: Malins, D. *Proceedings of the National Academy of Sciences*, 1996; 93(6):2557–2563.

6: BREAST IMPLANTS

Page 130   FDA suspects silicone causes cancer in humans: 1987 FDA task force report. *A Consideration of the Potential of Silicone to Cause Cancer in Humans.* Report by Dr. Tom Withrow based on internal FDA review. Attached to memorandum by Dr. M.E. Stratmeyer, Division of Life Sciences, FDA. August 9, 1988.

Page 130   Asian prostitutes began asking their doctors for implants following World War II: Epstein, S.S. "Implants pose poorly recognized risks of breast cancer." *International Journal of Occupational Medicine and Toxicology,* 1995;4(34):315–342.

Page 131   Silicone gel used in implants caused cancer in rats: Dow Corning Co. "Lifetime carcinogenicity study with TX-1028, TX-1029, TX-1210, and TX-211 in albino rats, IBT study no. 672-0811." Unpublished report, September 5, 1979; Dow Corning Co. (Rasmussen, C.R., and Ruhr, L.P.). "Revision of histopathology report (IBT Study No. 672-0811)." Hughes R&D, December, 1981.

Page 133   The report showed that silicone gel injected in rats induced tumors: Dow Corning Co. (Rasmussen, C., and Ruhr, L.P.). A two-year gel implant study of Dow Corning G7-2159A and Dow Corning MDF-0193 in rats." Unpublished report, October 21, 1988.

Page 134   Report finally emerges in *Federal Register.* "General and plastic surgery devices; effective date of requirement for premarket approval of silicone gel-filled breast prothesis." *Federal Register,* 1990;55(90):20568–20577.

Page 134   Silicone gel induced a high incidence of tumors in mice: Potter, M., *et al.* "Induction of plasmocytomas with silicone gel in genetically susceptible strains of mice." *Journal of the National Cancer Institute,* 1994;86(14):1058–1065.

Page 134   Silicone degrades in the body to carcinogenic crystalline silica: Shanklin, D.R., and Smalley, D.L. "Microscopic techniques and histologic findings in silicone mammary implant capsules and regional paranodal tissues." *Current Topics in Microbiologic Immunology,* 1995;210:253–261.

Page 134   Silicone gel acts like estrogen in rodents: Hayden, J.F. and Barlow, S.A. "Structure-activity relationships of organosiloxanes and the female reproductive system." *Toxicology and Applied Pharmacology,* 1972; 21:68–79.

Page 134   Hormones at implant site may cause cancer: Food and Drug
             Administration. *Risks and Benefits of Silicone-Gel-Filled Breast
             Implants: A Survey of Findings in the Literature.* Unpublished
             report, October 1989.

Page 135   Polyurethane foam degrades in the body: Hueper, W.C.
             "Polyurethane plastic foam for fractures." *Journal of the American
             Medical Association,* 1960;173:860; Hueper, W.C. "Carcinogenic
             studies on water-soluble polymers." *Pathology and Microbiology,*
             1961;24:77–106; Hueper; W.C. "Cancer induction by polyurethane
             and polysilicone plastics." *Journal of the National Cancer Institute,*
             1964;33:1005–1027.

Page 135   Both TDI and TDA induce breast and other cancers in rodents:
             National Cancer Institute. "Bioassay of 2,4-diaminotoluene in flex-
             ible urethane foams." *Analytical Chemistry,* 1977;49(12):
             1676–1680; Cardy, R.H. "Carcinogenicity and chronic toxicity of
             2,4-toluenediamine in F344 rats." *Journal of the National Cancer
             Institute,* 1979;62:1107–1116.

Page 135   TDA "probably carcinogenic to man": United States Enviromental
             Protection Agency. *Health and Environmental Effects Profile for 2,4-
             Toluenediamine.* Office of Health and Environmental Assessment,
             Cincinnati, OH, May, 1986; National Toxicology Program (NTP).
             "Silica, crystalline (respirable)." *Sixth Annual Report on
             Carcinogens.* U.S. Department of Health and Human Services,
             Public Health Service, Washington, D.C., 1991.

Page 135   Free TDA found in the urine and breast milk of women with PUF
             implants: Chan, S.C., *et al.* "Detection of toluenediamines in the
             urine of a patient with polyurethane-covered breast implants."
             Clinical Chemistry, 1991;37(5):756–758; Chan; S.C., *et al.* "Urinary
             excretion of free toluenediamines in a patient with polyurethane-cov-
             ered breast implants." *Clinical Chemistry,* 1991;37(12):2143–2145;
             Black, D.L. Aegis Analytical Laboratories, Inc. Press release. "2,4-TDA
             analysis with regards to PUF breast implants." June 4, 1991.

Page 136   The levels of the TDA in human urine "were extremely low": ENV-
             IRON International Corp., Confidential Report. "Assessment of
             potential excess lifetime risk of cancer posed by exposure to 2,4-
             toluenediamine at levels observed in Medical Engineering
             Corporation Clinical Study." March, 1995.

Page 136   Bristol-Myers Squibb study demonstrated "very small amounts" of
             TDA in 80 percent of women with implants: Bristol-Myers Squibb
             Pharmaceutical Research Institute. *Final Confidential Report on the*

Pilot Study of Urine and Serum Samples from Women with Meme and Replicon Breast Implants. July 14, 1995. Project 70010.

Page 136   Ethylene oxide persists on the surface of implants: FDA. "Institutional observations." *Cooper Surgical/Aesthetic,* 1988:1–13; International Agency for Research on Cancer. *Alkyl Compounds, Aldehydes, Epoxides, and Phenoxides Ethylene Oxide.* Lyon, France: World Health Organization, 1985;36:189–226; World Health Organization. *Environmental Health Criteria 55: Ethylene Oxide.* WHO, Geneva, Switzerland, 1985; United States Environmental Protection Agency. *Health Assessment Document for Ethylene Oxide.* Final Report, June 1985; Agency for Toxic Substances and Disease Registry (ATSDR). *Public Health Service Toxicological Profile for Ethylene Oxide.* 1990.

Page 136   This steriod induces breast and other cancers in rodents: International Agency for Research on Cancer. Monograph. *Ethylene Oxide.* Lyon, France: World Health Organization, 1987;7:205–207; National Toxicology Program. "Ethylene oxide." In *Sixth Annual Report on Carcinogens.* U.S. Department of Health and Human Services, Public Health Service, Washington, D.C., 1991:212–218; Stolley, P. A *Preliminary Report of Cancer Incidence in a Group of Workers Potentially Exposed to Ethylene Oxide.* Clinical Epidemiology Unit, University of Pennsylvania School of Medicine, April 25, 1986.

Page 136   More than 60 case reports: Brinton, L. "Protocol for a follow-up study of women with augmentation mammoplasty." National Cancer Institute, unpublished report, November, 1991; Epstein, S.S. "Women at risk are still in the dark." *Los Angeles Times,* September 9, 1994:B7.

Page 136   "All have in common a long latency period": Food and Drug Administration. "TDA and polyurethane breast implants." Press release, June 28, 1995.

Page 137   A 1986 study showed lower than expected breast cancer risks with implants: Deapen, D.M., *et al.* "The relationship between breast cancer and aumentation mammoplasty: An epidemiologic study." *Plastic and Reconstructive Surgery,* 1986;77:361–367.

Page 137   The follow-up period averaged only about ten years: Berkel, H., *et al.* "Breast augmentation: a risk factor for breast cancer?" *New England Journal of Medicine,* 1992;326(25):1649–1653.

Page 138   The follow-up report showed increasing numbers of breast cancers: Bryant, H., and Brasher, P. "Breast implants and breast cancer: Reanalysis of a linkage study." *New England Journal of Medicine,* 1995;332(23):1535–1539.

Page 138   Epidemiological studies had methodologic limitations: Brinton, L.A., *et al.* "Epidemiologic follow-up studies of breast augmentation patients." *Journal of Clinical Epidemiology*, 1995;48;4: 5570–5563.

Page 138   FDA and NCI establish breast implant/multiple myeloma registries: Food and Drug Administration. "FDA seeking referral of patients who have developed monoclonal gammopathy or myeloma after silicone implants or injections." Miller, F.W., Molecular Immunology Laboratory, Bethesda, MD, August 1995. Anderson, L.F. "Scientists grapple with silicone, breast implant research." *Journal of the National Cancer Institute*, 87(9):634–635.

Page 139   Evidence that the implant industry knew risks of implants: Anderson, J., and Krtiz, F. "Dow Corning releases research." *Medical Tribune*, February 27, 1992:4; Hilts, P.J. "Top manufacturer of breast implant replaces its chief." *The New York Times*, February 11, 1992:IY.

Page 139   Plastic surgeons joined in conspiracy of silence: Epstein, S.S. "Implants pose poorly recognized risks of breast cancer." *International Journal of Occupational Medicine and Toxicology*, 1995;4(3):315–342.

Page 139   Experimental evidence of PUF carcinogenicity: Epstein, S.S. "Women at risk are still in the dark." *Los Angeles Times*, September 9, 1994:B7; Gessner, D.M. "Trip report of meeting with Dr. Autian. May 28, 1971. General Electric."

Page 139   "Polyurethanes have no history of implantation without deterioration": Lynch, W. "Polyurethane cover on gel-filled mammaries." Memo to Rich Stolfa, August 15, 1985. Medical Engineering Co.; Wertke, L. "Natural Y aesthetic." Memo to Bob Wiles, August 20, 1985. Surgitek Co.; Gessner, D.M. "Trip report of meeting with Dr. Autian. May 28, 1971. General Electric."

Page 139   "How would anyone defend himself in a malpractice suit?": Wertke, L. "Natural Y Update," memo to Bob Wiles, Surgitek Co., August 20, 1985.

Page 140   "Foam could be a time-bomb": Lichty, L. "Summary of papers on polyurethane foam implants, ASAPS, April, 1985." April 22, 1985. L. McGhan Medical Co.

Page 140   Laboratory admits polyurethane's carcinogenicity in rats and mice: Batelle Laboratories. Fax to Gary Carter, October 26, 1988. Surgitek.

Page 140   Surgitek consultant noted in a private memorandum: Black, D. "Letter to Markham." July 10, 1990. Bristol-Myers Squibb.

Page 140 Evidence that diaminotoluene is carcinogenic in humans: Kushner, J. "Re: Ungar article, 1979." Memo to J. Bark, July 19,1990. Bristol-Myers Squibb.

Page 140 Surgitek consultant protested at rejection of findings: Black, D. "Letter to Dr. Gary Carter." May 31, 1991. Surgitek consultant.

Page 140 Consultant organizes opposition to claims against implants: Rosenbaum, J.T. "Lessons from litigation over silicone breast implants: A call for activism from scientists." *Science*, 1997; 276:1524–1525.

Page 141 Nearly 29,000 women had implants removed: "Implants on the rise." *Ms.*, March/April 1996:58–59.

Page 142 Insurance companies assert removal of implants unnecessary: Rigdon, J.E. "Women find it difficult to get breast implants removed." *Wall Street Journal*, March 20, 1992:B1.

Page 142 Breast Implant Accountability Act deems ruptured implants eligible for removal: Traficant, J.A., Jr. Press release. "Breast implant global settlement collapses! Support H.R. 2796, the breast implant accountability act." January 3, 1996.

Page 142 Dow Chemical's bankruptcy limits money available to women: "Latest settlement figures less than 5 percent." *Medical Legal Aspects of Breast Implants*, 1995;3(8):1.

7: CHEMOPREVENTION

Page 146 One million American breast cancer patients treated with tamoxifen: Marshall, E. "Reanalysis confirms results of 'tainted study.' Long-term tamoxifen trial halted." *Science*, 1995;270:1562.

Page 146 Women with breast cancer who take tamoxifen: Fisher, B., *et al.* "A randomized clinical trial evaluating tamoxifen in the treatment of patients with node-negative breast cancer who have estrogen-receptor-positive tumors." *New England Journal of Medicine*, 1989;320:479–484; Nayfield, S.G., *et al.* "Potential role of tamoxifen in prevention of breast disease." *Journal of the National Cancer Institute*, 1991;83:1450–1459.

Page 147 Dr. Susan Love protests the use of tamoxifen: Love, S.M. Introduction. In *Reducing Breast Cancer Risk in Women*, ed. B.A. Stoll. Dordrecht, Netherlands: Kluwer Academic Publishers, 1995.

Page 147 No basis for comparison between the breasts of healthy women and the unaffected breast of women with cancer: Fugh-Berman, A., and Epstein, S.S. "Should healthy women take tamoxifen?" *New England Journal of Medicine*, 1992;327(22):1596.

Page 147   Tamoxifen increased incidence of contralateral cancers: Baum, M., *et al.* "Results of the Cancer Research Campaign Adjuvant Trial for perioperative cyclophosphamide and long-term tamoxifen in early breast cancer reported on at the ten-year follow-up." *Acta Oncologica*, 1992;31(3):251–257.

Page 148   Tamoxifen provides "no advantage" for preventing contralateral breast cancer: Marshall, E. "Long-term tamoxifen trial halted." *Science*, 1995;270:1562.

Page 148   Tamoxifen fails to affect bone density: Fugh-Berman, A., and Epstein, S.S. "Should healthy women take tamoxifen?" *New England Journal of Medicine*, 1992:327(22):1596.

Page 148   Tamoxifen does appear to reduce total cholesterol: Bilimoria, M.M., *et al.* "Should adjuvant tamoxifen therapy be stopped at 5 years?" *Cancer Journal*, 1996;2(3):140–150.

Page 148   Tamoxifen's effect on levels of "good cholesterol" less certain: Rossner, S., *et al.* "Serum lipoproteins and proteins after breast cancer surgery and effects of tamoxifen." *Atherosclerosis*, 1984; 52:339–346; Love, R.R., *et al.* "Effects of tamoxifen on cardiovascular risk factors in postmenopausal women." *Annals of Internal Medicine*, 1991; 115:860–864; Bruning, P.F., *et al.* "Tamoxifen, serum lipoproteins, and cardiovascular risk." *British Journal of Cancer*, 1988;58:497–499; Bush, T.L., *et al.* "Cholesterol, lipoproteins, and coronary heart disease in women." *Clinical Chemistry*, 1988;34:B60–B70.

Page 148   Lack of benefit of tamoxifen prompts organization to reduce support: Lenvant, C. In Marshall, E. "Tamoxifen's trials and tribulations." *Science*, 1995;270:910.

Page 149   6 percent of women taking tamoxifen suffer damage to the retina: Kaiser-Kupfer, M.I., and Lippman, M.E. "Tamoxifen retinopathy." *Cancer Treatment Reports*, 1978;62:315–320; Pavlidis, N.A., *et al.* "Clear evidence that long-term, low-dose tamoxifen treatment can induce ocular toxicity. A prospective study of 63 patients." *Cancer*, 1992;69(12):2961–2964.

Page 149   Tamoxifen increases risk of blood clots about seven times: Lipton, A., *et al.* "Venous thrombosis as a side effect of tamoxifen treatment." *Cancer Treatment Reports*, 1984;68:887–889; Hendrick, A., and Subramanian, V.P. "Tamoxifen and thromboembolism." *Journal of the American Medical Association*, 1980;243:514–515; National Surgical Adjuvant Breast and Bowel Project. 1991b.

Protocol P-1, August 31 (earlier version presented before the FDA Oncological Drugs Advisory Committee, July 2, 1991).

Page 149   Tamoxifen is toxic to the liver: Epstein, S.S., and Rennie, S. "A travesty at women's expense." *Los Angeles Times*, June 22, 1992:B5.

Page 149   Tamoxifen is a "rip-roaring" liver carcinogen: Williams, G., medical director of the American Health Foundation Inc. *Ibid.*

Page 150   Contralateral cancers treated with tamoxifen often aggressive and fatal: Rutqvist, L.E., *et al.* "Contralateral primary tumors in breast cancer patients in a randomized trial of adjuvant tamoxifen therapy." *Journal of the National Cancer Institute*, 1991; 83:1299–1306.

Page 150   Leading tamoxifen proponent deigns risks of highly aggressive uterine cancers "no big deal": Fugh-Berman, A., and Epstein, S.S. "Tamoxifen: Disease prevention or disease substitution." *The Lancet*, 1992;340:1143–1145.

Page 150   Tamoxifen is unequivocally carcinogenic: Marshall, E. "Tamoxifen's trials and tribulations." *Science*, 1995;270:910; Jacobs, P. "Debate swirls over breast cancer drug." *Los Angeles Times*, November 8, 1995:A3.

Page 150   Sixfold increase in uterine cancer in tamoxifen-treated patients: California Environmental Protection Agency. *Evidence on the Carcinogenicity of Tamoxifen.* Reproductive and Cancer Hazard Assessment Section, Office of Environmental Health Hazard Assessment, March 1995.

Page 150   Tamoxifen clearly causes cancer in humans and animals: *Ibid.*

Page 151   NCI staffer challenges tamoxifen's carcinogenicity: Ford, L. "Letter to James W. Stratton, Interim Director, California Environmental Protection Agency, Sacramento, CA." Bethesda, MD, National Cancer Institute, June 23, 1995.

Page 152   Second generation of related SERM drugs under development: Smigel, K. "Next generaion of SERMs being seen in clinic." *Journal of the National Cancer Institute*, 1997;89:96.

Page 153   Aspirin three times a week for five years reduces breast cancer risk: Harris, R.E., *et al.* "Nonsteroidal anti-inflammatory drugs and breast cancer risk: Heterogeneity of effect in a case-control study." *Preventive Medicine*, 1995;24:119–120; Shreinemachers, D.M., and Everson, R.B. "Aspirin use and lung, colon, and breast cancer incidence in a prospective study." *Epidemiology*, 1994;5:138–146; Gridley, G., *et al.* "Incidence of cancer among patients with rheumatoid arthritis." *Journal of the National Cancer Institute,* 1993;85:307–311; Marnett, L.J. "Aspirin and the potential role of prostaglandins in colon cancer." *Cancer Research,* 1992;52: 5575–5589; Thun, M.J., *et al.* "Aspirin use and reduced risk of fatal colon cancer." *New England Journal of Medicine,* 1991;325: 1593–1596; Harris, R.E., *et al.* "Nonsteroidal anti-inflammatory drugs and breast cancer." *Epidemiology,* 1996;7(2):203–205.

Page 154 "Nonsteroidal anti-inflammatory drugs may have chemopreventive potential": Sternberg, S. "Aspirin users may trim breast cancer risk." *Science News,* 1996;149:118.

8: COMMON MEDICATIONS

Page 156 Reserpine treatment for 25 percent of hypertensives: Labarthe, D.R., and O'Fallon, W.M. "Resperine and breast cancer. A community-based longitudinal study of 2,000 hypertensive women." *Journal of the American Medical Association,* 1980;243(22):2304–2310.

Page 156 Studies establish links between reserpine and breast cancer: Boston Collaborative Drug Surveillance Program. "Reserpine and breast cancer." *The Lancet,* 1974;2:669–671; Armstrong, B., *et al.* "Retrospective study of the association between use of rauwolfa derivatives and breast cancer in English women." *The Lancet,* 1974;2:672–675; Heinonen, O.P., *et al.* "Reserpine use in relation to breast cancer." *The Lancet,* 1974;2:675–677.

Page 157 Significant association between breast cancer and rauwolfia derivatives: Williams R.R., *et al.* "Case-control study of antihypertensive and diuretic use by women with malignant and benign breast lesions detected in a mammography screening program." *Journal of the National Cancer Institute,* 1978;61:327–335.

Page 157 Reserpine increases blood concentration of prolactin: Martinez, A.J. "Prolactin and carcinoma of the breast." *Mayo Clinic Proceedings,* 1992;67:1011–1012; Haraguchi, S., *et al.* "Human prolactin regulates transfected MTV LTR-directed gene expression in a human breast carcinoma cell line through synergistic interaction with steroid hormones." *International Journal of Cancer,* 1992; 52:928–933.

Page 157 One-third of human breast cancers depend on the presence of prolactin: Smithline, F., *et al.* "Prolactin and breast carcinoma." *New England Journal of Medicine,* 1975;292(15):784–792; Martinez, A.J. "Prolactin and carcinoma of the breast." *Mayo Clinic Proceedings,* 1992;67:1011–1012; Adams, J.B. "Human breast cancer: Concerted role of diet, prolactin, and adrenal C19-delta 5-steroids in tumorigenesis." *International Journal of Cancer*, 1992;50(6):854–858; Ingram, D.M., *et al.* "Prolactin and breast cancer risk." *Medical Journal of Australia*, 1990;153(8):469–473; Olsson, H., *et al.* "Increased plasma prolactin levels in a group of men with breast cancer—a preliminary study." *Anticancer Research*, 1990;10(1):59–62.

Page 157   Women taking reserpine for five years have elevated prolactin levels: Ross, R.K., *et al.* "Effects of reserpine on prolactin levels and incidence of breast cancer in postmenopausal women." *Cancer Research*, 1984;44:3106–3108.

Page 157   Reserpine induced breast and other cancers in rodents: National Toxicology Program. "Bioassay of Reserpine for possible carcinogenicity." *National Institutes of Health*, 1980; Publication No. 80:1749.

Page 158   Taking Apresoline for more than five years doubles risk: Williams, R.R., *et al.* "Case-control study of antihypertensive and diuretic use by women with malignant and benign breast lesions detected in a mammography screening program." *Journal of the National Cancer Institute*, 1978;61:327–335.

Page 158   Authors of study admit long-term risks of breast cancer not evaluated: Kaufman, D.W., *et al.* "Hydrazaline and breast cancer." *Journal of the National Cancer Institute*, 1987;78:243–246.

Page 158   Spironolactone induces incidence of breast cancers in rodents and monkeys: *Physicians' Desk Reference*. Montvale, NJ: Medical Economics Data Production Company, 1996:2413–2416; Newman, T.B., and Hulley, S.B. "Carcinogencity of lipid-lowering drugs." *Journal of the American Medical Association*, 1996;275(1):55–60. International Agency for Research on Cancer. *Some Pharmaceutical Drugs*. Lyon, France: World Health Organization, 1980;24:264.

Page 158   "Carcinoma has been reported in patients taking spironolactone": *Physicians' Desk Reference*, Montvale, NJ: Medical Economics Data Production Company, 1996:2413–2416.

Page 159   Atenolol caused breast and pituitary cancers [in rats]: *Ibid.*: 2848–2851.

Page 159   Human studies show link between Flagyl and breast cancer: Danielson, D.A., *et al.* "Metronidazole and cancer." *Journal of the American Medical Association*, 1982;247(18):2498–2499; Beard, C.M., *et al.* "Lack of evidence for cancer due to metronidazole." *New England Journal of Medicine*, 1979;301(10):519–522.

Page 159   Flagyl causes excesses of breast cancer in male rodents: Rustia, M., and Shubik, P. "Experimental induction of hepatomas, mammary tumors, and other tumors with metronidazole in nobred Sas:MRC(WI)BR rats." *Journal of the National Cancer Institute*, 1979;63:863–868; Cavaliere, A., *et al.* "Induction of mammary tumors with metronidazole in female Sprague-Dawley rats." *Tumori*, 1984;70:307–311.

Page 160   Furacin significantly increases breast cancer in rodents: Erturk, E., *et al.* "Transplantable rat mammary tumors induced by 5-nitro-2-furaldehyde semicarbazone and by formic acid 2[4-(5-nitro-furyl)-2-thiazolyl]hydrazide." *Cancer Research*, 1970;30: 1409–1412. National Toxicology Program, *Toxicology and Carcinogenesis Studies of Nitrofurazone (CAS No.59-87-0) in F344/N rats and B6C3f1 Mice (Feed Studies).* NTP Technical Report 337, Research Triangle Park, NC. 1988;18–19, 160–164.

Page 160   Link between tranquilizer use and invasive breast cancer: "Psychosomatic factors and their growth" in Stoll, B.A. (ed). *Risk Factors in Breast Cancer.* Chicago: Yearbook Medical Publishers, 1976:193; Horrobon, D.F., *et al.* "Mind and cancer (letter)." *The Lancet*, May 5, 1979;1:978.

Page 161   Tranquilizers may accelerate cancer: Tudge, C. "Does valium promote cancer?" *New Scientist*, January 8, 1981:80.

Page 161   Elavil and Prozac promote the growth of breast cancer in rodents: Brandes, L.J. "Stimulation of malignant growth in rodents by anti-depressant drugs at clinically relevant doses." *Cancer Research*, 1992;52:3796–3800.

Page 161   Haldol triggers release of prolactin and increases risk in rodents: *Physicians' Desk Reference*, Montvale, NJ: Medical Economics Data Production Company, 1996:1577–1579.

Page 162   Cancer drugs increase risk of future breast cancer: National Cancer Institute. *Breast Cancer: Research and Programs*, June 1993.

Page 162   Procarbazine induces breast and other cancers in rats: International Agency for Research on Cancer. *Some Aziridines, N-, S- and 0-Mustards and Selenium.* Lyon, France: World Health Organization, 1975;9:193–207; International Agency for Research on Cancer. *Some Antineoplastic and Immunosuppressive Agency.* Lyon, France: World Health Organization, 1981;26:293–309; *Ibid.*, 311–339.

Page 162   Pravacol increases breast cancer rates twelve times: Associated Press. "Wider use seen for drugs to reduce cholesterol of heart patients." *The New York Times*, March 27, 1996:A1.

Page 162   Anticholesterol drugs cause breast and other cancers in rodents: Newman, T.B., and Hully, S.B. "Carcinogenicity of lipid-lowering drugs." *Journal of the American Medical Association,* 1996;275 (1):55–60.

Page 162   Tagamet may cause gynecomastia: Smedley, H.M. "Malignant breast change in man given two drugs associated with breast hyperplasia." *The Lancet,* 1981;2:638–639.

Page 164   Calcium, magnesium, and potassium protect the cardiovascular system: Lardinois, C.K. "Nutritional factors and hypertension." *Archives of Family Medicine,* 1995;4:707–713.

Page 164   Deglycyrrhizinate licorice good for ulcers: Montgomery, R.D., and Cookson, J.B. "The treatment of gastric ulcer. A comparative trial of carbenoxolone and a deglycyrrhizinated licorice preparation (Caved-S)." *Clinical Trials Journal,* 1972;1:33–38; Morgan, A.G., *et al.* "Comparison between cimetidine and Caved-S in the treatment of gastric ulceration, and subsequent maintenance therapy." *Gut,* 1982;23:545–551; Glick, L. "Deglycyrrhizinated licorice in peptic ulcer." *The Lancet,* 1982;ii:817.

Page 165   Changing behavior has biological effects: "Psychotherapy found to produce changes in brain function." *The New York Times,* February 15, 1996:C22.

9: EATING FOR HEALTH AND LONGEVITY

Page 170   33 percent of American men and women are obese: Kuczmarksi, R.J., *et al.* "Increasing prevalence of overweight among U.S. adults." *Journal of the American Medical Association,* 1994;272(3):205–211.

Page 170   Only 6 percent of French people are overweight: Levy, E., et al. "The economic cost of obesity: the French situation." *International Journal of Obesity,* 1995;19(11):788–792.

Page 170   Number of overweight American children has more than doubled: Associated Press. "Study finds soaring rate of obesity in children." *The New York Times.* October 9, 1995:Y14.

Page 171   Television increases risks of obesity: Specialty Journal Reports. "Kid couch potatoes more likely to be obese." American Medical Association. Press release. April 14, 1996.

Page 171   Obesity increases risk of postmenopausal breast cancer: Hershcopf, R.J., and Bradlow, H.L. "Obesity, diet, endogenous estrogens, and the risk of hormone-sensitive cancer." *American*

Journal of Clinical Nutrition, 1987;45:283–289; den Tonkelaar, I., *et al.* "A propective study on obesity and subcutaneous fat patterning in relation to breast cancer in postmenopausal women participating in the DOM project." *British Journal of Cancer,* 1994;69(2):352–357.

Page 171   With other risk factors, obesity increases risks up to 600 percent: Sellers, T.A., *et al.* "Effect of family history, body-fat distribution, and reproductive factors on the risk of postmenopausal breast cancer." *New England Journal of Medicine,* 1992;326(20):1323–1329.

Page 172   Overweight women more likely to die from breast cancer: Simopoulos, A.P. "Obesity and carcinogenesis: Historical perpective." *American Journal of Clinical Nutrition,* 1987;45:271–276; Lees, A.W., *et al.* "Risk factors and 10-year breast cancer survival in northern Alberta." *Breast Cancer Research and Treatment,* 1989;13:143–151; Greenberg, E.R., *et al.* "Body size and survival in premenopausal breast cancer." *British Journal of Cancer,* 1985;51:691–697; Eberlein, T., *et al.* "Height, weight, and risk of breast cancer relapse." *Breast Cancer Research and Treatment,* 1985;5:81–86; Hershcopf, R.J., and Bradlow, H.L. "Obesity, diet, endogenous estrogens, and the risk of hormone-sensitive cancer." *American Journal of Clinical Nutrition,* 1987;45:283–289.

Box

Page 172   A 1977 study in *Preventive Medicine*: Staszewski, J. "Breast cancer and body build." *Preventive Medicine,* 1977;6:410–415.

Page 172   A 1977 Netherlands report: de Waard, F., *et al.* "Breast cancer incidence according to weight and height in two cities of the Netherlands and in Aichi prefecture, Japan." *Cancer,* 1977;40: 1269–1275.

Page 172   In 1978, a report: Hirayama, T. "Epidemiology of breast cancer with special reference to the role of diet." *Preventive Medicine,* 1978;7:173–195.

Page 172   A 1978 Canadian study: Choi, N.W., *et al.* "An epidemiologic study of breast cancer." *American Journal of Epidemiology,* 1978;107: 510–521.

Page 172   A large-scale 1979 ACS study: Lew, E.A., and Garfinkel, L. "Variations in mortality by weight among 750,000 men and women." *Journal of Chronic Disease,* 1979;32:563–576.

Page 172   A 1979 study: Brinton, L.A., *et al.* "Breast cancer risk factors among screening program participants." *Journal of the National Cancer Institute,* 1979;62:37–44.

Page 172   A 1980 study: Paffenberger, R.S., *et al.* "Characteristics that predict risk of breast cancer before and after the menopause." *American Journal of Epidemiology*, 1980;112:258–268.

Page 172   A 1983 study: Helmrich, S.P., *et al.* "Risk factors for breast cancer." *American Journal of Epidemiology*, 1983;117:35–45.

Page 173   A 1988 study: Yuan, J.M., *et al.* "Risk factors for breast cancer in Chinese women in Shanghai." *Cancer Research*, 1988; 48:1949–1953.

Page 173   A 1994 Netherlands study: den Tonkelaar, I., *et al.* "A prospective study on obesity and subcutaneous fat patterning in relation to breast cancer in postmenopausal women participating in the DOM project." *British Journal of Cancer*, 1994;69(2):352–357.

Page 173   A 1996 study: Ziegler, R.G., *et al.* "Relative weight, weight change, height, and breast cancer risk in Asian-American women." *Journal of the National Cancer Institute*, 1996;88(10):650–660.

END BOX

Page 173   The more weight a woman carries, the higher her risk of breast cancer: Folsom, A.A., *et al.* "Increased incidence of carcinoma of the breast associated with abdominal adiposity in postmenopausal women." *American Journal of Epidemiology*, 1990;131(5):794–803; Schapira, D.V., *et al.* "Visceral obesity and breast cancer risk." *Cancer*, 1994;74(2):632–639.

Page 173   Obesity decreases premenopausal risk by 10 to 20 percent: Potischman, N., *et al.* "Reversal of relation between body mass and endogenous estrogen concentrations with menopausal status." *Journal of the National Cancer Institute*, 1996;88(11):756–758.

Page 174   Fat contains enzyme that converts testosterone to estrogen: Angier, N. "New respect for estrogen's influence." *The New York Times*, June 24, 1997:B8.

Page 175   Feeding laboratory animals high amounts of fat increased breast cancer rates: Sugiura, K. *The Publications of Kanematsu Sugiura: Memorial Edition.* New York: Sloan-Kettering Institute, 1965.

Page 175   Breast cancer rates of immigrants from Japan increase: Gori, G.B. "Dietary and nutritional implications in the multifactorial etiology of certain prevalent human cancers." *Cancer*, 1979;43(suppl. 5):2151–2161.

Page 175   No difference in the breast cancer rates with high-fat diet: Willett, W.C., *et al.* "Dietary fat and the risk of breast cancer." *New England Journal of Medicine*, 1987;316:22–28.

Page 175   Fat-breast cancer theory "bombs out": Marshall, E. "Search for a killer: Focus shifts from fat to hormones." *Science*, 1993;259: 618–621.

Page 175   No connection between low fat diets and decreased breast cancer risk: Hunter, D.J., *et al.* "Cohort studies of fat intake and the risk of breast cancer—a pooled analysis." *New England Journal of Medicine*, 1996;334:356–361.

Page 175   Conclusion of study: Further investigation of fatty diet is a dead end: Kolata, G. "Study finds no relationship between fat in diet and breast cancer." *The New York Times*, February 8, 1996:4.

Page 176   Low-fat, high-carbohydrate diet reduces breast density: Boyd, N.F., et al. "Effects at two years of a low-fat, high-carbohydrate diet on radiologic features of the breasts results from a randomized trial." *Journal of the National Cancer Institute*, 1997;89(7):488.

Page 183   Dietary contaminants increase breast cancer risk: Davis, D.L., and Bradlow, H.L. "Avoidable environmental links to breast cancer." *Reducing Breast Cancer in Women*. Dordrecht, Netherlands: Kluwer Academic Publishers, 1995:231–235; Dao, T.L. "The role of ovarian hormones in initiating the induction of mammary cancer in rats by polynuclear hydrocarbons." *Cancer Research*, 1962;22:973; Epstein, S.S. "Environmental and occupational pollutants are avoidable causes of breast cancer." *International Journal of Health Services*, 1994; 24(1):145–150.

Page 183   A 1993 study shows strong association between high blood concentrations of DDE in breast cancer patients: Wolff, M., *et al.*, "Blood levels of organochlorine residues and risk of breast cancer." *Journal of the National Cancer Institute*, 1993;85(8):648–652.

Box

Page 184   A 1976 World Health Organization study: Wasserman, M., *et al.* "Organochlorine compounds in neoplastic and adjacent apparently normal breast tissue." *Bulletin of Environmental Contamination and Toxicology*, 1976; 15:478–484.

Page 184   A small 1982 study: Altert, L., *et al.* "Chlorinated hydrocarbon residue concentrations in neoplastic human breast tissue, nonmalignant breast tumor tissue and adjacent adipose tissues." International Congress of Pesticides 5, Chemistry, Kyoto, Japan, 1982. IUPAC VII-34. Washington, D.C.: International Union for Pure and Applied Chemistry, 1982.

Page 184   Higher levels of benzene hexachloride found in breast cancers: Mussalo-Rauhamaa, H.E., *et al.* "Occurrence of beta-hexachlorocyclhexane in breast cancer patients." *Cancer*, 1990;66:2124–2128.

Page 184   A 1992 study: Falck, A., *et al.* "Pesticides and polychlorinated biphenyl residues in human breast lipids and their relation to breast cancer." *Archives of Environmental Health*, 1992;47:143–146.

Page 184   In 1993, researchers found: Wolff, M., *et al.* "Blood levels of organochlorine residues and risk of breast cancer." *Journal of the National Cancer Institute*, 1993;85(8)648–652.

Page 184   In 1994, Canadian researchers: Dewailly, É., *et al.* "High organochlorine body burden in women with estrogen receptor-positive breast cancer." *Journal of the National Cancer Institute*, 1994;86(3):232–234.

Page 184   A "strong, positive association": Krieger, N., *et al.* "Breast cancer and serum organochlorine: A study among white, black, and Asian women." *Journal of the National Cancer Institute*, 1994;(86): 589–599.

END BOX

Page 185   *USA Today* reports breast cancer link to pollutants: Tyson, R. "Breast cancer may have link to pollutants." *USA Today*, October 15, 1993:1A.

Page 185   Study showing DDT link to cancer had global implications: Hunter, D.J., and Kelsey, K.T. "Pesticide residues and breast cancer: The harvest of a silent spring?" *Journal of the National Cancer Institute*, 1993;85(8):598–599.

Page 185   Women with breast cancer have higher concentrations of pesticides in fat and blood: Dewailly, É., *et al.* "High organochlorine body burden in women with estrogen receptor-positive breast cancer." *Journal of the National Cancer Institute*, 1994;86(3):232–234.

Page 185   Relationship between concentrations of estrogen receptors in the cancers and DDE levels: Dewailley, É., *et al.* "Could the rising levels of estrogen receptor in breast cancer be due to estrogenic pollutants?" *Journal of the National Cancer Institute*, 1997;89(112):888.

Page 186   High emissions of fission material around Millstone I reactor, higher than Three Mile Island: Sternglass, E.J., and Gould, J.M. "Breast cancer: Evidence for a relation to fission products in the diet." *International Journal of Health Services*, 1993;23(4):783–804.

Page 186   Milk in Waterford contained high levels of strontium-90: Sternglass, E.J., and Gould, J.M. "Breast cancer: Evidence for a relation to fission products in the diet." *International Journal of Health Services*, 1993;23(4):783–804.

Page 186   Mortality rates for breast cancer rose with strontium-90 levels: Sternglass, E.J., and Gould, J.M. "Breast cancer: Evidence for a relation to fission products in the diet." *International Journal of Health Services*, 1993;23(4):783–804.

Page 186   The Florida panther is nearing extinction because of pollutants: Colborn, T., *et al.* "Development effects of endocrine-disrupting chemicals in wildlife and humans." *Environmental Health Perspectives*, 1993;101(5):378–384.

Page 187   The testicles of rooster chicks exposed to DDT became feminized: Burlington, H., and Lindeman, V.F. "Effect of DDT on testes and secondary sex characters of white leghorn cockerels." *Proceedings of the Society for Experimental Biology and Medicine*, 1950;74: 48–51.

Page 187   Methoxychlor increased uterine weight in mice: Yang, N.C., *et al.* "Polynuclear aromatic hydrocarbons, steroids and carcinogenesis." *Science*, 1961;134:386–387.

Page 187   Study confirms earlier ones: Colborn, T., *et al.* "Development effects of endocrine-disrupting chemicals in wildlife and humans." *Environmental Health Perspectives*, 1993;101(5):378–384.

Page 188   United States food industry imports food grown with illegal pesticides it exported: Weir, D., and Schapiro, M. *Circle of Poison*. San Francisco, CA: Institute for Food and Development Policy, 1981.

Page 188   Beef and dairy products are the most contaminated foods we eat: Steinman, D. *Diet for a Poisoned Planet*. New York: Ballantine, 1992:72–102; Steinman, D., and Epstein, S.S. *The Safe Shopper's Bible*, New York: Macmillan, 1995:325–334.

Page 188   Veal and lamb are also contaminated with pesticides: *Ibid.*

Page 189   Fish from industrialized waterways contain pseudoestrogens: Steinman, D. *Diet for a Poisoned Planet*. New York: Ballantine, 1992:103–120.

Page 189   White croaker contains high concentrations of DDT and other pollutants: Epstein, S.S., and Steinman, D. "All we're doing is rearranging the deck chairs on a seafood Titanic." *Los Angeles Times*, February 18, 1994.

Page 189   Tap water contains atrazine, a pseudoestrogenic herbicide: Kelley, R.D. "Pesticides in Iowa's drinking water." *Pesticides and Groundwater: A Health Concern in the Midwest*. Proceedings of a conference held October 16–17, 1986, Navarre, MN: Freshwater Foundation; Pintér, G., *et al.* "Long-term carcinogenicity bioassay of the herbicide atrazine in F344 rats" *Neoplasia*, 1990;37:533–544; International Agency for Research on Cancer Monograph, Vol. 52.

"Occupational exposures in insecticide application, and some pesticides: Atrazine," 1991:441–466; Donna, A., *et al.* "Ovarian mesothelial tumors and herbicides: A case-control study." *Carcinogenesis,* 1984;5(7):941–942; Donna, A., *et al.* "Triazine herbicides and ovarian epithelian neoplasms." *Scandinavian Journal of Work and Environmental Health,* 1989;15:47–53.

Page 190   Contamination of water is associated with high rates of breast cancer: Salig, J. "Cancer mortality rates and drinking water in 346 counties of the Ohio River Valley Basin." U.S. Environmental Protection Agency, PO-5-03-4528, 1977; Gottlieb, M.S. and Carr, J.K. "Case-control cancer mortality study and chlorination of drinking water in Louisiana." *Environmental Health Perspectives,* 1982;46:169–177.

Page 190   Excess of breast cancer where creosote taints drinking water: Dusich, K., *et al.* "Cancer rates in a community exposed to low levels of creosote components in municipal water." *Minnesota Medicine,* 1980;63(11):803–806; Dean, A.G., *et al.* "Adjusting morbidity ratios in two communities using risk factor prevalence in cases." *American Journal of Epidemiology,* 1988;127:654–662; *Ibid.*; Gottlieb, M.S., and Carr, J.K. "Case-control cancer mortality study and chlorination of drinking water in Louisiana." *Environmental Health Perspectives,* 1982;46:169–177.

Page 190   Endosulfan is the seventh most commonly detected pesticide: Cox, C. "Prevention is crucial." *Journal of Pesticide Reform,* 1996; 16(1):2–7.

Page 190   United States allows California to use DDT-containing dicofol: Steinman, D. *Diet for a Poisoned Planet.* New York: Ballantine, 1992. Steinman, D., and Epstein, S.S. *The Safe Shopper's Bible,* New York: Macmillan, 1995.

Page 190   Baby food is contaminated with carcinogenic and estrogenic chemicals: *Ibid.*

Page 190   Risk of cancer increases with childhood exposure to carcinogens: Hiatt, R.A., *et al.* "Exogenous estrogen and breast cancer after bilateral oophorectomy." *Cancer,* 1984:139–144.

Page 191   Alkylphenols, nonylphenol, and bisphenol A migrate into foods: Soto, A.M., *et al.* "P-Nonyl-phenol: An estrogenic xenobiotic released from 'modified' polystyrene." *Environmental Health Perspectives,* 1991;92:167–173.

Page 191   Red Dye No. 3 binds to estrogen receptors on breast cells: Dees, C., *et al.* "Estrogenic-damaging activity of Red No. 3 in human breast cancer cells." *Environmental Health Perspectives*, 1997;103 (suppl.3):625–632.

Page 192   Use of DES resulted in high residues in meat: Schell, O. *Modern Meat.* New York: Vintage Books, 1985:254–256.

Page 192   Inspectors discovered DES-contamination in nearly 1,500 veal calves: *Ibid.*

Page 193   Profound physiological effects with hormones in meat: Hertz, R. "The estrogen-cancer hypothesis with special emphasis on DES." In: *Origins of Human Cancer,* ed. H.H. Hiatt and J.D. Watson, *Cold Spring Harbor Conference on Cell Proliferation,* Vol. 4. Cold Spring Harbor, NY: Cold Spring Harbor Laboratory, 1977: 1665–1682.

Page 193   American children entering puberty years earlier: Giddens-Herman, M.E., *et al.* "Secondary sexual characteristics and menses in young girls seen in office practice." *Pediatrics,* 1997;88 (4):505–511.

Page 194   Up to half of all cattle sampled in feedlots had hormone pellets illegally implanted: Herrin, A. "FDA investigates 17 feedlots for improper hormone use." *Food Chemical News,* July 28, 1986:37–38

Page 194   Pellets found in crowns of cattles' heads: United States Department of Agriculture. Herrin, A. "FDA evaluating health hazards of cattle hormone implant's misuses." *Food Chemical News,* July 28, 1986:37–38.

Page 194   Syntex petitioned the FDA to allow repeated ear implants: Syntex Animal Health, Inc. "Environmental assessment. Synovex S. NADA 9-576." Freedom of information summary. U.S. Food and Drug Administration, Washington, D.C.: October 1989.

Page 194   Cattle today receive more hormones: Graves, M. Personal communication from Mack Graves, former Chief Executive Officer and President of the Coleman Meat Company, of Denver, Colorado, August 1993, and former executive of Armour Food and Perdue companies, 1985–1988.

Box

Page 194   An October 1983 FDA report: Freedom of information summary for Synovex-S. U.S. Food and Drug Administration, Washington, D.C.: October 5, 1983:2–3.

Page 195   A November 1991 FDA report: Freedom of information summary for REVALOR-S (trenbolone acetate and estradiol). U.S. Food and Drug Administration, Washington, D.C.: November 27, 1991:5–6.

Page 195   Melengestrol acetate is fed to cows: Mark, J.H., Acting Director of the Bureau of Veterinary Medicine to Tuco Products Company, Division of the Upjohn Company, Kalamazoo, MI. Briefing memorandum. November 28, 1967.

END BOX

Page 196   World Trade Organization ban vigorously challenged: Blackburn. P. "Scientists back EU meat hormone ban." Reuters, May 21, 1997; Epstein, S.S. "None of us should eat extra estrogen." *Los Angeles Times*, March 24, 1997:B5.

Page 197   FDA approves milk from cows injected with rBGH: Epstein, S.S. "Needless new risk of breast cancer." *Los Angeles Times*, March 20, 1994:M5.

Page 197   IGF-I regulates cell division and growth: Epstein, S.S. "Potential public health hazards of biosynthetic milk hormones." Letter and report to FDA Commissioner Frank Young, July 19, 1989; Epstein, S.S. "Needless new risk of breast cancer." *Los Angeles Times*, March 20, 1994:M5.

Page 197   Pasteurization increases IGF-I levels: Epstein, S.S. "Unlabeled milk from cows treated with biosynthetic growth hormones: A case of regulatory abdication." *International Journal of Health Services*, 1996;26(1):1730–1185.

Page 197   IGF-I major problem with milk contaminated with rBGH: American Medical Association Council on Scientific Affairs. "Biotechnology and the American agricultural industry." *Journal of the American Medical Association*, 1991;265:1429–1436; Schneider, K. "Congressmen seek inquiry of milk hormone approval." *The New York Times*, April 18, 1994:A8; Epstein, S.S. "Unlabeled milk from cows treated with biosynthetic growth hormones: A case of regulatory abdication." *International Journal of Health Services*, 1996;26(1):1730–1185.

Page 198   IGF-I causes cells of the gut to grow and divide abnormally: Lippman, M.E. "The development of biological therapies for breast cancer." *Science*, 1993;259:631–632; Resnicoff, M., *et al.* "The insulin-like growth factor-I receptor protects tumor cells from apoptosis *in vivo*." *Cancer Research*, 1995;55:2463–2469. Geler, A. "Insulin-like growth factor-I inhibits cell death induced by anti-cancer drugs in the MCF-7 cells: Involvement of growth factors in drug resistance." *Cancer Investigation*, 1995;13(5):480–486.

Page 198   AMA concerned over increased IGF-1 levels in milk: American Medical Association Council on Scientific Affairs. "Biotechnology and the American agricultural industry." *Journal of the American Medical Association,* 1991;265:1429–1436.

Page 199   Labels identifying hormones in milk would be "false and misleading": Epstein, S.S. "Potential public health hazards of biosynthetic milk hormones." Letter and report to FDA Commissioner Frank Young, July 19, 1989; Epstein, S.S. "Potential public health of hazards of biosynthetic milk hormones." *International Journal of Health Services,* 1990;20:73–84.

Page 199   Former head legal counsel to Monsanto joins FDA: Schneider, K. "Congressmen seek inquiry of milk-hormone approval." *The New York Times,* April 18, 1994:A8.

Page 202   Diet drugs dangerous in other ways: Finerty, A. "Despite warnings, the sales of diet drugs soar." *The New York Times,* June 24, 1997:B1; Kolata, G. "Diet-pill combination linked to heart ailment." *The New York Times,* July 9, 1997:A1.

Page 207   Diets rich in soy foods increase urine concentrations of phytoestrogens: Adlercreutz, H., *et al.* "Dietary phytoestrogens and the menopause in Japan." *The Lancet,* 1992;339:1233.

Page 207   Genistein, an isoflavonoid phytoestrogen, competes against estradiol: Zava, D.T. and Duwe, G. "Estrogenic and antiproliferative properties of genistein and other flavonoids in human breast cells *in vitro.*" *Nutrition and Cancer,* 1997;27(8):31–40; Angier, N. "New respect for estrogen's influence." *The New York Times,* June 24, 1997:B8.

Page 211   Vitamin C and flavonoids lower lower breast cancer mortality: Howe, G.R., *et al.* "Dietary factors and risk of breast cancer: Combined analysis of 12 case-control studies." *Journal of the National Cancer Institute,* 1990;82(7):561–569.

Page 211   High-fiber diets lower overall estrogen levels: *Ibid.*

Page 213   *Laminaria* is a factor in low breast cancer rates: Teas, J. "The dietary intake of Laminaria, a brown seaweed, and breast cancer prevention." *Nutrition and Cancer,* 1983;4(3):217–223.

Page 214   Indole-3-carbonyl stimulates production of "good" cholesterol: Michnovic, J.J., *et al.* "Changes in levels of urinary estrogen metabolites after oral indole-3-carbinol treatment in humans." *Journal of the National Cancer Institute,* 1997;89(10):718–722.

Page 214   Indole-3-carbinol stimulates products of normal CYP1 gene: Michnovicz, J.J., *et al., Ibid.*

Page 215   Diet high in carotenoids result in a 50 percent reduction in risk: Freudenheim, J.L., *et al.* "Premenopausal breast cancer risk and intake of vegetables, fruits, and related nutrients." *Journal of the National Cancer Institute,* 1996;88;6:340–348.

Page 215 Study confirms protective effect of vitamen E: Omer, B., *et al.* "Inhibition of mammary carcinogenesis in rats by parenteral high-dose vitamin E." *Journal of the National Cancer Institute,* 1997; 89(13):972–973.

Page 216 Selenium has a protective effect: Shamberger, R.J., *et al.* "Antioxidants and cancer. VI: Selenium and age-adjusted human cancer mortality." *Archives of Environmental Health,* 1976;31:231–235; Clark, L.C. "The epidemicology of selenium and cancer." *Federal Proceedings,* 1985;44:2584–2589; Schrauzer, G.N., *et al.* "Cancer mortality correlation studies, III: statistical association with dietary selenium intakes." *Bioinorganic Chemistry,* 1977;7:23–35; Hardell, L., *et al.* "Levels of selenium in plasma and glutathione peroxidase in erythrocytes and the risk of breast cancer: A case-control study." *Biological Trace Element Research,* 1993;36:99–108.

10: LIFESTYLE RISK FACTORS AND COPING STRATEGIES

Page 218 A series of well-controlled studies shows significant associations between breast cancer and smoking: Schechter, M.T., *et al.* "Cigarette smoking and breast cancer: A case control study of screening program participants." *American Journal of Epidemiology,* 1985;121:479–487; Brinton, L.A., *et al.* "Cigarette smoking and breast cancer." *American Journal of Epidemiology,* 1986;123:614–622; Brownson, R.C., *et al.* "Risk of breast cancer in relation to cigarette smoking." *Archives of Internal Medicine,* 1988;148:140–144; Rohan, T.E., and Baron, J.A. "Cigarette smoking and breast cancer." *American Journal of Epidemiology,* 1989;129:36–42; Meara, J., *et al.* "Alcohol, cigarette smoking, and breast cancer." *British Journal of Cancer,* 1989;60:70–73; Chu, S.Y., *et al.* "Cigarette smoking and the risk of breast cancer." *American Journal of Epidemiology,* 1990;131:242–253; Palmer, J.R., *et al.* "Cigarette smoking and breast cancer: A hypothesis." *American Journal of Epidemiology,* 1991;134:1–13; Smith, S.J., *et al.* "Alcohol, smoking, passive smoking, and caffeine in relation to breast cancer in young women." *British Journal of Cancer,* 1994;70:112–119; Hiatt, R.A., and Fireman, B.H. "Smoking, menopause, and breast cancer." *Journal of the National Cancer Institute,* 1986;76:833–838; London, S.J., *et al.* "Prospective study of smoking and risk of fatal breast cancer." *Journal of the National Cancer Institute,* 1989;81:1625–1631; Calle,

E.E., *et al.* "Cigarette smoking and risk of fatal breast cancer." *American Journal of Epidemiology*, 1994;139:1001–10007.

Page 219   Teenage smoking is on the rise: "Use laws to save our kids." *USA Today*, July 21, 1995:6A.

Page 219   Secondhand smoke contains up to 150 times higher levels of carcinogens: Horton, A.W. "Epidemiologic evidence for the role of indoor tobacco smoke as an initiator of human breast carcinogenesis." *Cancer Detection and Prevention*, 1992;16(2):119–127.

Page 219   Secondhand smoke and breast cancer risk: Smith, S.J., *et al.* "Alcohol, smoking, passive smoking and caffeine in relation to breast cancer in young women." *British Journal of Cancer*, 1994;70:112–119.

Page 219   "The prevalence of smoking among substance abusers": Hurt, R.D., *et al.* "Mortality following inpatient addictions treatment. Role of tobacco use in a community-based cohort." *Journal of the American Medical Association*, 1996;275(14):1097–1103.

Page 220   Fewer than three percent of women have two or more drinks daily: Hurly, J., and Horowitz, J. *Alcohol and Health*, New York: Hemisphere, 1990:3.

Page 220   Alcohol increases the level of HDLs and helps prevent heart disease: Gaziano, U.S., *et al.* "Moderate alcohol intake, increased levels of high-density lipoprotein and its subfractions, and decreased risk of myocardial infarction." *New England Journal of Medicine*, 1993;329(25):1829–1834.

Page 220   Three to nine drinks per week reduce risk of heart disease by half: Fuchs, C.S., *et al.* "Alcohol consumption and mortality among women." *New England Journal of Medicine*, 1995;332(19):1245–1250.

Page 220   Protective effect of moderate alcohol consumption reduces postmenopausal cardiovascular risk: Gavaler, J.S., and Van Thiel, D.H. "The association between moderate alcoholic beverage consumption and serum estradiol and testosterone levels in normal postmenopausal women: Relationship to literature." *Clinical and Experimental Research*, 1992;16(1):87–92.

Page 221   Chronic alcoholism and risk of cancer of esophagus, mouth, and liver: International Agency for Research on Cancer. *Alcohol Drinking.* Lyon, France: World Health Organization, 1988;44:153–250.

Page 221   Researchers have explored relationship between alcohol and breast cancer: Longnecker, M.P., *et al.* "A metaanalysis of alcohol consumption in relation to risk of breast cancer." *Journal of the American Medical Association*, 1988;260(5):652–656.

Page 221   One drink daily increases risk by 11 percent: Longnecker, M.P., "Alcoholic beverage consumption in relation to risk of breast cancer: metaanalysis and review." *Cancer Causes and Control*, 1994;5:73–82.

Page 221   Consuming one to two drinks daily increases risk by 37 percent: Fuchs, C.S., *et al.* "Alcohol consumption and mortality among women." *New England Journal of Medicine*, 1995;332(19): 1245–1250.

Page 221   One drink a day raises risk of breast cancer: Longnecker, M.P., *et al.* "Risk of breast cancer in relation to lifetime alcohol consumption." *Journal of the National Cancer Institute*, 1995;87(12):923–929.

Page 221   Women who did most of their drinking in youth doubled risk compared to later life drinking: Hiatt, R.A., *et al.* "Alcohol consumption and the risk of breast cancer in a prepaid health plan." *Cancer Research* 1988;48:2284–2287.

Page 221   Women drinking before 25 experienced an 80 percent increase in risk: Vant Veer, P., *et al.* "Alcohol dose, frequency, and age at first exposure in relation to risk of breast cancer." *International Journal of Epidemiology* 1989;18:511–517.

Page 222   80 percent of sorority women are now binge drinkers: "Study ties binge drinking to fraternity house life." *The New York Times*, December 6, 1995:B8.

Page 222   If onset of drinking delayed, could mean reduced risk of breast cancer: Frazier, A.L., and Colditz, G.A. "Models of breast cancer show that risk is set by events of early life: Prevention efforts must shift focus." *Cancer Epidemiology, Biomarkers, and Prevention*, 1995;4:567–571.

Page 222   Levels of estrogen raised by alcohol, especially in women on ERT: Ginsburg, E., *et al.* "Effects of alcohol ingestion on estrogen in postmenopausal women." *Journal of the American Medical Association*, 1996;276:1747–1751.

Page 222   Alcohol increases overall estrogen levels: Gavaler, J.S., and Van Thiel, D.H. "The association between moderate alcoholic beverage consumption and serum estradiol and testosterone levels in normal postmenopausal women: Relationship to literature." *Clinical and Experimental Research*, 1992;16(1):87–92; Reichman, M.E., *et al.* "Effects of alcohol consumption on plasma and urinary hormone concentrations in premenopausal women." *Journal of the National Cancer Institute*, 1993;85(9):722–727.

Page 223   Alcohol causes liver to metabolize more "bad" estrogen: Welsch, C.W. "Host factors affecting the growth of carcinogen-induced rat mammary carcinomas: A review and tribute to Charles Brenton Huggins." *Cancer Research*, 1976;45:3415–3443.

Page 223   Alcohol inhibits release of melatonin: Raloff, J. "Ecocancers: Do environmental factors underlie a breast cancer epidemic?" *Science News* 1993;144:10–13.

Page 223   Urethane causes breast tumors in 100 percent of dosed animals: Mitchell, C.P., and Jacobsen, M.F. *Tainted Booze.* Washington, D.C.: Center for Science in the Public Interest, 1987:9–22.

Page 223   Urethane exacerbates carcinogenic effects of X rays: International Agency for Research on Cancer. *Some Anti-Thyroid and Related Substances, Nitrofans and Industrial Chemicals.* Lyon, France: World Health Organization, 1974;111–140.

Page 224   Manufacturers can reduce urethane levels sharply by eliminating urea additives: Mitchell, C.P., and Jacobsen, M.F. *Tainted Booze.* Washington, D.C.: Center for Science in the Public Interest, 1987:9–22.

Page 224   United States liquor industry trivializes risk of urethane: *Ibid.*

Page 224   DDVP increases breast cancer in rodents: International Agency for Research on Cancer. *Alcohol Drinking.* Lyon, France: World Health Organization, 1988;44:98–99.

Page 224   Prolonged binge-drinking linked to immune system depletion: Ben-Eliyahu, S. *Nature Medicine*, 1996:2(4):457–460; United Press International. "Study shows alcohol-cancer link." March 28, 1996.

Page 224   Single incident of binge drinking may spread cancer: *Ibid.*

Page 225   Alcohol stimulates production of enzymes that raise "bad" estrogen: Westin, J.B., and Richter, E. "The Israeli breast cancer anomaly." *Annals of the New York Academy of Sciences*, 1990;609:269–279.

Page 225   Annual sales of hair dyes over $1 billion: International Agency for Research on Cancer. *Occupational Exposures of Hairdressers and Barbers, and Personal Use of Hair Colorants; Some Hair Dyes, Cosmetic Colorants, Industrial Dyestuffs, and Aromatic Amines.* Lyon, France: World Health Organization, 1993;57:63.

Page 226   ACS and FDA claim no connection between hair dyes and cancer: Thun, M.J., *et al.* "Hair dye use and risk of fatal cancers in U.S. women." *Journal of the National Cancer Institute*, 1994;86 (3):310–215.

Page 226   The body rapidly absorbs chemicals in hair dyes: International
Agency for Research on Cancer. *Occupational Exposures of
Hairdressers and Barbers, and Personal Use of Hair Colorants, Some
Hair Dyes, Cosmetic Colorants, Industrial Dyestuffs, and Aromatic
Amines.* Lyon, France: World Health Organization. 1993;57:93–94.

Page 226   Permanent and semipermanent colors contain carcinogenic ingre-
dients and contaminants: National Cancer Institute. "Bioassay of
2,4-diaminoanisole sulfate for possible carcinogenicity."
Carcinogenesis Technical Report Series, no. 84, 1978; *Federal
Register* August 30, 1988;53(168):33110–33121; U.S. Food and
Drug Administration, Washington, D.C. *Cosmetic Handbook.* 1996.

Page 227   Temporary dyes and rinses contain carcinogenic metals and petrochemicals: "Are hair dyes safe?" *Consumer Reports,* August 1979:
455–460.

Page 227   Dye TDA induces liver, breast, and other cancers in rodents:
Ibid.: 455–460; National Cancer Institute. "Bioassay of 2,4-
diaminoanisole sulfate for possible carcinogenicity." Carcinogenesis Technical Report Series, no. 84, 1978; Van Duren, B. Quoted in
"Are hair dyes safe?" *Consumer Reports,* August 1979; 455–460.

Page 227   Diaminoanisole was shown to induce breast cancer: National
Cancer Institute, "Bioassay of 2,4-diaminoansole sulfate for possible carcinogenicity." Carcinogenesis Technical Report Series, no.
84, 1978.

Page 229   When women start to use hair dye affects risk: Nisbet, I.C.T., and
Rosenblatt, K. *Carcinogenic Risk Estimates for 2,4-DAA.* A report
prepared by Clement Associates, Inc. (undated):22.

Box

Page 230   A 1976 study: Shafer, N., and Shafer, R.W. "Potential of carcinogenic effects of hair dyes." *New York State Journal of Medicine.*
1976;76:394–396.

Page 230   A 1977 United Kingdom study: Kinlen, L.J., *et al.* "Use of hair dyes
by patients with breast cancer: A case-control study." *British
Medical Journal,* 1977;ii:366–368.

Page 230   A 1979 United States Study: Shore, R.E., *et al.* "A case-control study
of hair dye use and breast cancer." *Journal of the National Cancer
Institute,* 1979;62:277–283.

Page 230   Another 1979 study: Hennekens, C.H., *et al.* "Use of permanent
hair dyes and cancer among registered nurses." *The Lancet,*
1979;1(1831):1390–1393.

Page 230   A well-controlled 1980 study: Nasca, P.C., et al. "Relationship of hair dye use, benign breast disease, and breast cancer." *Journal of the National Cancer Institute*, 1980;64:23–28.

END BOX

Page 230   ACS/FDA report admitted hair dyes linked to rare cancers, including multiple myeloma: Thun, M.J., et al. "Hair dye use and risk of fatal cancers in U.S. women." *Journal of the National Cancer Institute*, 1994;86(3):215–310.

Page 231   NIH panel emphasizes physical inactivity: Brody, J.E. "Heart experts urge even easier, softer exercise to counter sedentary habits." *The New York Times*, December 21, 1995:A15

Page 231   Fewer than 20 percent of high school girls get adequate exercise: Anonymous. "Participation of high school students in school physical education—United States, 1990." *Morbidity Mortality Weekly Report* 1992;41:613–615.

Page 232   Risk of breast cancer 70 percent greater in inactive than active women: Albanes, D., et al. "Physical activity and risk of cancer in the NHANES I population." *American Journal of Public Health*, 1989;79(6):744–750.

Page 232   Women with high-activity jobs have lower rates of breast cancer: Zheng, W., et al."Occupational physical activity and incidence of the breast, corpus uteri, and ovary in Shanghai." *Cancer*, 1993; 71(11):3620–3624.

Page 233   Lower cancer risk in athletic women: Associated Press. "Lower cancer risk found in athletic women." *The New York Times*, January 10, 1986:7Y; Frisch, R.E., et al. "Lower prevalence of breast cancer and cancers of the reproductive system among college athletes compared to non-athletes." *British Journal of Cancer*, 1985; 52:885–891; Frisch, R.E., et al. "Lower lifetime occurrence of breast cancer and cancers of the reproductive system among former college athletes." *American Journal of Clinical Nutrition*, 1987;45: 328–335.

Page 233   Exercising four hours per week cuts risk by 60 percent: Berstein, L., et al. "Physical exercise and reduced risk of breast cancer in young women." *Journal of the National Cancer Institute*, 1994;86: 1403–1408.

Page 234   Vigorous exercise reduces risk by 37 percent: Kolata, G. "Study suggests exercise fights breast cancer." *The New York Times*, May 1, 1997: A1.

Page 235   Exercise may be more protective than low-fat diet: Cohen, L.A., *et al.* "Modulation of N-nitrosomethylurea induced mammary tumorigenesis by dietary fat and voluntary exercise." *In Vivo*, 1991;5(4):333–344.

Page 235   Moderate to intense exercise "highly protective against tumors": Thompson, H.J., *et al.* "Inhibition of mammary carcinogenesis by treadmill exercise." *Journal of the National Cancer Institute*, 1995;87(6):453–455.

Page 236   Exercise reduces body fat and delays menarche: Frisch, R.E., and McArthur, J.W. "Menstrual cycles: Fatness as a determinant of minimum weight for height necessary for their maintenance or onset." *Science*, 1974;185:949–951; Sherman, B., *et al.* "Relationship of body weight to menarcheal and menopausal age: Implications for breast cancer risk." *Journal of Clinical Endocrinology and Metabolism*, 1981;52:488–493; Warren, M.P. "The effects of exercise on pubertal progression and reproductive function in girls." *Journal of Clinical Endocrinology and Metabolism*, 1989;51(5): 1150–1157.

Page 236   Exercise enhances protective effects of breast feeding: *Ibid.*

Page 237   Active women eat less beef and dairy products: Frisch, R.E., *et al.* "Lower prevalence of breast cancer and cancers of the reproductive system among college athletes compared to non-athletes." *British Journal of Cancer*, 1985;52:885–891.

Page 238   Stress triggers release of hormones that impair immunity: Henry, J.P., *et al.* "Force breeding, social disorder, and mammary tumor formation in CBA/UC mouse colonies: A pilot study." *Psychosomatic Medicine*, 1975;37(3):277–283; Peteet, J.R. "Psychological factors in the causation and course of cancer." In *Cancer, Stress, and Death*, 2nd ed., ed. S.B. Day. New York: Plenum, 1987:63–77.

Page 238   Forcible removal of baby mice causes increased breast cancer: Henry, J.P., *et al.* "Force breeding, social disorder, and mammary tumor formation in CBA/UC mouse colonies: A pilot study." *Psychosomatic Medicine*, 1975;37(3):277–283.

Page 238   Stress directly increases risk of breast cancer: Visintainer, M.A., *et al.* "Helplessness, chronic stress, and tumor development." *Psychosomatic Medicine*, 1983;45:75–79.

Page 239   High stress increases breast cancer: Riley, V. "Psychoneuroendocrine influences on immunocompetence and neoplasia." *Science*, 1981;212:1100–1108.

Page 241   Health considerations slightly favor not drinking: Friedman, G.D.,
              and Klatsky, A.L. "Is alcohol good for your health?" *New England
              Journal of Medicine*, 1993;329(25):1882–1883.

Page 244   More than half of Americans do not get enough activity: Brody, J.E.
              "Heart experts urge even easier, softer exercise to counter sedentary
              habits." *The New York Times*, December 21, 1995:A15.

11: WHERE YOU LIVE

Page 248   Immigrants slowly assume risks similar to native-born women:
              Kliewer, E.V., and Smith, K.R. "Breast cancer mortality among
              immigrants in Australia and Canada." *Journal of the National
              Cancer Institute*, 1995;87(15):1154–1161.

Page 249   Women in the West and Northeast have higher risk than southern
              women: Blot, W.J., *et al.* "Geographic patterns of breast cancer in
              the U.S." *Journal of the National Cancer Institute*, 1977;59(5):
              1407–1411.

Page 249   NCI claims excess Northeast cancers due to reproductive risk fac-
              tors: Sturgeon, S.L., *et al.* "Geographic variation in mortality from
              breast cancer among white women in the United States." *Journal of
              the National Cancer Institute*, 1995;87(24):1846–1852.

Page 250   "Findings of NCI should help allay fears": *Ibid.*: 1819–1820.

Page 251   High vitamin D levels protective against cancer: "Diet of teenage
              girls may increase their risk of breast cancer: Inadequate levels of
              dietary calcium and vitamin D may increase the risk of breast and
              other cancers for young females and the elderly." *Primary Care and
              Cancer*, 1994;14(2):8; Anderson, J.J.B., and Toverud, S.U. "Diet and
              vitamin D: A review with an emphasis on human function."
              Journal of Nutritional Biochemistry, 1994;5:58–65.

Page 251   Women in North eat more meat and fewer vegetables: Blot, W.J., *et
              al.* "Geographic patterns of breast cancer in the U.S." *Journal of the
              National Cancer Institute*, 1977;59(5):1407–1411.

Page 251   Long Island counties' breast cancer rates higher than elsewhere:
              Goldman, B.A. *The Truth about Where You Live: An Atlas for Action
              on Toxins and Mortality*. New York: Times Books, Random House,
              1991.

Page 253   New Jersey's high breast cancer rates related to hazardous waste:
              Najem, G.R., and Greer, T.W. "Female reproductive organs and
              breast cancer mortality in New Jersey counties and the relationship
              with certain environmental variables." *Preventive Medicine*,
              1985;14:620–635.

Page 253   Counties with high breast cancer rates house four to thirteen times more hazardous waste facilities: Griffith, J., *et al.* "Cancer mortality in U.S. counties with hazardous waste sites and ground water pollution." *Archives of Environmental Health,* 1989;44 (2):69–74.

Page 253   High breast cancer incidence related to environmental factors: Kay, J., and Flinn, J. "Alarming results for Bay women in cancer study." *San Francisco Press,* November 11, 1994.

Page 253   Chevron discharges 57,000 pounds of methylene chloride annually: Brady, J. "Chevron: Good guys?" *Women's Cancer Resource Center,* Winter 1996:5–6.

Page 253   Difficulty in identifying environmental risk factors: Robbins, Anthony S. *et al.* "Regional differences in known risk factors and the higher incidence of breast cancer in San Francisco." *Journal of the National Cancer Institute,* 1997;39(13):960–965.

Page 254   People exposed to estrogen chemicals by breathing air and drinking contaminated water: Davis, D.L., and Bradlow, H.L. "Can environmental estrogens cause breast cancer?" In *Scientific American,* 1995:273(4):167–172.

Page 255   Women living on Cape Cod near military base at higher risk: Aschengrau, A., and Ozonoff, D.M. "Upper Cape cancer incidence study. Final report." Boston: Boston University School of Public Health, September, 1991.

Page 256   Living near chemical plants increased breast cancer rates about equal to having family history: New York State Department of Health. *Residence Near Industries and High Traffic Areas and the Risk of Breast Cancer on Long Island,* April 1994. Division of Occupational Health and Environmental Epidemiology, Bureau of Environmental and Occupational Epidemiology.

Page 256   Link between cancer and industrial pollution cited: Schemo, D.J. "Chemical plants seen as factor in breast cancer." *The New York Times,* April 13, 1994:A1.

Page 257   Radioactive emissions from nuclear plants linked to breast cancer: Gould, J.M., *et al. The Enemy Within: The High Cost of Living Near Nuclear Reactors.* New York: Four Walls, Eight Windows, Greenpeace Edition, 1996.

Page 257   Plants operating on Long Island since the 1950s: Sternglass, E.J., and Gould, J.M. "Breast cancer: Evidence for a relation to fission products in the diet." *International Journal of Health Services,* 1993;23(4):783–804.

Page 257   Breast cancer rates rise in direct connection to peak plant emissions: *Ibid.*: 783–804.

Page 257   Emissions from Millstone plant caused shutdown: Wald, M.L. "3rd Connecticut A-plant cited for long-standing problems." *The New York Times,* April 5, 1996:8.

Page 258   In counties downwind from the reactor in Hanford: Sternglass, E.J., and Gould, J.M. "Breast cancer: Evidence for a relation to fission products in the diet." *International Journal of Health Services,* 1993;23(4):783–804.

Page 258   Rates increased 15 percent downwind from the Savannah River plant: *Ibid.*: 783–804.

Page 259   20 million Americans exposed to EMFs: Pinsky, M.A. *The EMF Book.* New York: Warner Books, 1994.

Page 259   EMFs can damage the immune system: Alvin, L., *et al.* "Electrical and magnetic fields: Measurements and possible effects on human health from appliances, powerlines, and other common sources: What we know, what we don't know in 1990." Berkeley: Special Epidemiological Studies Program, California Department of Health Services, 1991.

Page 259   Women exposed to EMFs deliver children who later develop cancers: Wertheimer, N., and Leeper, E. "Electric wiring configurations and childhood cancer." *American Journal of Epidemiology,* 1979;109:273–284; Spitz, M.R., and Johnson, C.C. "Neuroblastoma and paternal occupation: A case-control analysis." *American Journal of Epidemiology,* 1985;121:924–929; Tomenius, L. "50-Hz electromagnetic environment and the incidence of childhood tumors in Stockholm County." *Bioelectromagnetics,* 1986;7:191–207; Savitz, D.A., *et al.* "Case control study of study of childhood cancer and exposure to 60-Hz magnetic fields." *American Journal of Epidemiology,* 1988;128:21–38; Wilkins, J.R., and Koutras, R.A. "Paternal occupation and brain cancer in off-spring—a mortality-based case-control study." *American Journal of Industrial Medicine,* 1988;14:299–318; Johnson, C.C., and Spitz, M.R. "Childhood nervous system tumors: An assessment of risk associated with paternal occupations involving use, repair, or manufacture of electrical and electronic equipment." *International Journal of Epidemiology,* 1989;18:756–762; London, S.J., *et al.* "Exposure to residential electric and magnetic fields and risk of childhood leukemia." *American Journal of Epidemiology,* 1991;134:923–937; Kuitjen, R.R., *et al.* "Parental occupation and childhood astrocytoma: Results of a case-control study." *Cancer Research,* 1992; 52:782–786; Feychting,

M., and Ahlbom, A. "Magnetic fields and cancer in people residing near Swedish high-voltage power lines." *American Journal of Epidemiology*, 1993;138(7):467–481.

Page 259   Increased rates of premenopausal breast cancer in women living near transmission lines in Colorado: Wertheimer, N., and Leeper, E. "Magnetic field exposure related to cancer subtypes." *Annals of the New York Academy of Sciences*, 1987;502:43–54.

Page 260   Increased risk of breast cancer in women living within 500 feet of electric power substations: Aschengrau, A., and Ozonoff, D.M. *Upper Cape Cancer Incidence Study. Final Report.* Boston: Boston University School of Public Health, September, 1991.

Page 260   ACS denies EMF relationship to cancer: Heath, C.W. "Electromagnetic field exposure and cancer: A review of epidemiologic evidence." *CA: A Cancer Journal for Clinicians*, 1996;46(1): 29–44.

Page 260   Indoor concentrations of pollution 500 time higher than outside: Wallace, L., cited in Stammer, L.B. "Clean air quest—an inside job: When it comes to human health, pollution in homes and offices may be the greatest threat." *Los Angeles Times* December 26, 1989:A1.

Page 262   Aerosol paints and paint strippers contain carcinogenic methylene chloride: Steinman, D.S. and Epstein, S.S. *The Safe Shopper's Bible.* New York: Macmillan, 1995:93–101.

Page 262   Lawn pesticides applied at a rate of 5 to 11 pounds per acre: National Academy of Sciences. *Urban Pest Management.* Washington, D.C., 1971.

Page 262   EPA study found indoor levels of pesticides up to ten times higher than outside: Environmental Protection Agency. *Nonoccupational Pesticide Exposure Study.* Atmospheric Research and Exposure Assessment Laboratory, Research Triangle Park, NC: U.S. Environmental Protection Agency, EPA/699/3-90//003, January 1990.

Page 262   EPA estimates No-Pest Strips pose cancer risks ten times greater than for pest control workers who apply DDVP: "No-Pest Strip insecticide poses an unacceptably high risk of cancer in people and pets. . . ." *Journal of Pesticide Reform*, Spring 1988:29.

Page 263   Carcinogenic solvents and contaminants become gases at room temperatures and are easily inhaled: Bronaugh, R.L., *et al.* "Extent of cutaneous metabolism during percutaneous absorption of xenobiotics." *Toxicology and Applied Pharmacology*, 1989;99:

534–543; Brown, H., *et al.* "The role of skin absorption as a route for volatile organic compounds (VOCs) in drinking water." *American Journal of Public Health*, 1984;74(5):479–484; Andelman, J.B. "Human exposures to volatile halogenated organic chemicals in indoor and outdoor air." *Environmental Health Perspectives*, 1985;62:313–318.

Page 263   Inhaled volatiles provide same exposure as drinking eight glasses of contaminated water: Brown, H., *et al.* "The role of skin aborption as a route of exposure for volatile organic compounds in drinking water." *American Journal of Public Health*, 1984;74:479; Andelman, J.B. "Human exposures to volatile halogenated organic chemicals in indoor and outdoor air." *Environmental Health Perspectives*, 1985;62:313–318.

Page 263   Kerosene heaters, gas burners, and natural gas cooking and heating emit carcinogenic pollutants: International Agency for Research on Cancer. *Diesel and Gasoline Engine Exhausts and Some Nitroarenes.* Lyon, France: World Health Organization, 1989;46:231–246, 277–289; Southern California Gas Company. "Proposition 65 Warning." March 1993.

Page 263   Contamined clothing source of exposure to carcinogens of families, raising risk of cancer: National Institute for Occupational Safety and Health. *Report to Congress on Workers' Home Contamination Study Conducted Under the Workers' Family Protection Act (29 U.S. C 671a).* Cincinnati, OH: NIOSH, September, 1995.

Page 264   Home appliances emit EMFs: Raloff, J. "EMFs run aground. Mapping magnetic fields from water pipes and other homely sources" *Science News*, 1993;144:124.

Page 264   Higher exposure to indoor EMFs than outdoor: Sanders, B. "Field trip." *Green Alternatives*, July/August 1993:21.

Page 264   Increased risk of breast cancer with EMFs from electric blankets: Vena, J.E., *et al.* "Use of electric blankets and risk of postmenopausal breast cancer." *American Journal of Epidemiology*, 1991;134(2):180–185.

Page 264   The National Institute of Environmental Health funding research on EMFs: "EMFs and breast cancer." *Environmental Health Letter*, January 29, 1996:26.

Page 265   The ACS denies risks of EMFs: Heath, C.W. "Electromagnetic field exposure and cancer: A review of epidemiologic evidence." *CA: A Cancer Journal for Clinicians*, 1996;46(1):29–44.

Page 266   Exposure to near-constant electric light inhibits melatonin levels; increases estrogen: Stevens, R.G. "Electric power use and breast cancer. A hypothesis." *American Journal of Epidemiology*, 1987;125:556–561; Hahn, R.A., *et al.* "Nulliparity, decade of first birth, and breast cancer in Connecticut cohorts, 1855–1945, an ecological study." *American Journal of Public Health*, 1989;79(11):1503–1507; Stevens, R.G., *et al.* "Electric power, pineal function, and the risk of breast cancer." *FASEB Journal*, 1992;6:853–860; Lewy, A.J., *et al.* "Light suppresses melatonin secretion in humans." *Science*, 1980;210:1267–1269; McIntyre, I.M., *et al.* "Melatonin supersensitivity to dim light in seasonal affective disorder." *The Lancet*, 1990;335:488.

Page 267   Blind women have lower rates of breast cancer: Hahn, R.A. "Profound bilateral blindness and the incidence of breast cancer." *Epidemiology*, 1991; 2:208–210.

Page 267   Light expert writes of dangers of electric lights: Harrell, B.B. "Cancer and light." Letter to the editor. *The New York Times*, August 8, 1995:A10.

Page 268   Court ruling forces chemical companies to disclose emissions: Cushman, J.H., Jr. "Court backs E.P.A. authority on disclosure of toxic agents." *The New York Times*, May 2, 1996:A12; Federal judge upholds TRI expansion; ruling clears way for further actions." *Environmental Health Letter*, May 2, 1996:92.

12: HAZARDS IN THE WORKPLACE

Page 273   Little is known about workplace risks for breast cancer: Vena, J.E., *et al.* "Breast cancer and lifetime occupation." Baltimore, MD: International Conference on Women's Health: Occupation and Cancer, November 1–2, 1993, National Institutes of Health:36.

Page 274   Only 14 percent of 1,200 publications on occupational cancer: Zham, S.H. "Inclusion of women and minorities in occupational cancer epidemiological research." Baltimore, MD: International Conference on Women's Health: Occupation and Cancer, November 1–2, 1993, National Institutes of Health:14.

Page 274   Few ocupational studies focus on women: Labreche, F.P. and Goldberg, M.S. "Exposure to organic solvents and breast cancer in women: A hypothesis." *American Journal of Industrial Medicine*, 1997; 32:1–14.

Page 282   Women working in petrochemical, manufacturing, and cosmetics industries have high breast cancer rates: Hall, N.E.L., and Rosenman, K.D. "Cancer by industry: Analysis of a population-based cancer registry with an emphasis on blue-collar workers." *American Journal of Industrial Medicine*, 1991;19:145–159.

Page 282 Polyvinyl chloride poses breast cancer risk: Chiazze, L., *et al.* "Mortality among employees of PVC fabricators." *Journal of Occupational Medicine*, 1977;19(9):623–628.

Page 282 Breast cancer among women exposed to vinyl chloride is plausible: Maltoni, C., *et al.* "Carcinogenicity bioassays of vinyl chloride monomer: A model of risk assessment on an experimental basis." *Environmental Health Perspectives*, 1981;41:3–30; Feron, V.J., *et al.* "Life-span oral toxicity study of vinyl chloride in rats." *Food Cosmetics Toxicology*, 1981;19:317–333; Infante, P.F., and Peasak, J. "A historical perspective of some occupationally-related diseases of women." *Journal of Occupational Medicine*, 1994;36(8):826–831.

Page 282 Textile workers at high risk: Cantor, K.P., *et al.* "Associations of occupation and industry from death certificates with breast cancer mortality in case-control analysis." Baltimore: International Conference on Women's Health: Occupation and Cancer, November 1–2, 1993, National Institutes of Health:43; Morton, W.E. "Major differences in breast cancer risks among occupations." *Ibid.*: 14.

Page 282 Methylene chloride and breast cancer among women manufacturing lamps: Shannon, H.S., *et al.* "Cancer morbidity in lamp manufacturing workers." *American Journal of Industrial Medicine*, 1988;14:281–290.

Page 282 Breast cancer increases in women working in electrical equipment and printing industries: Hall, N.E.L., and Rosenman, K.D. "Cancer by industry: An analysis of a population-based cancer registry with an emphasis on blue-collar workers." *American Journal of Industrial Medicine*, 1991;19:145–159; MacCubbin, P.A., *et al.* "Mortality in New York State, 1980–1982: A report by occupation and industry." Albany: New York State Department of Health (Monograph No. 21), 1986.

Page 283 Breast cancer increases in workers exposed to chlorinated organic solvents and Freons: Spritas, R., *et al.* "Retrospective cohort mortality study of workers at an aircraft maintenance facility. I Epidemiological results." *Journal of Industrial Medicine*, 1991;48: 515–530.

Page 283 Health care workers exposed to ethylene oxide at risk: Stolley, P. "A preliminary report of cancer incidence in a group of workers potentially exposed to ethylene oxide." Clinical Epidemiology Unit, University of Pennsylvania School of Medicine, April 25, 1986.

Page 283   Carcinogenic solvents collect in breast tissue and become activated by enzymes. Labreche, F.P., and Goldberg, S.M. "Exposure to organic solvents and breast cancer in women: A hypothesis." *American Journal of Industrial Medicine*, 1997;32:1–14.

Page 283   Atrazine causes breast cancer in rodents: Wiles, R., *et al. Tap Water Blues: Herbicides in Drinking Water*. Washington, D.C.: Environmental Working Group, 1994; Epstein, S.S. "Environmental and occupational pollutants are avoidable causes of breast cancer." *International Journal of Health Services*, 1994;24(1):145–149.

Page 283   Of 400 German women exposed to dioxin, four developed breast cancer: Manz, A., *et al.* "Cancer mortality among workers in a chemical plant contaminated with dioxin." *The Lancet*, 1991;338:959–964.

Box

Page 284   Several studies from Great Britain: Registrar General. *The Registrar General's Decennial Supplement, England and Wales, 1951. Occupational Mortality*, 1958: Part II, Vol. 2, *Tables*, London: Her Majesty's Stationery Office, as cited in *International Agency for Research on Cancer Monographs, Volume 57*; Office of Population Censuses and Surveys, *Occupational Mortality Decennial Supplement*, 1979–80, 1982–83, 1986. London: Her Majesty's Stationery Office, as cited in *International Agency for Research on Cancer Monographs*, Vol. 57.

Page 284   In 1972: International Agency for Research on Cancer. *Occupational Exposures of Hairdressers and Barbers and Personal Use of Hair Colorants; Some Hair Dyes, Cosmetic Colorants, Industrial Dyestuffs and Aromatic Amines*. Lyon, France: World Health Organization, 1993;57.

Page 284   A 1990 Japanese study: Kato, I., *et al.* "An epidemiological study on occupation and cancer risk." *Japanese Journal of Clinical Oncology*, 1990;20:121–127.

Page 284   A 1992 Finnish study: Pukkala, E., *et al.* "Changing cancer risk patterns among Finnish hairdressers." *International Archives of Occupational Environnmental Health*, 1992;64:39–42.

Page 284   A 1993 Washington State study: Habel, L.A., *et al.* "Occupational exposures and risk of breast cancer in middle-aged women." Baltimore: International Conference on Women's Health: Occupation and Cancer, November 1–2, 1993, National Institutes of Health.

End Box

Page 284   Pharmaceutical workers suffer from excess rates of breast cancer: Hall, N.E.L., and Rosenman, K.D. "Cancer by industry: An analysis of a population-based cancer registry with an emphasis on blue-collar workers." *American Journal of Industrial Medicine,* 1991;19:145–159; Thomas, T.L., and Decoufle, P. "Mortality among workers employed in the pharmaceutical industry: A preliminary investigation." *Journal of Occupational Medicine,* 1979;21:619–623, as cited in Hall and Rosenman, *Ibid.*

Page 285   Acute hormonal effects in women manufacturing contraceptives: Anonymous. "Occupational exposure to synthetic estrogens—Puerto Rico." *Morbidity and Mortality Weekly Report,* Centers for Disease Control, 1977;26(13):101.

Page 285   Exposure to overlapping combinations of metals poses risk: Cantor, K.P., *et al.* "Occupational exposures and female breast cancer mortality in the United States." *Journal of Occupational and Environmental Medicine,* 1995;37(3):336–348.

Page 285   Workers exposed to solder at risk: Spritas, R., *et al.* "Retrospective cohort mortality study of workers at an aircraft maintenance facility. I. Epidemiological results." *British Journal of Industrial Medicine,* 1991;48:515–530.

Page 285   High rates of breast cancer among 700 asbestos workers: Newhouse, M.L., and Wagner, J.C. "Mortality of factory workers in East London 1933–1980." *British Journal of Industrial Medicine,* 1985;42: 4–11.

Page 285   High concentrations of asbestos in women with breast cancer: Doniach, I., *et al.* "Prevalence of asbestos bodies in necropsy series in East London: Association with disease, occupation, and domiciliary address." *British Journal of Industrial Medicine,* 1975;32: 16–30.

Page 286   Chemicals found in oil paints are carcinogenic and concentrate in the breast: Grumbacher Corporation. Cranbury, N.J.: Material Safety Data Sheets, 1995; Davis, D.L., and Bradlow, H.L. "Avoidable environmental links to breast cancer." In: *Reducing Breast Cancer Risk in Women,* ed. B.A. Stoll. Dordrecht, Netherlands: Kluwer Academic Publishers, 1995:231–235; Falck, F.A., *et al.* "Pesticides and polychlorinated biphenyl residues in human breast lipids and their relation to breast cancer." *Archives of Environmental Health,* 1992;47:143–146.

Page 286   A preliminary NCI study of 16,000 artists: Miller, B.A., *et al.* "Cancer risk among artistic painters." *American Journal of Industrial Medicine,* 1986;9:281–287.

Page 286   Women painting luminous radium on instrument dials ran high risk: Gofman, J. *Radiation-Induced Cancer from Low-Dose Exposure: An Iindependent Analysis.* San Francisco, CA: Committee for Nuclear Responsibility, 1990; Baverstock, K.F., *et al.* "Risk of radiation at low dose rates." *The Lancet,* 1981;1:430–433; Baverstock, K.F., and Vennart, J. "A note on radium body content and breast cancers in U.K. radium luminizers." *Health Physics,* 1983;44, suppl. 1:575–577; Baverstock, K.F. "UK luminizer survey misrepresented." *Journal of Occupational Medicine,* 1985;27(9):613; Baverstock, K.F., and Papworth, D.G. "The UK radium luminizer survey." *British Journal of Radiology,* 1987, Supplemental British Institute of Radiology Report 21:71–76.

Page 286   Significant excess in breast cancer among X-ray workers in China: Wang, J.X., *et al.* "Cancer among medical diagnostic x-ray workers in China." *Journal of the National Cancer Institute,* 1988;80: 344–350.

Page 287   Small excess of breast cancer among nuclear weapons plant workers: Vaughan, T.L., *et al.* "Breast cancer incidence at a nuclear facility: Demonstration of a morbidity surveillance system." *Health Physics,* 1993;64(4):349–354.

Page 287   Significantly higher risks of breast and bone cancer among airline cabin attendants: Pukkala, E., *et al.* "Incidence of cancer among Finnish airline cabin attendants, 1967–1992." *British Medical Journal,* 1992;311:649–652.

Page 288   Two studies find no excess risk with EMF exposure: Guenel, P., *et al.* "Incidence of cancer in persons with occupational exposure to electromagnetic fields in Denmark." *British Journal of Industrial Medicine,* 1993;50:758–764; Vågerö, D. *et al.* "Incidence of cancer in the electronics industry; Using the new Swedish Cancer Environment Registry as a screening instrument." *British Journal of Industrial Medicine,* 1983;40:188–192; Vågerö, D., *et al.* "Cancer morbidity among workers in the telecommunications industry." *British Journal of Industrial Medicine,* 1985;42:191–195.

Page 288   Exposure to modern telephone industry may account for excess risk: Dosmeci, M., and Blair, A. "Occupational cancer mortality among women employed in the telephone industry." Baltimore: International Conference on Women's Health: Occupation and Cancer, November 1–2, 1993, National Institutes of Health.

Page 288   Women in electrical occupations with high EMF exposure were nearly 40 percent more likely to die of breast cancer: Loomis, D.P., *et al.* "Breast cancer mortality among female electrical workers in the United States." *Journal of the National Cancer Institute,* 1994; 86(12):921–925.

Page 288   ACS admits link between EMFs and breast cancer risk: Heath, C.W.
                  "Electromagnetic field exposure and cancer: A review of epidemiolog-
                  ic evidence." *CA: A Cancer Journal for Clinicians*, 1996;46 (1):29–44.

Page 288   Excess breast cancers among women workers exposed to EMFS:
                  Pinsky, M. *The EMF Book: What You Need to Know about
                  Electromagnetic Fields, Electromagnetic Radiation, and Your Health.*
                  New York: Warner Books, 1995; Matanoski, G.M., *et al.*
                  "Electromagnetic field exposure and male breast cancer." *The
                  Lancet*, 1991;337:737; Deamers, P.A., *et al.* "Occupational exposure
                  to electromagnetic fields and breast cancer in men." *American
                  Journal of Epidemiology*, 1991;134:340–347; Tynes, T., *et al.*
                  "Incidence of cancer in Norwegian workers potentially exposed to
                  electromagnetic fields." *American Journal of Epidemiology*, 1992;
                  136:81–88; Loomis, D.P. "Cancer of the breast among men in elec-
                  trical occupations." *The Lancet*, 1992;339:1482–1483; Anonymous.
                  "Epidemiologists call for study of EMFs and female breast cancer."
                  Micro Wave News, 1991;XI(1):1,14; Trichopoulos, D. "Are electric
                  or magnetic fields affecting mortality from breast cancer in
                  women?" *Journal of the National Cancer Institute*, 1994;86
                  (12):885–886.

Page 288   EMFs suppress melatonin production: Pool, R. "Electromagnetic
                  fields: The biological evidence." *Science*, 1990;249(4975):1378–1381.

Page 290   Teachers and other professionals at special risk: Cantor, K.P., *et al.*
                  "Associations of occupation and industry from death certificates
                  with breast cancer mortality in case-control analysis." Baltimore:
                  International Conference on Women's Health: Occupation and
                  Cancer, November 1–2, 1993, National Institutes of Health;
                  Gunnarsdottir, H., and Ranfnsoon, V. "Cancer incidence among
                  nurses." Baltimore: International Conference on Women's Health:
                  Occupation & Cancer, November 1–2, 1993, National Institutes of
                  Health; Katz, R.M. "Causes of death among registered nurses."
                  Journal of Occupational Medicine, 1993;25(10):760–762; Kato, I., *et
                  al.* "An epidemiological study on occupation and cancer risk."
                  Japanese Journal of Clinical Oncology, 1990;20:121–127; Zheng, W.,
                  et al. "Occupational physical activity and the incidence of cancer of
                  the breast, corpus uteri, and ovary in Shanghai." *Cancer*,
                  1993;71(11):3620–3624; Williams, R.R., *et al.* "Associations of can-
                  cer site and type with occupation and industry from third nation-
                  al cancer survey interview." *Journal of the National Cancer Institute*,
                  1977;59(4):1147–1185;

Page 290   Teachers in U.S. and Canada have excess breast cancer: Rubin, C.,
                  et al. "Occupation as a risk identifier for breast cancer." *American
                  Journal of Public Health*, 1993;83(9):1311–1315.

Page 290   Intensive application of carcinogenic pesticides in schools: Cooper, S. "Getting pesticides expelled from schools." *Pesticides and You,* August, 1992:22–23;

Page 290   Clergywomen, mathematicians, computer scientists, and dieticians also have increased risk: Williams, R.R., *et al.* "Associations of cancer site and type with occupation and industry from the third national cancer survey interview." *Journal of the National Cancer Institute,* 1977;59(4):1147–1185; Rubin, C., *et al.* "Occupation as a risk identifier for breast cancer." *American Journal of Public Health,* 1993;83(9):1311–1315; Sankila, R., *et al.* "Cancer risk among health care personnel in Finland, 1971–1980." *Scandinavian Journal of Work and Environmental Health,* 1990;16:252–257.

Page 290   Increased breast cancer related to sedentary work: Vena, J.E., *et al.* "Occupational exercise and risk of cancer." *American Journal of Clinical Nutrition,* 1987;45:318–327.

Page 290   Low physical activity and higher risk of breast cancer: Zheng, W., *et al.* "Occupational physical activity and the incidence of cancer of the breast, corpus uteri, and ovary in Shanghai." *Cancer,* 1993;71(11):3620–3624.

13: THE POLITICS OF BREAST CANCER

Page 299   NCI spends less than 5 percent of its money on prevention: Epstein, S.S. "Evaluation of the National Cancer Program and proposed reforms." *International Journal of Health Services,* 1993; 23(1):15–44.

Page 299   Federal GAO warns that no progress has been made in preventing breast cancer: General Accounting Office. *Breast Cancer, 1971–1991, Prevention, Treatment, and Research.* GAO/PEMD-92-12. Report to the Committee on Government Operations. Washington, D.C., December 1991.

Page 299   Scientists urge shift in cancer establishment priorities: Epstein, S.S. "Losing the 'war against cancer': A need for public policy reforms." *International Journal of Health Services,* 1992;22(3):455–469.

Page 300   NCI admits loss of war against preventing cancer: National Cancer Advisory Board. *Cancer at a Crossroads: A Report to Congress for the Nation.* Bethesda, MD: September, 1994.

Page 301   Biologist admits lack of knowledge and interest in prevention: Angier, N. *Natural Obsessions: The Search for the Oncogene,* Boston: Houghton, Mifflin, 1988:12.

Page 301   Harold Varmus reveals NCI priorities: *Ibid.*: 13.

Page 302   NCI Advisory Board remains devoid of environmental experts: Landrigan, P.J. Testimony before National Cancer Advisory Board, Publication Participation Hearings, Philadelphia, April 19, 1988.

Page 302   NCI consistently refuses to provide guidance to Congress and agencies: Epstein, S.S. "Evaluation of the National Cancer Program and proposed reforms." *International Journal of Health Services,* 1993;23(1):15–44.

Page 302   Ex-NCI scientist urges shift from treatment to prevention: Smeltz, K.J. "Common ground found: Overall cancer mortality rates are falling." *Journal of National Cancer Industry,* 1997;89(4):1001.

Page 303   Basic conflict of interest within NCI: Moss, R.W. *The Cancer Industry: Unraveling the Politics.* New York: Paragon House, 1989.

Page 303   Sloan-Kettering board members have conflicts of interest: Epstein, S.S. "Losing the war against cancer: Who's to blame and what to do about it." *International Journal of Health Services,* 1990;20:53–71; Epstein, S.S. "Evaluation of the National Cancer Program and proposed reforms." *International Journal of Health Services,* 1993; 23(1):15–44.

Page 303   Employment revolving door: *Ibid.*

Page 303   NCI Director, Samuel Broder, M.D., resigned: Eliot, M. "Broder to join exodus from NCI." *Science,* 1995;267:24.

Page 304   Dr. Frank Rauscher resigned in 1976: Mahaney, F.S., Jr. "Dr. Frank J. Rausher, Jr.: An appreciation." *Journal of the National Cancer Institute,* 1993;85(3);174–175.

Page 304   NCI allowed Bristol-Myers to sell Taxol at inflated price: Bleifuss, J. "Cancer politics." *In These Times,* May 1, 1995; Love, J.P. "Comments on the need for better federal government oversight of taxpayer supported research and development." Center for Study of Responsive Law, Washington, D.C. Testimony before the Subcommittee on Regulation, Business Opportunities, and Technology of the Committee on Small Business, U.S. House of Representatives, July 11, 1994:8–9.

Page 304   Bristol-Myers Squibb sells nearly one-third of cancer drugs: Alexander, R. "First reform welfare for corporations." Letter to the editor. *The New York Times,* January 13, 1995:A14.

Page 305   James P. Love protests against conflicts of interest: Bleifuss, J. "Cancer politics." *In These Times,* May 1, 1995; Love, J.P. "Comments on the need for better federal government oversight of taxpayer supported research and development." Center for Study of Responsive Law, Washington, D.C. Testimony before the Subcommittee on Regulation, Business Opportunities, and Technology of the Committee on Small Business, U.S. House of Representatives, July 11, 1994:8–9.

Page 305 ACS is the tail that wags the dog of the NCI: Epstein, S.S. "Losing the war against cancer: Who's to blame and what to do about it." *International Journal of Health Services,* 1990;20:53–71; Epstein, S.S. "Evaluation of the National Cancer Program and proposed reforms." *International Journal of Health Services,* 1993;23(1):15–44.

Page 306 ACS ignores requests from Congress to provide information: Greenberg, D.S., and Randal, J.E. "Waging the wrong war on cancer." *Washington Post,* May 1, 1977:C1.

Page 306 Representative of major union admits no support for safety standards from ACS: Mazzocchi, T., cited in Public Interest Roundtable with American Cancer Society Representative Joseph H. Young, chairman of the board, Dr. Benjamin Byrd, cochairman, and others. Washington, D.C.: October 26, 1978.

Page 307 ACS memo about documentary discounts environmental hazards: American Cancer Society. "Upcoming television special on pesticides in food." March 22, 1993. Memorandum from Dickinson, S., Vice-President Public Relations and Health, to Clark W. Heath, Jr., M.D., Vice-President, Epidemiology and Statistics.

Page 307 Former director of National Academy of Sciences Board of Agriculture calls ACS actions "unconscionable": Kaplan, S. "Lobby-PR giant makes hay from client 'cross-pollination.' Porter/Novelli plays all sides." *PR Watch,* First Quarter 1994:4.

Page 307 Reporter calls ACS actions a major conflict of interest: Kaplan, S. "Porter-Novelli plays all sides." *Legal Times,* November 23, 1993;16(27):1.

Page 308 ACS refuses to testify on DES: Greenberg, D.S., and Randal, J.E. "Waging the wrong war on cancer." *Washington Post,* May 1, 1977:C1.

Page 308 ACS vice-president dismisses evidence of risk of organochlorine pesticides: Heath, C. quoted in "Chlorine Institute issues response to the report on breast cancer issued this week by Greenpeace." Press release. Chlorine Institute, Washington, D.C., November 13, 1992.

Page 309 ACS balance in 1988 more than $400 million: Bennett, J.T. "Health research charities: Doing little in research but emphasizing politics." Manchester (New Hampshire) *Union Leader,* September 20, 1990:10.

Page 309   By 1989 ACS cash reserves at $700 million: Bennett, J.T., and DiLorenzo, T.J. *Unhealthy Charities: Hazardous to Your Health and Wealth.* New York: Basic Books, 1994.

Page 309   Americans increase cancer contributions in 1991: Flach, J. "ACS mobilizes forces to keep record straight." *Journal of the National Cancer Institute,* 1992;84(14):1071–1073.

Page 309   Philanthropy organization claims ACS interested in accumulating wealth: Hall, H., and Williams, G. "Professor vs. Cancer Society." *The Chronicle of Philanthropy,* January 28, 1992:26.

Page 310   Article cites evidence of ACS wealth and lack of community service in Texas, Arizona, California, and Missouri: DiLorenzo, T.J. "One charity's uneconomic war on cancer." *Wall Street Journal,* March 15, 1992: A10.

Page 312   ACS ad promises early detection means cure 100 percent: Dempsey, K., *et al.* "Screening mammography: What the cancer establishment never told you." The Women's Community Cancer Project, Cambridge, MA, May 5, 1992:33.

Page 312   ACS fails to tell women limits of baseline studies: Center for Devices and Radiologic Health. "Center supporting efforts to improve mammography quality." *Radiologic Health Bulletin,* 1987;21(4):1–4.

Page 314   NABCO retains close links with cancer establishment: National Association of Breast Cancer Organizations. "NABCO calendar for October." *NABCO News,* October 1995;9(3).

Page 314   Coalition persuades Congress to add $200 million for breast cancer: Erikson, J. "Breast cancer activists seek voice in research decisions." *Science,* 1995; 269:1508–1509.

Page 315   NABCO claims little is known about breast cancer causes: The National Breast Cancer Coalition. *Research Agenda.* Washington, D.C..

Page 319   Women need to participate in informed consent: Soffa, V.M. *The Journey Beyond Breast Cancer.* Rochester, VT: Healing Arts Press, 1994:109.

Page 320   Scientists urge shift in cancer establishment priorities: Epstein, S.S. "Losing the 'war against cancer': A need for public policy reforms." *International Journal of Health Services,* 1992;22(3):455–469.

Page 321   NCI asks Congress that requirement for prevention program spending be dropped: Marshall, E. "A new phase in the war on cancer." *Science*, 1995;256:1415.

Page 322   The political is personal: Steinem, G. *Revolution from Within: A Book of Self-Esteem.* Boston: Little, Brown, 1992.

Glossary

Abortion: Spontaneous or deliberate termination of pregnancy.

Adrenal gland: Located above kidney; secretes chemicals that trigger body to produce sex hormones including estrogen, progesterone, and testosterone.

Aldactone: Drug used to treat blood pressure.

Antihypertensive: Drug used to lower blood pressure.

Antimalignin Antibody in Serum Test (AMAS): Simple, noninvasive urine test for screening for earliest signs of cancer.

Antioxidant: Nutrient that helps to protect cells against damage by harmful chemicals and natural body processes, such as those that occurs in aging.

Apresoline (hydralazine): Drug used to treat blood pressure.

Ataxia-telongiectasia (A-T): Uncommon genetic disease that causes skin lesions and damages nervous system; heightens sensitivity to radiation.

Autoimmune disease: Disease in which the immune system produces antibodies against the body's own cells, destroying healthy tissue.

Benzene: Common pollutant to the breast carcinogenic.

Bovine growth synthetic hormone: Animal drug used to stimulate cows to produce more milk; known to cause infections in animals, requiring antibiotics and other drugs that end up in milk; consumption by humans results in higher levels of tumor-stimulating insulinlike growth factor.

Breast cancer: A malignant tumor of breast tissue, and the second most common form of cancer among women in the United States.

Calcium: The most common mineral on earth and the fifth most common in the human body; found mainly in the bones and teeth and essential for several body functions including metabolism of bone.

Carcinogen: Substance that can cause the growth of cancer.

Carcinogenic: Having the effect of causing and promoting cancer.

Carotenoids: Any of a group of red, yellow, or orange pigments found in fruits and vegetables that help protect the body against cancer and other diseases; beta-carotene and canthaxanthin, among many others, are carotenoids.

Catalase: An enzyme found in most living cells that speeds up the breakdown of hydrogen peroxide (a chemical that can damage cells) to water and oxygen.

Chemoprevention: The use of chemicals (usually medications or vitamins) to prevent cancer.

Cholesterol: Waxy fatty chemical the body uses to make hormones. Too much of certain types can clog arteries and contribute to heart disease risk.

Contaminants: Harmful substances that taint food, cosmetics, and other consumer products; may come from natural or artificial sources.

CYP1: A gene that controls estrogen production; a variation of the gene increases risk of breast cancer.

Cytochromes P450: Family of enzymes produced in response to toxic chemicals.

DDE: Chemical breakdown product of the pesticide DDT.

DDT: Chemical of the organochlorine family used after World War II to control insect pests.

Desogen: *See* "Morning-After Pill"

Desogesterol: *See* "Morning-After Pill"

Depo-Provera: Injectable form of hormonal birth control.

Diabetes: Disease characterized by the body's inability to metabolize and use sugar.

2,4-diaminotoluene (TDA): Contaminant in hair dyes and polyurethane foam breast implants.

Diethylstilbestrol (DES): Hormone used in veterinary and human medicine known to be carcinogenic to the breast and other organs.

Digitized mammography: Computer-enhanced mammography.

Dioxane: Contaminant found in hair dyes and other cosmetics with certain families of chemical ingredients.

DNA: Large molecule found mainly in the chromosomes of the nucleus of a cell; carrier of genetic information that is the body's "master blueprint."

Ductal carcinoma *in situ* (DCIS): A type of breast cancer confined to the milk ducts.

Elavil (amitryptiline): Antidepressant drug.

Electromagnetic fields (EMFs): Long-wave radiation emitted naturally and by appliances, electrical equipment, and power lines and stations.

Enovid-10: Early oral contraceptive.

Estrace: Type of hormone replacement therapy for menopausal symptoms.

Estradiol: The most powerful of the natural estrogen hormones; the body produces "good" and "bad" types of estradiol.

Estriol: The weakest of the primary estrogen hormones.

Estrogen: The primary feminizing hormones, including estradiol, estrone, and estriol; there are also synthetic, plant, and animal estrogens.

Estrogen-binding proteins: Substances that bind to and help eliminate estrogen from the body.

Estrogen-dependent breast cancer: Breast cancer that depends on estrogen to fuel its growth; now most common type of breast cancer.

Estrogen replacement therapy (ERT): Use of estrogens derived from plants or horse urine (*see* Premarin) to treat effects of menopause.

Estrone: The most readily used form of estrogen circulating in the bloodstream.

Ethinyl estradiol: Synthetic estrogen that is highly potent.

Ethylene oxide: Chemical used to sterilize breast implants; residues remain after implants are placed in women's breasts; breast carcinogen.

False-negative: An incorrect failure to diagnose breast cancer; common among premenopausal women who are screened with mammography.

False-positive: A diagnosis of cancer where none exists.

Fiber: Substance found in plant foods; stuff of which food is made and held together; forms our dietary roughage.

First-degree relative: Parent or blood-related sibling.

Flagyl (metronidazole): Drug used to treat yeast infections.

Flavonoids: Substances in plants that provide color, flavor, and odor; act as antioxidants to prevent harmful substances from destroying cells.

Fluoroscopy: Extended examination of body with X rays; involves high doses of radiation.

Free radicals: Substances found in food and the environment that cause damage to cells in the body and that could lead to cancer or other degenerative diseases; neutralized by antioxidants.

Gynecomastia: A disease causing breast enlargement in men.

Haldol (haloperidol): Antipsychotic drug.

High-density lipoprotein (HDL): The "good" cholesterol that helps to prevent damage to arteries.

Hormone: A chemical messenger secreted by a gland into the bloodstream.

2-hydroxyestrone (2-HE): The "good" estrogen that is easily broken down by liver and eliminated by the body.

16-hydroxyestrone (16-HE): The "bad" estrogen that remains in the body and may trigger breast cancer development.

Hypothalamus: Portion of the brain that helps activate, control, and integrate the nervous system, endocrine process (including the release of sex hormones), and many other body functions.

Implant: In livestock, a hormone drug stuck in animals' ears and elsewhere in the muscle to stimulate growth. In breast implant surgery, a bag containing silicone gel or saline for breast enlargement and reconstruction.

Indole-3-carbinol: Plant chemical that helps the body maintain high levels of "good" estrogen; found in crucifers such as cauliflower and cabbage.

Insulinlike growth factor-I (IGF-I): Chemical that stimulates the growth and division of human cells.

Interval cancer: Breast cancer that is diagnosed between mammograms.

Low-density lipoprotein (LDL): The "bad" cholesterol that causes blood vessel damage.

Magnetic resonance imaging: Use of electromagnetic fields for producing images of breast tissues and diagnosing breast cancer.

Mammography: Method of detecting breast cancer by use of a machine that emits X rays that provide an image of the breast.

Mastitis: Pain, swelling, and inflammation of the breast.

Medroxyprogesterone acetate: Active hormone in the contraceptives Depo-Provera, Amen, and Curretabs.

Megestrol acetate: Synthetic hormone for contraceptive use in Megace, Delalutin, and other drugs.

Melatonin: Hormone produced by pineal gland; believed to protect against breast cancer.

Melengestrol: Synthetic hormone for fattening cattle.

Meme: Type of breast implant covered with polyurethane foam.

Metaanalysis: Pooling together many studies for an overall analysis.

Methylene chloride: Chemical commonly used in paint strippers, spray paints, and decaffeinated coffee; carcinogenic to breast.

Mifepristone: *See* RU-486.

Miscarriage: Spontaneous end of pregnancy due to defects of the fetus or womb.

Morning-After Pill: Medication used to prevent pregnancy by inducing abortion of potential embryo; taken shortly after intercourse, it consists of high dosages of synthetic estrogen and progestins.

Multiple myeloma: Bone marrow cancer.

Mutation: Change in the cell's function caused by damage to its DNA.

Non-estrogen-dependent breast cancer: Type of cancer that is not "fueled" by the hormone estrogen.

Norplant: Implantable form of birth control.

Organochlorine: Family of chemicals containing chlorine, such as DDT. Highly persistent in environment and to humans; breast carcinogen.

Osteoporosis: A disease characterized by the loss of bone density; most common in postmenopausal women.

Perimenopausal: Period just before and during menopause, usually occurring around age 48 to 51.

Pesticides: Chemicals used to kill pests; some are safe, others are dangerous and can cause breast and other cancer. *See* DDT, for example.

Phytoestrogen: Plant-based estrogenic chemical that promotes breast health.

Pituitary gland: Cherry-shaped structure at base of brain known as the "master" endocrine gland.

Polyurethane foam (PUF): A material used to cover silicone breast implants; contains impurities and degradation products shown to cause breast cancer.

Polyvinyl chloride (PVC): Chemical commonly used in the manufacturing and chemical industries that is known to cause breast cancer.

Pravachol (pravastatin): Cholesterol-lowering drug.

Premarin: The most popular postmenopausal estrogen drug, derived from urine of pregnant mare.

Progesterone: Hormone produced during the second half of the menstrual cycle.

Progestin: Synthetic form of progesterone.

Prolactin: Pituitary hormone that promotes lactation and growth of both healthy and cancerous breast cells.

Prostaglandins: Hormonelike substances that act in small amounts on certain organs; used in some abortion procedures.

Prostate cancer: Malignancy of the prostate gland.

Prozac: Antidepressant drug.

Pseudoestrogen: A substance that acts like estrogen in the body such as a pesticide (DDT) or industrial food packaging chemical (bisphenol).

Radiation absorbed dose (rad): Unit of measurement for radiation; usually expressed as millirad, or a thousandth of a rad.

Radiology: Medical specialty that uses radiation to diagnose and treat disease.

Ralgro: Veterinary growth-stimulating sex hormone drug used to fatten cattle.

Replicon: Type of silicone gel breast implant wrapped in polyurethane foam.

Risk factor: A condition or behavior that increases one's likelihood of developing a disease; exposure to pesticides is a "risk factor" for breast cancer.

RU-486 (mifepristone): A drug used to induce abortion that contains steroids and prostaglandins.

Second-degree relative: Cousins, aunts, and further distant relations.

Selenium: Important dietary mineral that acts to protect cells. *See* antioxidant.

Serpasil (reserpine): Drug used to treat blood pressure.

Silicone gel: A material used inside breast implants; known to be carcinogenic.

Stroke: A blood clot or bleeding in the brain resulting in a loss of oxygen to brain tissues.

Sulforaphane: Protective nutrient found in crucifers.

Tagamet: Drug to treat indigestion and ulcers.

Tamoxifen: An estrogenic drug being tested for preventing breast cancer.

Tenormin (atenolol): Drug used to treat hypertension.

Testosterone: Primary masculinizing hormone.

Thermography: Method of detecting breast cancer using body heat patterns, successful because cancer emit more heat than healthy tissue.

Thymus gland: The primary central gland of the lymphatic system, the immune system that scouts for "enemies"; located in frontal upper chest area.

Tocopherols: The vitamin E family of plant chemicals.

Toluene diisocyanate (TDI): Industrial chemical contaminating hair coloring products and polyurethane foam breast implants; breast carcinogen.

Traditional risk factors: Familial, genetic, and reproductive influences on the development of breast cancer.

Transillumination with infrared light scanning: A method of detecting breast cancer that involves shining a special light through the breast to identify abnormal tissue; not yet approved by the FDA.

Ultrasonography: Use of sound waves for diagnosing breast cancer.

Urethane: Highly carcinogenic contaminant found in some brands of alcoholic beverages.

Valium: Tranquilizing drug.

Zearalenone: Fungal toxin; carcinogenic.

Zeranol: A toxic estrogenic chemical, from fungus, used for fattening cattle.

Zinc: Beneficial dietary mineral.

Index

411